Enabling Technologies: Body Image and Body Function

For Churchill Livingstone

Commissioning Editor: Mary Law
Design Direction: Judith Wright
Project Development Manager: Dinah Thom
Project Manager: Morven Dean
Illustration Manager: Bruce Hogarth

Enabling Technologies: Body Image and Body Function

Edited by

Malcolm MacLachlan BSc MSc MA PhD DipBA FPSI FTCD
Associate Professor, Department of Psychology, Trinity College, University of Dublin, Ireland

Pamela Gallagher BAMod DipStat PhD
Lecturer in Psychology, Faculty of Science and Health, School of Nursing, Dublin City University, Dublin, Ireland

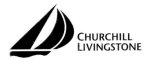

EDINBURGH LONDON NEW YORK OXFORD PHILADELPHIA ST LOUIS SYDNEY TORONTO 2004

CHURCHILL LIVINGSTONE
An imprint of Elsevier Science Limited

First published 2004

ISBN 0 443 07247 7

British Library Cataloguing in Publication Data
A catalogue record for this book is available from the British Library

Library of Congress Cataloging in Publication Data
A catalog record for this book is available from the Library of Congress

Notice
Medical knowledge is constantly changing. Standard safety precautions must be followed, but as new research and clinical experience broaden our knowledge, changes in treatment and drug therapy may become necessary or appropriate. Readers are advised to check the most current product information provided by the manufacturer of each drug to be administered to verify the recommended dose, the method and duration of administration, and contraindications. It is the responsibility of the practitioner, relying on experience and knowledge of the patient, to determine dosages and the best treatment for each individual patient. Neither the Publisher nor the editors and contributors assume any liability for any injury and/or damage to persons or property arising from this publication.

The Publisher

your source for books,
journals and multimedia
in the health sciences

www.elsevierhealth.com

The
publisher's
policy is to use
**paper manufactured
from sustainable forests**

Printed in China

Contents

Contributors

For full biographical information on the authors please go to pages 265–274.

Campbell Aird
Moffat, Scotland

Ned Augenblick HDipMaths
Dublin, Ireland

Danièle Bachmann MD
Lyon, France

Ian Bennun BSocSci(Hons) MPhil PhD
Devon, UK

Niels Birbaumer PhD
Tübingen, Germany

Gabriel Burloux MD
Lyon, France

Verna Cain RN
Seattle, USA

James Condron BScEng
Dublin, Ireland

Robert D. Dowling BSc MD
Louisville, USA

Phil Ellis PhD MA ARCM CertEd
Sunderland, UK

Pamela Gallagher BAMod PhD DipStat
Dublin, Ireland

Azucena Garcia-Palacios PhD
Seattle, USA

David Gow BSc PG Dip
Edinburgh, UK

Hunter G. Hoffman PhD
Seattle, USA

Darran Hughes BScEng MScEng
Dublin, Ireland

Bodil Jönsson PhD MA
Lund, Sweden

Thierry Keller MS PhD
Zurich, Switzerland

Andrea Kübler PhD MSc Msc
Tübingen, Germany

Malcolm MacLachlan BSc MSc MA PhD DipBA FPSI FTCD
Dublin, Ireland

Gary McDarby BE MengSc PhD
Dublin, Ireland

Aoife Moran DipHE BNS(Hons)
Dublin, Ireland

David R. Patterson PhD ABPP ABPH
Seattle, USA

Milos R. Popovic PhD
Toronto, Canada

Anne Schmidt BA
Seattle, USA

John Sharry D Psych MSc(Mod)
Dublin, Ireland

Richard A. Sherman PhD
Suquamish, USA

Emma K. Stokes BSc MSc MISCP MCSP
Dublin, Ireland

Jennifer Tininenko BA
Seattle, USA

Helena Villa-Martín
Castellon, Spain

Preface

This volume is concerned with understanding the enormous potential of enabling technologies in the field of rehabilitation. Central to many of these technologies is the idea of providing people with more effective body functioning. However, the effects of enabling technologies on the person's body image, social functioning, self-esteem and other psychosocial variables, are poorly understood. This volume seeks to combine the excitement of technological innovations that enable people to overcome disabling conditions and disability, with the challenge of understanding how these innovations influence the user's relationship to their own sense of self and how they interact with other people.

The contributors to this volume are leading international authorities in their areas of specialization and are from multidisciplinary backgrounds. They include psychologists, physicians, surgeons, psychiatrists, engineers, prosthetists, physiotherapists, bioengineers, nurses and musicians. The content reflects the myriad of enabling technologies available and their potentially wide applicability across a number of disabling conditions. Of necessity, choice of content was made because of the extraordinary breadth and depth of this field. Selected for inclusion was content considered to be the latest cutting-edge technology in healthcare and rehabilitation and also technology whose effects are not only powerful but also intriguing.

Contributors were encouraged to structure their contributions around a common framework, which we believe makes the book easier to read, and to dip in and out of. The chapters can be read as stand-alone entities, but there are also many fascinating and exciting interplays to be uncovered throughout the book. The use of case studies provides not only a means of bringing the technology to life, but also a practicality that is appropriate for the novice and the expert. This is further supplemented with the inclusion of a glossary of terms and websites of interest in each chapter. In addition to being asked to give a description of the technology and its development, application, effectiveness and advantages, contributors were asked to address the psychological impact of the technology they describe on the people for whom it was developed, and not just the functions it enables. A discussion of potentially contentious, ethical and cultural factors, where appropriate, was also encouraged. Finally, contributors were asked to comment on the future prospects of the technology, that is, to identify upcoming research and practice issues and speculations on the development of the area.

Chapter 1 places the purpose of the book in context and summarizes the content of each of the subsequent chapters. Chapters 2–14 showcase the intriguing and innovative developments in the field of enabling technologies and are organized into four sections. The first of these sections, Interacting with Technology, refers to technology that acts as an adjunct to our usual experiences; for example, the use of virtual reality as a psychological analgesic (*Spiderworld, Snow World*), the 'pictures as language' concept to enable communication (*Isaac*), sound therapy, which enables expression through sound (*Soundbeam*) and robot-mediated therapy (*GENTLE/s*). The second section, Listening to the Body, relates to the use of technologies that provide us with feedback about, and raises our awareness of what is going on in our own bodies, thus enabling us to use this information for our own therapeutic advantage; for example, *biofeedback* enables the recognition and control of levels of physiological functioning, *affective feedback* helps people achieve and maintain internal states through the innovative use of computer games (*Relax to Win, Brainchild*), and behavioral neuroprostheses use psychophysiological training to teach a new behavioral response (*Thought Translation Device*). The third section, Technology of Replacement, is concerned with the ways in which parts of the body can be replaced; for example, externally powered whole limb prostheses (*Edinburgh Arm*), *limb transplantation*, and artificial hearts (*AbioCor™ implantable replacement heart*). The fourth section, Living Through Technology, describes the way in which technology can 'take over' bodily functioning. This includes a discussion of neuroprostheses for grasping (*Compex Motion*), *hemodialysis*, and the technological environment found in the intensive care unit (*ICU Syndrome*). We conclude the volume with a chapter where we draw on the implicit and explicit themes emerging throughout the book, and provide what we consider could be used as a guiding framework for the development and implementation of enabling technologies.

This book will have considerable utility for practitioners, researchers and scholars in a variety of health, social and engineering sciences. For example, this volume will be applicable to a large number of advanced undergraduate and postgraduate students, and qualified practitioners such as physiotherapists, occupational therapists, prosthetists, orthotists, nurses, physicians, surgeons, rehabilitation specialists, and psychologists working in the area of rehabilitation or at the person/technology interface. The volume will also be of interest to a broad array of social scientists interested in disability and embodiment. Overall, the book aims to help those who encounter enabling technologies and biotechnological innovations as part of their research, scholarly work or professional practice to better understand their potential, the psychosocial responses of the user, and how to use the technology to ensure faster and more effective rehabilitation and functioning.

On a final note, we would like to acknowledge those people who have played a role in facilitating this venture. Firstly, we would like to thank all at Elsevier Science for their vision, encouragement and assistance. In particular we would like to thank the commissioning editor Mary Emmerson Law, and the project development managers Morven Dean and Dinah Thom. We are also indebted to all the contributors whose time and expertise in contributing to the book is greatly appreciated. Lastly, we would like to thank our families, friends and colleagues who have all helped us enormously in this endeavor.

Malcolm MacLachlan
Pamela Gallagher

Introduction

CONTENT

1

Imagining the body

Malcolm MacLachlan   Pamela Gallagher

SUMMARY

In this introductory chapter to the volume we consider the ways in which body image may be affected by enabling technologies. Body image is a complex multifaceted concept that includes both perceptual and evaluative components that are influenced by a range of physical, cognitive and sociocultural factors. While the cortex of the brain 'maps out' the body in terms of sensory and motor function, not only is this 'map' different from our phenomenological experience, it is also dynamic and capable of changing in response to loss of body function and environmental changes. If sociocultural, cognitive and neurological perspectives give us alternative ways in which we can imagine – provide different images of – the body, so do the plethora of intriguing and innovative technologies described in this volume. We briefly review the forthcoming chapters illustrating how technologies may enable people to live better lives and have alternative forms of embodied experience. We conclude by emphasizing the importance of the user's perspective and of considering not just the technological marvel of alleviating impaired functioning, but also the psychological challenge of imagining and coping with alternative ways of living with ourselves.

INTRODUCTION

Your heart lies at the centre of a 96 000 km (60 000 miles) network of blood vessels. If all these vessels were laid out end to end, they would stretch almost two and a half times around the earth's circumference.[1]

The human heart pumps an amazing 7200 litres (1600 gallons) of blood around the body each day – enough to fill a small swimming pool.[1]

Popular books and, indeed, textbooks on human anatomy and physiology are replete with staggering statistics on our anatomy, physiology and biochemistry. How can you possibly mentally stretch yourself once around the world, never mind your innards making it two and a half times! It is undeniable that the human body is not only fantastically complex, but also that in our everyday existence, we are estranged from its workings. For instance, it is hard to resist the metaphor of the heart as a brilliant *machine* – what else could fill a swimming pool with your blood in just a day? The sweat and tears that we are certainly more aware of, would take a lifetime to do the same job, if, that is, your heart held out.

When the body fails to allow us to live the lives we wish for, at times we can be enabled to do so, through the use of technology. With the likes of organ transplants, robotic therapists, genetic engineering, neuroprostheses, renal dialysis and thought-transfer devices, it is tempting to think of the human body as a sort of master computer, with numerous 'ports' and gadgets and gismos that can be plugged into it, in series, or in parallel, in order to enhance or enable 'the various parts of you'. In an age of accelerating technological sophistication, when we can experience 'virtual' or 'augmented' worlds, when people can continue to exist for years on 'life support' machines, what that 'you' is, is increasingly difficult to say.

A nurse walks into a patient's private room and checks the monitors above the bed and to each side of it, and on striding toward the door, the 'thing' which these machines have some sense of, gruffly announces; 'Hey, I'm fine too'! While consumerism has had a strong impact on many aspects of life, and the value of exploring people's views about their experience of health services is now clear, the realm of biotechnology has remained largely cloaked in the impenetrable nomenclature and lore of scientists, engineers, technicians, and specialized clinicians. Much of the technology used today is beyond the ken of most of us using it. One could imagine a situation where to ask a patient how they feel about their dialysis machine could be almost as ridiculous as asking them how they feel about the 96 000 km of blood vessels busily at work inside of them: sure how would they know! Taken to extremes the person – you – becomes only an interface between a biological wonder, on the one hand, and a technological wonder, on the other hand.

In this volume we have set out to bring together some of the most exciting and innovative examples of enabling technology currently in use, or about to come into use. Chapters in this volume come from internationally renowned researchers and clinicians, and describe truly leading edge, state of the art technology. However, as the subtitle of the volume indicates – *Body Image and Body Function* – we have also asked contributors to address the psychological impact of the technology they describe, on the people for whom it was developed, and not just the functions (e.g. pumping or filtering blood) of the body that it may cleverly replace or enhance. It is our belief that the promise of enabling technologies is prohibited, not by our imaginations, but by our ability to integrate that technology into a life worth living and a view of the self worth living for.

BODY IMAGES

Paul Schilder[2] was the first to consider the broader psychological and social context in which our experience of the body occurs. He defined body image as 'the picture of the body which we form in our mind'.[2] He was also interested in what he called the 'elasticity' of the body image; how its properties of size and heaviness and its influence on interactions with others could all fluctuate. Over the decades the term 'body image' has subsequently been used to refer to attractiveness, size, distorted body perceptions, perceptions of body boundaries and perception of internal body states. These are all legitimate aspects of bodily experience, and can perhaps be included within Grogan's use of the term 'body image': 'a person's perceptions, thoughts and feelings about his or her body'.[3] However, at the most fundamental level it is useful to recognize a division between purely perceptual aspects of the body and evaluative aspects of the body.

Cash and Pruzinsky[4] identified seven integrative themes from the body image literature:

1. *Body images are multifaceted:* there is no one single dimension on which body image can be measured (e.g. size) that conveys the complexity of the concept.

2. *Body image refers to perceptions, thoughts, and feelings about the body and bodily processes:* thus, estimation of one's own and idealized physical attributes involves many and complex processes.

3. *Body-image experiences are intertwined with feelings about the self:* the sense of self and of the physical self are developmentally and reciprocally interrelated. Thus, a vulnerable sense of self can undermine one's body image.

4. *Body images are socially determined:* physical esthetics and personal ideas about the body occur in a social and cultural context that influences the sorts of meanings we attribute to different types of bodies.

5. *Body images are not entirely fixed or static:* we do not feel the same way about our bodies all the time. These feelings fluctuate across different social situations, across the age span, between health and illness, and so on.

6. *Body images influence information processing:* people who are strongly focused on their body image process implicit information about their bodies in a different manner to those for who their body image is more incidental.

7. *Body images influence behavior:* a belief that one is attractive may foster approach behaviors, such as self-grooming, exercise, socializing. A belief that one is unattractive may foster attempts to avoid certain people, activities, poses and so on.

It is clear from Cash and Pruzinsky's review of the body image literature that body image is a multifaceted phenomenon, which, unless understood and taken into consideration, may impact on the integration of technology into our sense of self. The idea of understanding just how the body is 'imaged', or 'imagined' becomes even more complex and fascinating when we consider neurological factors. Within hours or even minutes of delivery, newborn babies can imitate orofacial and head movements performed in front of them.[5] This ability to identify specific bodily movement and then produce the same action with the corresponding part of their own body, suggests that neonates have some sense of their own body. Such an idea would tie in well with Ronald Melzack's neuromatrix theory that suggests we innately inherit a type of 'neurosignature' of our bodies.[6] This 'matrix', or network, is comprised of somatosensory cortex, posterior parietal lobe and the limbic system, and together it is argued they produce an implicit sense of the body.

Wilder Penfield, a Canadian neurosurgeon working in the 1940s and 1950s, opportunistically stimulated specific regions of the brain that were exposed during operations. These patients were conscious because only local anesthesia was used and since there are no pain receptors in the brain, such stimulation is painless. He simply touched an area with an electrode and asked people what they felt. Elicited sensations ranged from images and memories to physical sensations.[7] By tracing sensations experienced down one strip of the brain Penfield 'mapped' out where the different parts of the body are represented. This strip, now known as the somatosensory cortex (or sensory homunculus – meaning 'little man') reconfigures the body and allots greater space on the cortex to those body parts that are more sensitive (there is a similar pattern in the motor cortex). The area given over to the hands, for instance, is much larger than that given over to the back or the trunk. In effect, the somatosensory cortex is a map of how we *physically* sense the world, but importantly, this is very different from how we actually (emotionally) experience it. Furthermore, this 'map' is not fixed; it changes depending on our experience of the world.

A dramatic example of this comes from the treatment of 'webbed-finger-syndrome' (or syndactyly) where people are born with fingers webbed together with the result that they do not move independently of each other. Rather than the fingers having – as they usually do – their own distinct area on the somatosensory cortex, the somatosensory representation for people with 'webbed-finger-syndrome' clumps all the fingers together as a 'whole hand'. For example, the distance between the sites of representation of the thumb and little finger is significantly smaller than normal. However, when fingers are surgically separated from each other so that they can move independently, within a month of this happening, the somatosensory representation of the fingers has changed so that they each have their own 'patch' on the cortex and the distance between representation of the thumb and little finger has increased.[8]

It would seem that a genetically inherited condition that webs the fingers together and has associated morphology in the brain, is not only treatable in the sense of separating the fingers, but also in the sense of changing brain structure, or brain image, *how the brain images the body*. This is just one example of what is referred to as brain, or neural, plasticity. It is in this sense that Robertson[9] talks about 'sculpturing the brain', where people's experience of their world is *inscribed* upon their brain. It is this very ability of the brain to restructure itself, to *re-imagine* the world, that may account for the body's ability to recover function in a limb paralyzed by stroke, after being schooled through repeated movements by a robot (see Chapter 5, this volume). This also relates to one of the points made by Burloux and Bachmann (see Chapter 10 of this volume) in relation to accepting a grafted hand as one's 'own'. An element important in the psychological integration of the grafted hand was magnetic resonance imaging (MRI) showing activity in the associated cortical areas as the patient recovered motility with the grafted hand. According to Burloux and Bachmann, MRI shows the cerebral flexibility on a scientific level, but it also has a major psychological impact: in the case reported, the patient uses the imagery as a sign that the hands are becoming his own, since he can see that his brain now activates them.

While the homunculi in our brain offer a representation of our human body, they are very clearly not the only representations, and, indeed, not the ones that we are consciously aware of. The fact that these neurological homunculi are so strange and foreign to us, testifies to the fact that they (usually) play a limited role – if one at all – in our sense of the physical self. Indeed, our phenomenological experience of self often differs from any account we can muster from even the most compelling scientific evidence. In a recent National Geographic article on skin, Joel Swerdlow[10] describes in fascinating detail how the skin 'works' and how it can be re-worked in the case of people who suffer with burns or various skin disorders. In amongst the glossy Disney-like figures of the skin's structure and function that inform and bewilder, Swerdlow also sensitively and lovingly tells us of the visit he made to his 86-year-old mother who was in hospital after collapsing. The doctors had informed him that she may not be able to see or hear and he tried to comfort her by talking, singing songs from his childhood, or just sitting quietly. 'I'm not sure what she can sense, but her skin feels warm and normal. I keep my fingers on her arm or cheek, anything to let her know that she is not alone and that she is loved. I realize that our only unbroken connection now is through touch. We are skin to skin, warmth to warmth. According to the textbooks, transduction within the skin is transforming physical energy to neural energy. But something far more important is occurring. Love and memory are flowing through my skin and into her dreams'.[10] For the very reason that it is difficult to reconcile the sophisticated biotechnology that is the human body, with the need of human beings to express feelings, it is important that when we build enabling technologies that they do not obscure the perennial need for a life of emotional meaning.

THE USERS OF TECHNOLOGIES

While we offer this volume as a celebration of the potential of technology, and have asked contributors to write in that vein, we wish to pause, just momentarily, to reflect somewhat critically on the social implications of biotechnological innovation. There has been a veritable explosion of technologies that assist and enable over the past decade. Here we make no fundamental distinction between terms such as 'assistive technology' or 'enabling technology' or other similar terms. While these terms may have their puritanical supporters, in practice their use often overlaps; for instance, a single form of technology can legitimately be described as assisting, enabling and biological. We use the term *enabling technologies* because many of the technologies reported in this volume are not strictly 'biological' and many go beyond 'assisting' in that they effectively provide an ability that the person was devoid of prior to it. However, we would not wish to overstate this argument, for whatever technology is being adopted we recognize that it is *the person* who is being assisted or enabled, and that the focus should be on the person rather than on the technology.

The Institute on Disability and Rehabilitation Research within the US Department of Education lists over 18 000 types of assistive technology that are currently available. However, Scherer and Galvin[11] suggest that about one in three of all devices provided are abandoned by their intended users, primarily because there is a lack of consumer involvement in the selection of the technology. In her now classic book, *Living in the State of Stuck (3rd Edition)*, Scherer[12] calls for a greater focus on the unique user of a particular device. If the 20th century's ethos of technology was 'people-focused', meaning that it was directed at providing technology to meet the needs of people with different types of 'collective problems' (e.g. wheel chairs for immobility), then 21st century's technology should be 'person-focused', where more attention is given to the unique circumstances and needs of particular users.[13]

Thus, assistive technology should be targeted at enabling people to overcome the restrictions experienced, the consumer's perspective becoming the driving force in device selection. The difference in user and provider perspectives is noted by Scherer: 'Professionals have tended to define goals achieved (e.g. independence) in terms of *physical functioning*, where as consumers more often equate independence with *social and personal freedoms*' (italic added).[13] We are perhaps too used to thinking of biotechnology as 'fixing' physical problems, rather than as 'overcoming' social problems. According to Craddock and McCormack[14] the social model is concerned with how society responds to disability; the emphasis is not on the disability but on the barriers that exist in society that prevents the person from achieving his or her potential. 'This approach reverses the medical model focus from the disability to the client. Disability researchers have challenged this (medical) model, arguing that it does not usefully explain disability and that it has a profound effect on the self-identity of many people with disabilities who have considered themselves to be ill, rather than merely living with one or more functional limitations'.[14] It is clear that there is great importance in recognizing that, for instance, a thought transfer device for people with locked-in syndrome is about enabling their communication – their ability to participate 'verbally' in a social world – rather than overcoming a physical deficiency. On the other hand, other technologies, such as dialysis for end-stage renal disease, are about directly influencing physiological processes that make people ill.

In its basic message, however, the social model of rehabilitation challenges what could be called 'technological-innovation-led rehabilitation' to be responsive to 'consumer-needs-led rehabilitation'. In this volume we have tried to emphasize the solutions offered by technology, by leading off each chapter with a case study. Nonetheless, it would be naïve to think that creative and opportunistic researchers and clinicians do not become excited by new technological possibilities and then think how these possibilities can be translated into realizing the potential of people with disabilities. Some of the technologies reported in these chapters are only in their initial stages and will need further development through consumer feedback and, ultimately, these technologies will need to be adaptable to the circumstances of individual's needs. The way in which people feel about themselves is also likely to influence how they think about enabling technologies. Furthermore, Lupton and Seymour[15] found that for some people with physical disabilities the use of technology actually interfered with them presenting their preferred identity. Thus, while a device may indeed lower environmental barriers and thereby enhance independence and control, it may also threaten a user's self-image and preferred identity.[16]

Once the individual's social context and needs are admitted to the technology equation; once the importance of understanding personal appraisals and the personal meanings assigned to technology is recognized, the role of cultural factors becomes apparent. Although technologies may be developed on the assumption of providing solutions to universal – often biologically based – problems, the relevance of these technologies is always a local matter. While it is well recognized that cultural factors influence health,[17,18] the influence of cultural factors on technology use is only now becoming recognized.

According to Pape et al.[16] the acceptance of disability is related to the manner in which people view themselves as well as their relations with others. 'Cultural norms, in other words, influence incorporating a disability into one's self-concept and in turn affect disability acceptance and decisions about use or abandonment of assistive devices. Cultural norms often dictate social roles and activities in which persons are expected to function and these expectations may influence device use'.[16] In a recent major review of factors influencing the abandonment of assistive technologies, Pape et al.[16] found that psychosocial and cultural issues had an important influence on the meanings that individuals ascribed to their devices. The sort of enabling technologies described in this volume are primarily developed within Western societies, are often costly and resonate with the scientific, technocratic and biomedical discourses that dominate Western thinking, at least in the health field. Yet there are ways in which our own innovativeness in this regard has come to challenge many of the assumptions that underpin our very existence. That is, some enabling technologies, question the assumptions of the culture that has produced the technology.

TECHNOLOGIES AND EMBODIMENTS

Biotechnologies create opportunities for increased medicalization of problems because they offer more possibilities for expert interventions into the human body. Yet it is important to recognize that biotechnology is not synonymous with a single ideological stance and that it is necessary to reach beyond a simplistic technophilia vs. technophobia clash: 'The celebratory rhetoric about biotechnology fits the 'philia' slot: the confident hope that technologies will ameliorate the human condition and decrease pain and suffering. Unfortunately, the critique of ideology can easily slip into the phobia, that is, the dystopian fear that technology uniformly strengthens certain forms of domination and destroys the subject's autonomy'.[19] Brodwin goes on to suggest that those of us caught up in the 'biotechnological embrace' have some of our most implicit assumptions questioned: distinctions between humans and machines; between kin and non-kin; between male and female; and between nature and culture. Our chapters in this volume on transplanting human organs and limbs, on kidney dialysis, on the implantation of a wholly synthetic heart and on developing fully myo-electrically powered limbs, are exciting not just because of their description of technological innovations, but because they raise our natural anxieties over being able to distinguish what is me from what is not me; what is human from what is not human.

Enabling technologies also empower certain understandings of the disabled experience. Nelson[20] describes the case of a 5½-month-old boy with nemaline rod myopathy – a rare and progressive neuromuscular disease that renders a person immobile. Breathing off a ventilator and being fed directly through a tube into his stomach, Michael had been transferred from the intensive care unit to the 'low tech' ward where the family would be trained in managing his home-ventilation unit. Subsequently, Michael's mother wanted him to be taken off the ventilator; she interpreted his tears as a sign of his suffering and the ventilator as 'something other than Michael: as a threat, as an invasion of his body, as something foreign'.[20] On the other hand, the staff on the ward saw his tears as a natural result of his inability to close his eyes and believed that there were other indications that he was able to experience pleasure and contentment.

The staff saw Michael as simultaneously body and machine and in refusing to turn it off, claimed greater authority over how to 'read' Michael's experience. This heart-wrenching case illustrates how enabling technologies may, indeed, privilege certain interpretations of experience and how the boundary between 'me-and-machine' can become obscured. It also sadly illustrates that technological capability may bring us no closer to 'truth', no more able to identify 'right' and 'wrong'. Indeed, enabling life often intensifies the anguish of its loss, symbolic or physical. The chapter in this volume on so-called 'ICU syndrome' also illustrates how peoples' experience of technology is not neutral; it is often confusing, sometimes threatening and always emotional, at least in the context of an Intensive Care Unit.

We conclude this chapter with a brief review of what follows. While all these technologies influence body functioning in some form or other, and this is obvious; what is perhaps less obvious is how they influence how we see ourselves. In offering alternative ways in which people can function or overcome different problems (e.g. pain), enabling technologies offer different images of not just these issues, but also the people who encounter them. This volume, showcasing some of the most imaginative technologies developed in order to benefit people, seeks to live in that space too rarely visited: between the fascinations of scientific ingenuity and the consequence for how the users of such technology experience their resulting self.

ENABLING TECHNOLOGIES

Following this introduction, the volume is divided into four sections. While these sections each have a common theme they also overlap and there are other ways they could have been arranged, thus this configuration is neither definitive nor exclusive. The chapters can be read as stand-alone pieces of work, but there are many interesting interconnections between them and many exciting interplays the careful reader can uncover.

The first section, *Interacting with technology*, deals with various ways in which people can use technology whilst retaining their bodily independence. The technology is an adjunct to their usual experience. For example, the development and application of virtual reality has burgeoned in recent times and the first chapter by Garcia-Palacios from Universidad Jaume 1, Spain, and Hoffman and colleagues from the University of Washington, USA, outlines their innovative use of virtual reality as a psychological analgesic for burn patients. The analgesic effect is achieved by blocking the patient's view of the real world and completely immersing them in a computer-generated virtual 3-D world (e.g. Spiderworld or Snow World). This attention-grabbing experience reduces the amount of attention available to process the excruciating pain normally engendered by wound care and physical therapy; the adherence to both of which are essential for successful rehabilitation of burn patients. Hoffman and colleagues exemplify this through the discussion of a man who suffered burns on 42% of his body surface area and who experienced a reduction in pain while immersed in Spiderworld. The psychological analgesic effects of virtual reality act as an invaluable supplement to opioids, which are often unable to adequately control the level of acute pain experienced during wound care. Although the findings presented are preliminary, this technology holds exciting prospects for being generalized to other clinical problems.

Technology by its very nature can be complex and often times this translates into complexity in its usage. One of the challenges for innovators of technology is its successful independent use by people with a cognitive or intellectual disability. One of the fascinating aspects of *Isaac* and the 'pictures as language' concept to enable communication discussed by Bodil Jönsson of Certec, Lund University, Sweden, is its simplicity, and yet its effects are both powerful and empowering to the user. The individual parts that constitute Isaac are standard pieces of equipment, but collectively they provide an effective means of communication in a group of people for whom acquisition of a language and, therefore, communication and learning, is very difficult and often virtually impossible. In effect, Isaac utilizes personal digital photographs as an active language and mode of communication. Jönsson's chapter introduces us to Abdulkader, a 10-year-old boy with autism, and Thomas and Stig who have cognitive limitations, each of whom with the use of Isaac has not only been enabled to develop a two-way channel of communication, but has also improved their personal development and learning. Despite the powerful effects – or perhaps because of them – identifying a theoretical framework on which to 'hang' and understand the workings of Isaac has, to date, eluded its creators. This has not, however, prevented its ongoing development in meeting the emerging needs of its users and the chapter concludes with the new phase of Isaac, which will facilitate the management of the multitude of photographs being taken and used to communicate.

Soundbeam as developed by Phil Ellis, of the University of Sunderland, UK, is one of the technologies used in *sound therapy*, which enables expression through sound in children with profound and multiple learning difficulties and also in the elderly 'mentally infirm'. The Soundbeam is a device, which emits an ultrasonic beam, which will trigger sound if any physical movement is made within the beam itself. This sound can vary depending on the movement. Initially, its purpose and benefit is not apparent. However, consider the case study of Mary who has cerebral palsy, epilepsy, diabetes, has almost no speech – apart from being able to say a kind of 'hello' – has no communication skills, cannot walk, has no self-help skills and generally has an attention span of only a few seconds. In this type of world where personal expression through the use of words/language is practically impossible, the ability to progress from unintentional to intentional movement, as a way of eliciting sounds that are independently chosen and enjoyed, may have enormous impact on the individual. It stimulates curiosity through exploration and enables self-expression. Originally developed for the dance community, it is an exemplar of how the potential use of technology is only constrained by our inability to think creatively about its usage and application. What is of importance is not the technology, which in itself cannot achieve anything, but rather the way in which it is used.

Emma Stokes of Trinity College Dublin, Ireland, discusses the development of the exciting new European *GENTLE/s* project, which is a system designed to deliver robot-mediated therapy to the upper limb for people with stroke. The purpose of robot-mediated therapy in stroke rehabilitation is to deliver exercise-based interventions that enable the patient to carry out repetitive and meaningful movements individually tailored and set up in the GENTLE/s system by the therapist. Part of this technology is the use of virtual rooms where everyday tasks are simulated as a means of stimulating movement that mirrors everyday requirements. Preliminary results are favorable and given the high incidence of stroke and the associated acquired disability, such robotic developments would be an integral augmentation to the rehabilitation process, as it would allow the person to continue exercises in the absence of a therapist. However, this concept presents the interesting scenario of a robot replacing the therapist and raises questions about how the person will react to and interact with the robot in place of the therapist. Issues of note emerging from the discussion in this chapter include the important role education plays in integrating new technologies into the workplace, and the necessity of their implementation being evidence based. Overall, we are left with the impression that the scope of robotics in rehabilitation is vast and their potential application manifold.

The second section, *Listening to the body*, concerns the use of technologies to monitor what is naturally going on in the body and then to use this activity for therapeutic advantage. The chapter by Richard Sherman from the Behavioral Medicine Research and Training Foundation and the Madigan Army Medical Center in Tacoma, Washington, USA, on *biofeedback* surveys the tools available to people to control their own physiology. Biofeedback enhances people's awareness of their psychophysiological functioning by recording what is going on inside the body and representing this outside the body, usually on a screen as visual feedback or as auditory feedback. Sherman follows a man referred for treatment of headaches, non-cardiac chest pain, and anxiety, as he participates in diagnostic procedures enhanced by psychophysiological recordings, learns to recognize how his body is (mis)behaving, and learns to use biofeedback devices to help control the systems. Today biofeedback is used in a broad range of conditions from tension headaches to irritable bowel syndrome to drug addiction and alcoholism.

It is a curious technology in that it at once makes us very familiar with our body's functioning and how this links to our thoughts and feelings, yet at the same time it 'objectifies' the body. The effective use of biofeedback requires not just clinical skill in its physical application, explanation, and interpretation, but also sensitivity to the experience of the biofeedback user – *psychofeedback* if you will.

The chapter by the McDarby group from Media Lab Europe, Ireland, in Dublin, presents an innovative application of biofeedback technology that they refer to as *affective feedback*. This involves using biofeedback in combination with sensory immersion, novel signal processing and compelling computer game playing. They incorporate narrative and intelligent technology into the biofeedback loop from which people can learn about their responses. They describe the case of Peter, a 9-year-old boy disabled by anxiety attacks who, as part of his therapy, was taught to relax by playing the 'Relax to Win' game. In this game your dragon races against another dragon, either another person or your previous best time. What is intriguing about this game is that while competitive racing is intuitively associated with tension – both physical and psychological – to win here you have to be the most relaxed competitor. The speed of the dragon presented on an engrossing screen with impressive graphics is determined through galvanic skin response (GSR): the more relaxed you are the lower the GSR and the *faster* your dragon goes. It is hard to describe the calm satisfaction derived from watching your dragon take flight and glide to the finishing line, over the head of the other poor fellow who is simply trying too hard! By emotionally engaging people in fun applications and augmentations of biofeedback, affective feedback holds the potential of making psychophysiological regulation more appealing to more and younger people.

The third chapter in this section, *The Thought Translation Device*, by Andrea Kübler (Trinity College Dublin, Ireland) and Niels Birbaumer (Universität Tübingen, Germany), also utilizes biofeedback technology, which they refer to as 'behavioral neuroprostheses or brain–computer interfaces'. Such devices can be used to treat chronic pain, tinnitus, Parkinson's disease, and epilepsy; however, Kübler and Birbaumer describe the case of a man diagnosed with amyotrophic lateral sclerosis (ALS) for 8 years (a neurological disorder, which involves progressive degeneration of central and peripheral motoneurons leading to severe or total motor paralysis – the evocatively so-called 'locked-in syndrome'). To salvage a means for him to communicate, he was taught, using EEG biofeedback, to discriminate the difference between the experience of producing negative and positive slow cortical potentials. A brain–computer interface uses the electrical, magnetic or metabolic activity of the brain to control an external application, for example, a cursor to select letters, words or icons on a computer screen. Based on this 'inner distinction' – imagined personalized scenarios that produce different sorts of cortical potentials, and can be made to move a cursor up or down, for instance – a binary distinction is made, and this 'Yes/No' ability is built on to allow him out of his constricting bodily shell. In a body that is no longer able to embody his needs, this man interfaces with the world through cursors. The thought translation device is effectively his vocal cord that allows him to *be-in-the-world* in Merleau-Ponty's terms (see below) and to be heard.

The third section, *Technology of replacement*, is concerned with the ways in which parts or functions of the body can be replaced and incorporated into a new body image. Gow (Eastern General Hospital, Edinburgh, Scotland) MacLachlan (Trinity College Dublin, Ireland) and Aird (a prosthesis user from Moffat, Scotland) in their chapter on *Reaching with electricity*, explore the relationship between prosthetic use and self-identity. David Gow's team in Edinburgh developed the world's first externally powered whole-limb prosthesis, which has been crowned the 'Bionic Arm' by the media because of a faint similarity to Hollywood portrayals of the same. To watch Cambell Aird control the prosthetic arm (via minute contractions of the remaining musculature in his shoulder stimulating pressure-sensitive electrodes) one is struck by the skill and dexterity he is able to achieve. Without its cosmetic cover this high-tech prosthesis embodies the wonder of modern prosthetic engineering. Yet for Campbell, the prosthetic arm he was first fitted with, which is controlled purely by muscle power, feels more 'a part of him'. For Campbell the essence of being embodied in a prosthesis is when it becomes possible to use it without being aware that you are doing so, as in gesticulating. Gow et al. consider how further technological developments, such as touch-sensitive prosthetics or the possibility of directly wiring a prosthesis into the nervous system, may not only facilitate prosthetic users, but also provide insight into some of the most profound questions about mind–body relationships.

A radical example of technology of replacement is the relatively recent but absorbing area of *limb transplantation* that is outlined by Gabriel Burloux and Danièle Bachmann (both Hospices Civils de Lyon, France). The idea of another person's body part being attached to our own and being clearly visible is quite difficult to comprehend. Unlike an internal organ transplant, a hand transplant is clearly visible both to the receiver and to those around them. Furthermore, as touch is such an intimate and personal act, the hand plays a huge role in developing a sense of who we are and what is around us. Consequently, the potentially differing skin texture, color and, indeed, initial clear demarcation lines between the recipient's arm and the new hand, poses questions about the recipient's capacity to integrate the new hand(s) into their sense of self and the way in which this can be achieved. There are ethical, social and psychological implications not only for the recipient, but also the families of both the recipient and the donor. In addition, the rehabilitation process is long and functionality is non-existent or limited for a long period of time following the transplant. This is clearly portrayed in the case study of GH who received a double-hand graft. Burloux and Bachmann, each psychiatrists and psychoanalysts, explore the myriad of issues that are evaluated prior to, during and subsequent to the limb transplant, and provide us with personal insights into the process from the perspective of their own clinical experiences.

Cardiac-replacement therapy is considered for people with advanced heart failure, but it is limited by the number of available donor hearts. Therefore, the quest to develop a mechanical device that could function as an artificial heart has been ongoing for decades. The chapter on *Implantable replacement hearts* by Robert D. Dowling (University of Louisville, USA) describes the AbioCor™ implantable replacement heart system, currently undergoing clinical trials, which was first implanted in a human in 2001. Given the symbolism of the heart, how an individual responds to such a device and what effect, if any, it has on their body and self-image would provide fascinating insights into mind–body problems. The case study included in the chapter depicts the experience of the second individual to have the AbioCor™ implanted from the point of being in the intensive care unit with near organ failure to being discharged home and resuming normal activities, such as fishing trips and card games. Unlike other artificial hearts there is no need for percutaneous lines or access, which can lead to infection and a negative impact on mobility and quality of life. Rather, energy transfer across the skin to power the device has been accomplished with inductive coupling. Furthermore, radiofrequency transmission from the internal controller in the AbioCor™ allows the close monitoring of the device performance. The initial results of the clinical trials have been impressive and the potential uptake on a successful form of cardiac-replacement therapy is indicative of the importance of this development.

The fourth section, *Living through technology*, has three chapters each describing ways in which technology 'takes over' bodily functioning and especially in the latter two cases, people have to, quite literally, 'live-through' the technology.

A neuroprosthesis is a device that applies short, low-intensity electrical pulses to the paralyzed muscles to cause the muscles to contract on demand. By stimulating a desired group of muscles and by properly sequencing their contractions, a neuroprosthesis can generate functions such as hand opening and closing, standing up, walking, etc. Such technology is a lifeline of hope for people who experience paralysis and a significant research effort is currently being expended in the area. The chapter by Milos Popovic (University of Toronto and Toronto Rehabilitation Institute, Canada) and Thierry Keller (Swiss Federal Institute of Technology, Zurich, Switzerland) discusses *Neuroprostheses for grasping*, and in particular delineates the inspiring new development of *Compex Motion*, a versatile electrical stimulation system with surface-stimulation technology that can be used, inter alia, to develop various custom-made neuroprostheses. The Compex Motion system is especially designed for treatments administered during early rehabilitation (for example, immediately after stroke or spinal cord injury), although it can also be applied as a neuroprosthetic system for patients to use in activities of daily living. This innovative technology is specially designed to encourage sharing of stimulation protocols, sensors, and user interfaces, a heretofore impossibility thereby limiting the impact of functional electrical stimulation technology. Consequently, it is anticipated that it will play an instrumental role in accelerating technological developments in the neuroprostheses field, facilitate the availability of neuroprostheses and promote greater usage. Popovic and Keller also provide us with some intriguing insights into the impact of neuroprosthesis for grasping on people with spinal cord injuries.

Aoife Moran and Pamela Gallagher (both Dublin City University, Ireland) in their chapter on *hemodialysis* provide a case in point of the interface between the person and technology for life-giving purposes. Hemodialysis has been in existence for significantly longer than many of the other technologies discussed in this volume and yet while the technical aspects continue to be advanced, our understanding of the psychosocial effects the technology has on the individual is still playing catch-up with what we know about the functional outcomes. The case study of Doreen is an informative demonstration of the potential to become infatuated with the technology that surrounds us, almost to the point of being dehumanizing and being detrimental to who we are. The person and machine are no longer separate. The technology becomes the focus instead of the person; it takes center stage and becomes all-consuming. This can be accentuated by the physical environment and culture, which surround the technology. The chapter raises the question of the price paid by the individual for this dependency on technology. Indeed, the chapter puts forward Heiddeger's notion of technological enframing, a concept which may facilitate our understanding of the way in which technology impinges on our being, and emphasizes the importance of familiarizing ourselves with the issues involved in psychosocial adjustment.

The last chapter in section four by Ian Bennun of the University of Exeter, UK, on critical care sheds an intriguing light on the potentially profound effects of being in a technologically sophisticated environment such as an *Intensive care unit* (ICU). This is an environment steeped in technology that is crucial in providing physiological support for the patient with an acute life-threatening condition. The chapter commences with a vivid illustration of the ICU environment experienced by Clifford who required respiratory support, monitoring of tissue oxygenation, fluid administration, cardiovascular monitoring, nutritional feed and intravenous drug lines, following surgery for the removal of two aneurysms. Such technology assumes an omnipotence that detracts from the person, and how the patient is doing is ascertained from the machinery, which speaks on the patient's behalf both in a visual and auditory fashion. This technological feedback is extremely important and necessarily works on the patient's behalf, particularly during critical periods, but there are also psychological implications. The chapter explores the complex relationship between technology and those benefiting and operating it, and the effect that the ICU environment has on the patients' psychological status.

We conclude the volume with a chapter by ourselves (Gallagher and MacLachlan) where we try and distill guidelines in the development of enabling technologies. Many of the chapters in the volume not only illustrate the fascinating content of the technology described, but also offer implicit and sometimes quite explicit guidance on the process of technology development. We would obviously endorse the importance of Scherer's 'matching technology to person' perspective and, as such, the views and needs of the 'end user' should often be the starting point. Yet at times technologies can come into existence and be applied to an existing need when that need has never been contemplated during the development of the technology. An example of this would be Hoffman's group who insightfully applied virtual reality technology to the treatment of the excruciating pain experienced by burns patients. So both in terms of 'user-needs-led' and 'technology-opportunity-led' enabling technologies, several important guidelines for the development and trialing of such technologies are offered in the hope that the potential benefits of technologies for both body image and body function can be more fully realized.

EMBODIMENT

Some of the technologies described above must surely question the certainty and clarity of our identity. Plato (5th century BC) and Descartes (17th century) split the mind from the body, a conception that still has influence today, at least in some quarters: 'people often think that the human (self) owns the body, and that the body is separate from the self'.[21] However, an alternative conception to this, one that is now becoming widely accepted in the social sciences, is that people exist through their embodiment. Embodiment may be defined as *'the identification of an abstract idea with a physical entity'*.[17] The French philosopher Merleau-Ponty[22] has been one of the leading advocates of the embodied perspective. If Descartes philosophy can be characterized by his famous *Cognito* (I think, therefore I am), then Merleau-Ponty's philosophy could possibly be characterized as; *I can only think through what I am*. As Carey[23] puts it: 'only a being with eyes to see and ears to hear can perceive the visible or hear the audible'. Our experience of the world is grounded in our physical being: 'our bodies express existence just in the same way that language expresses thought'[24] (see MacLachlan[17] for a fuller discussion).

If our sense of being is, indeed, so tied to the conduit of our body, what happens when the body is disabled and then re-enabled by technology? To what extent does that technology become a 'concrete expression of an abstract idea', where that idea is the idea of self? Do artificial hearts, transplanted limbs, ventilators and the like, remain 'foreign' objects that the body is connected to like a computer with various 'ports', or do they become such a familiar part of the way in which we live, solve problems and communicate with each other, that they effectively become a part of our *being-in-the-world*, as Merleau-Ponty put it.

If they do, then they offer us new ways of being-in-the-world, new eyes to see with and ears to hear with, new augmented and virtual worlds to live through. Technology can re-enable us and perhaps even super-enable us. However, the excitement and anxiety of such technological re-definition of the self should be guided by remembering that technologies, like skin, can be a barrier. Technologies, like skin, should not just be seen as a way of facilitating transduction when two people touch. We must aim for technologies that take us closer to Joel Swedlow's experience with his mother: 'Love and memory are flowing through my skin and into her dreams'. Enabling technologies that allow for a person's emotional and affectionate embodiment will allow them to feel, as the rest of us intuitively do, that they are always more than the technological marvel of their body(s). Different ways of understanding and/or presenting the body gives us different images of the body. If technology is to allow us to reach beyond ourselves, it must reach beyond *technological imaging*, into the realm of a more *humanistic imagining* of how the sense of self and communication with others can be integrated into its functional achievements.

REFERENCES

1. 2001 The heart and circulatory system. Readers Digest: p. 9, 12
2. Schilder P 1935 Image and appearance of the human body. Kegan Paul, London, p. 11
3. Grogan S 1999 Body image: understanding body dissatisfaction in men, woman and children. Routledge, London, p. 1
4. Cash TF, Pruzinsky T 1990 Body images: development, deviance and change. Guilford Press, New York
5. Meltzoff AN 1990 Towards a developmental cognitive science. The implications of cross-modal matching and imitation for the development of representation and memory in infancy. Annals of the New York Academy of Science 608: 1–37
6. Melzack R 1990 Phantom limbs and the concept of a neuromatrix. Trends in Neuroscience 13(3): 88–92
7. Penfield W, Rasmussen T 1950 The cerebral cortex of man: a clinical study of localisation of function. McMillan, New York
8. Mogilner A, Grosman JA, Ribary U et al. 1993 Somatosensory cortical plasticity in adult humans revealed by magnetoencephalography. Proceedings of the National Academy of Sciences 90: 3593–3597
9. Robertson I 1999 Mind sculpture. Bantam Books, London
10. Swerdlow JL 2002 Unmasking Skin. National Geographic 36–63: p. 61
11. Scherer MJ, Galvin JC 1996 An outcomes perspective of quality pathways to the most appropriate technology. In: Galvin JC, Scherer MJ eds. Evaluating, selecting and using appropriate assistive technology. Aspen, Gathersburg, MD, 1–26
12. Scherer MJ 2000 Living in the state of stuck: how assistive technology impacts the lives of people with disabilities. 3rd edn. Brookline Books, Cambridge, MA

13. Scherer MJ 2002 The change in emphasis from people to person: introduction to the special issue on Assistive Technology. Disability and Rehabilitation 24(1–3): 1–4, p. 3
14. Craddock G, McCormack L 2002 Delivering an AT service: client-focused, social and participatory service delivery model in assistive technology in Ireland. Disability and Rehabilitation 24(1–3): 160–170, p. 160
15. Lupton D, Seymour W 2000 Technology, selfhood and physical disability. Social Science and Medicine 50: 1851–1862
16. Pape TLB, Kim J, Weiner B 2002 The shaping of individual meanings assigned to Assistive technology: a review of personal factors. Disability and Rehabilitation 24(1–3): 5–20
17. MacLachlan M 2004 Embodiment: clinical, critical and cultural perspectives. Open University Press, Milton Keynes, p. 2
18. Helman CG 2001 Culture, illness and health. Arnold, London
19. Brodwin PE 2000 Introduction. In: Brodwin PE ed. Biotechnology and culture: bodies, anxieties, ethics. Indiana University Press, 3–23: p. 5
20. Nelson RM 2000 The Ventilator/Baby as Cyborg. A case study in technology and medical ethics. In: Brodwin PE ed. Biotechnology and culture: bodies, anxieties, ethics. Indiana University Press, Bloomington, 209–223: p. 211
21. Wilde MH 1999 Why embodiment now? Journal of Advanced Nursing Science 22: 25–38, p. 36
22. Merleau-Ponty M 1962 Phenomenology of perception. C. Smith (translation). Routledge, London
23. Carey S 2000 Cultivating ethos through the body. Human Studies 23: 23–42, p. 29
24. Mathews E 2002 The philosophy of Merleau-Ponty. Acumen, Chesham, Bucks, p. 84

WEBSITE OF INTEREST

Institute for Matching Person & Technology: http://members.aol.com/IMPT97/html

PART 1

Interacting with technology

PART CONTENTS

2

Using virtual reality to help reduce pain during severe burn wound-care procedures

Azucena Garcia-Palacios   Hunter G. Hoffman
Verna Cain   Jennifer Tininenko   Anne Schmidt
Helena Villa-Martín   David R. Patterson

SUMMARY

Despite aggressive use of opioid pain medications, the majority of severe burn patients suffer severe to excruciating pain during wound care. At Harborview Burn Center in Seattle, a regional burn center, we have recently shown that immersive virtual reality has promise as a powerful new supplementary psychological analgesic that can be used in addition to traditional pharmacologies during wound care and physical therapy. Our results have shown 50% reductions in subjective pain ratings for burn patients in virtual reality (VR). The present chapter describes the logic for how VR works to control pain (within the context of a gate-control heuristic), summarizes preliminary data showing how VR works for procedural pain of severe burn patients, and briefly discusses future directions for VR pain-control research.

CASE STUDY

A 32-year-old patient (J.P.) was injured from ignited gasoline while lying under his car repairing it. He had suffered deep burns on his face, neck, shoulder, chest, and legs, covering 42% of his body surface area and was having trouble with his pain. He was experiencing severe to excruciating pain during dressing changes most mornings and during physical-therapy

23

sessions two times each day. During his one month stay at Harborview Medical Center in Seattle, Washington, he underwent extensive skin grafting, approximately 30 wound-care sessions and 60 physical-therapy sessions.

The patient spent varying amounts of time (5 minutes on day one, 3 minutes on day two, 5 minutes on day three, 10 minutes on day four, and 15 minutes on day five) doing physical therapy in virtual reality (VR) and an equal amount of time in the same session undergoing physical therapy without VR. The order of the presentation of the treatments (VR vs. no VR) was counterbalanced. Treatment effectiveness for pain reduction was measured using 100-mm visual analog subjective pain rating scales (VAS[1,2]). J.P. gave pain ratings immediately after the VR segment, as well

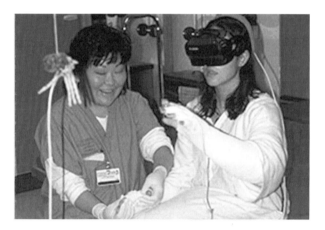

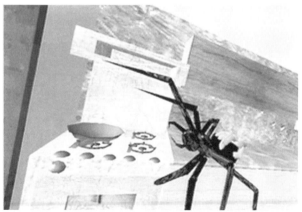

Figure 2.1 (Top) A female burn patient interacting with a mixed-reality spider during physical therapy (© Gretchen Carrougher, RN, Harborview). (Bottom) Image of what patients see in 3-D in SpiderWorld (© reproduced with permission from Duff Hendrickson, U.W. HITLab).

as immediately after the 'no distraction' control segment of the physical therapy session. The patient's doses of pharmacologic analgesics were not affected by his participation in the VR study (i.e. VR was administered in addition to any pharmacologic analgesics he typically received).

J.P. experienced the virtual world named 'Spider World', originally designed for treating spider phobics.[3] Spiderworld (Fig. 2.1) consists of a virtual kitchen where the patients can interact with virtual objects and virtual spiders. The patient could 'pick up' virtual objects with his cyberhand. He could find more than 20 virtual objects on the counter, pull objects out one by one and try to guess and identify them. Also, using tactile augmentation,[3,4] J.P. could 'physically' touch the furry body of a virtual tarantula, and could physically eat a virtual candy bar. The patient could drop a virtual spider out of a 'spider bucket' with sound effects, push it into a sink, fill the sink with water, and turn on the virtual garbage disposal. The patient explored a two-story virtual house during the last VR session, which lasted 15 minutes. Compared to pain during physical therapy with no VR, the results showed that the patient's pain was considerably reduced while in VR. The patient also reported spending 85% less time thinking about pain/wound care while in VR compared to no VR.[5]

THE NEED FOR BETTER PAIN-CONTROL TECHNIQUES

Although opioid analgesics form the cornerstone of any burn-pain-reduction plan,[6,7] the use of opioids is limited by side effects like nausea, constipation, sedation, itchiness, urinary retention, cognitive impairment, hallucinations, delirium, respiratory depression and dependence.[8,9] Opioids are highly effective for controlling background pain, but are much less effective for treating procedural pain. Carrougher et al.[10] recently reported that 74% of a 57 patient sample studied at Harborview Burn Center still rated their worst pain during wound care as severe to excruciating despite aggressive use of opioid analgesics. These data are even more disturbing because in addition to opioids, adjunctive 'anxiety reduction' anxiolytics were used for approximately 13% of Carrougher et al.'s patients, and psychological adjuncts, such as deep breathing and distraction were used in over 47% of the patients in their sample. Their finding that the majority of burn patients suffered severe to excruciating pain during wound care is consistent with other studies on pain levels during burn wound procedures.[11–13] The recovery of physical and psychological function in burn patients depends on successful wound care. Given the fact that opioid analgesics are often unable to adequately control the level of acute pain experienced during wound care, new, more powerful supplementary psychological analgesics would be valuable.[14,15]

VR AS A NEW TECHNIQUE FOR SUPPLEMENTARY PAIN CONTROL

An immersive VR system consists of 1) special 3-D graphics software, 2) head tracking sensors, 3) helmet-mounted visual display that blocks the patient's view of the real world, 4) 3-D sound effects and 5) a means for patients to interact with the environment (to navigate through it, affect it, blow things up, and/or to pick up or influence virtual objects). In a typical immersive VR setup, participants wear a VR helmet that positions two goggle-sized miniature computer monitor screens near their eyes, focused at infinity. Electromagnetic position-tracking devices communicate changes in the user's head (and sometimes hand) location to the computer. The scenery in the virtual world changes as the user moves their head orientation (e.g. virtual objects in front of the patient in VR get closer as the user, wearing their VR helmet, leans forward in the real world). Sometimes the patients can physically touch the virtual objects, using real object props, or computer-generated force feedback devices like the pHanTom. The converging multi-sensory combination of sight, sound, touch and sometimes taste[16] and smell helps give users a uniquely compelling experience of 'being there' in the virtual world. The essence of immersive VR is the illusion it gives users that they are inside the computer-generated environment. Immersive VR is different from related technologies, such as watching a video through a VR helmet; looking at 3-D objects through shutterglasses or 3-D glasses; augmented reality, where people see virtual images without blocking their view of the real world; and CAVES, where people go into rooms with rear-projection walls, where VR images are projected onto the walls.

The logic for how VR works to reduce pain is as follows. Attention involves the selection of relevant information. Each human has a finite amount of attention that can be divided between tasks.[17,18] Immersive VR (involving a head-mounted display that blocks the user's view of the real world) gives patients the illusion of 'going into' the 3-D computer-generated environment. The strength of the illusion of presence is thought to reflect the amount of attention drawn into the virtual world.[19] Because it is by nature a highly attention-grabbing experience, VR may prove to be an especially effective psychological pain-control technique, reducing the amount of attention available to process pain. Less attention to pain can result in a reduction in pain intensity, reduction in pain unpleasantness, and can reduce the amount of time patients spend thinking about their pain.

Hoffman et al.[20] presented a case report providing the first evidence of the effectiveness of VR as a powerful pain-control technique. They compared the amount of pain experienced during two different kinds of distraction: playing a video game vs. going into VR. The patients were two adolescent males (16 and 17 years old). One had a severe gasoline burn on 5% of his body (his leg). The second patient had deep flash burns on 33.5% of his body surface

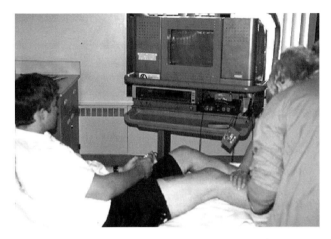

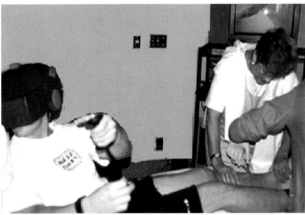

Figure 2.2   (Top) Patient playing Nintendo during wound care. (Bottom) Patient in VR during wound care (© reproduced with permission from Hunter Hoffman, U.W. HITLab).

including his face, neck, back, arms, hands and legs. Much of the second patient's uninjured skin was harvested as donor skin for his skin grafts. Both patients received skin graft surgery and staple placement. After the grafts healed sufficiently, both patients had their staples removed from their skin grafts during the study. They spent 3 minutes in VR and 3 minutes playing a video game (Fig. 2.2). The order of administering the treatments was randomized and counterbalanced, such that each distraction treatment had an equal chance of occurring first or second for each patient. The effectiveness was measured using subjective presence and pain ratings in 100-mm visual analog scales.[1,2] Patients were asked to rate their worst pain, average pain, anxiety, unpleasantness, bothersomeness, and time spent thinking about their pain/burn wound during the relevant wound care. They were also asked to rate how much nausea (if any) they experienced while in each condition. Finally, they were asked; 'To what extent did you feel you went into the computer-generated environment?' and 'How real did the objects in the virtual world seem to you?' The virtual world used was SpiderWorld. For the video game condition, Nintendo 64 video games (Wave Race 64 and Mario Kart 64) were used. Results showed that for both burn patients, VR was more effective in reducing pain than the video game on all measures of pain and anxiety (Fig. 2.3).

The effectiveness of distraction techniques is usually explained within the context of a gate-control heuristic.[21,22] According to Melzack and Wall,[22] higher-order thought processes can change the way incoming pain signals are interpreted, and can even change the intensity of incoming pain signals that make it into the brain.[23]

In addition to daily wound care, most burn patients must also perform frequent physical therapy to maintain range of motion and elasticity of the skin. Physical therapy increases the flexibility of the healing tissues, and helps maintain a normal degree of motion and function.[24] However, the pain experienced during these exercises can discourage patients from engaging in physical therapy.[25] This non-adherence can lead to additional surgery or permanent reduction in mobility and function.

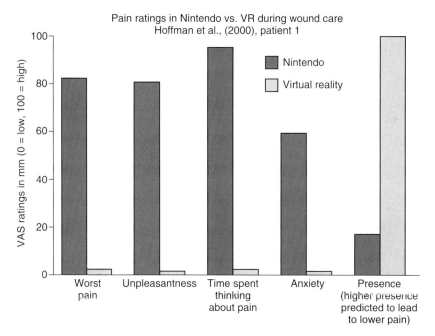

Figure 2.3   Drops in pain during VR wound care compared to Nintendo wound care (data from Hoffman et al.,[20] © reproduced with permission from Hunter Hoffman, U.W. HITLab).

Hoffman et al.[26] explored the use of immersive VR to distract patients from pain during physical therapy. Twelve patients aged 19–47 years (average of 21% total body surface area burned) performed range of motion exercises of their injured limb with assistance from an occupational therapist. Each patient performed physical therapy with no distraction for 3 minutes and physical therapy in VR for 3 minutes (condition order randomized and counterbalanced). All patients reported lower pain and less time thinking about pain when in VR, compared with no distraction (e.g. time spent thinking about pain during physical therapy dropped from 60 mm to 14 mm on a 100 mm visual analog scale). Furthermore, the amount of VR analgesia was statistically significant.

For the above-mentioned VR studies, patients received only one short VR session. It is theoretically possible that VR only works well the first time the patient tries it, while it is a novel experience. If so, its practical medical value would be limited. However, as demonstrated in the case study at the start of the chapter, researchers have found that immersive VR continues to work when used more than once.[5] Those findings have recently been replicated in a larger study. Hoffman et al.[27] studied seven patients aged 9–32 years, mean age 21.9 years (average of 23.7% total body surface area burned, range 3–60%), performing a range of motion exercises of their injured limb with help from an occupational therapist. Patients had the illusion of flying through SnowWorld (Fig. 2.4). SnowWorld depicts an icy 3-D virtual canyon with a river and waterfalls. Patients shot snowballs at snowmen and igloos. They aimed by looking at whatever they wanted to shoot, and pressing the spacebar on a keyboard. The snowballs exploded on impact with animations and 3-D sound

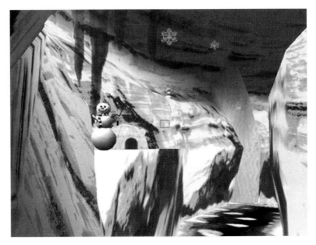

Figure 2.4   An image of what patients see in SnowWorld (© reproduced with permission from Hunter Hoffman, U.W. HITLab).

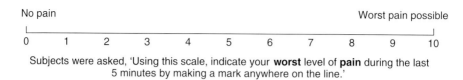

No pain   Worst pain possible

0   1   2   3   4   5   6   7   8   9   10

Subjects were asked, 'Using this scale, indicate your **worst** level of **pain** during the last 5 minutes by making a mark anywhere on the line.'

Figure 2.5   Visual analog scale.

effects. Each patient participated in the VR condition, during which they performed active, assisted physical-therapy exercises. The occupational therapist moved the patient's limb through a pre-determined sequence of ranging exercises while the patient was in VR (e.g. raising the patients arm as if they were asking a question, or crossing the injured arm across the patient's chest).

Each patient participated on at least three separate days. As before, they received VR for part of their physical therapy, and no distraction during another part of the same physical therapy session. Condition order was randomized and counterbalanced. The mean amount of time spent performing physical therapy in VR was 3.5, 4.9 and 6.4 minutes for the first, second and third session, respectively. Pain ratings (Fig. 2.5) were statistically lower when patients were in VR, and the amount of VR pain reduction did not get smaller with repeated use of VR. Although the small sample size limits generalizability, the results of that study suggest that VR retains its analgesic properties with multiple treatments. This finding is encouraging for the wound-care field, given the fact that burn patients usually need multiple wound-care and physical-therapy sessions during their recovery.

CONCLUSIONS AND FUTURE DIRECTIONS

Because recovering from burn injuries is especially painful, adjunctive psychological pain control techniques that prove effective with burn patients will likely prove effective for other painful procedures (e.g. pain from brief painful cancer procedures, physical therapy for cerebral palsy, recovery from knee injuries, etc). Consistent with this claim that VR analgesia will generalize to other pain populations, researchers recently reported in a case study that VR can reduce dental pain.[28] Although the findings summarized in the present chapter are preliminary, they suggest that VR is a promising technique for adjunctive pain reduction during wound-care procedures. More studies are needed with larger samples and including blind conditions to minimize demand characteristics and placebo effects. Ideally, future studies will lead to a better understanding of the mechanism of VR analgesia, and will inform the design of increasingly effective VR analgesia experiences.

ACKNOWLEDGEMENTS

The research was supported by NIH Grant GM42725-07, NIH Grant HD37683-02, NIDRR Grant H133A970014 and the Paul Allen Foundation.

REFERENCES

1. Gift AG 1989 Visual Analogue Scales: measurement of subjective phenomena. Nursing Research 38: 286–288
2. Huskisson DC 1994 Measurement of pain. The Lancet 2: 1127–1131
3. Garcia-Palacios A, Hoffman HG, Carlin A et al. 2002 Virtual reality in the treatment of spider phobia: a controlled study. Behavioural Research Therapy 40: 983–993
4. Carlin A, Hoffman HG, Weghorst S 1997 Virtual Reality and tactile augmentation in the treatment of spider phobia: a case study. Behavioural Research Therapy 35: 153–158
5. Hoffman HG, Patterson DR, Carrougher GJ et al. 2001 The effectiveness of virtual reality pain control with multiple treatments of longer durations: a case study. International Journal of Human-Computer Interaction 13: 1–12
6. Patterson DR 1992 Practical applications of psychological techniques in controlling burn pain. Journal of Burn Care Rehabilitation 13: 13–18
7. Patterson DR 1995 Non-opioid-based approaches to burn pain. Journal of Burn Care Rehabilitation 16: 372–376
8. Brown C, Albrecht R, Pettit H et al. 2000 Opioid and benzodiazepine withdrawal syndrome in adult burn patients. American Surgery 66: 367–370
9. Cherny N, Ripamonti C, Pereira J et al. 2001 Strategies to manage the adverse effects of oral morphine: an evidence-based report. Journal of Clinical Oncology 19: 2542–2554
10. Carrougher GJ, Ptacek JT, Sharar SR et al. 2002 A comparison of patient satisfaction and self-reports of pain in adult burn-injured patients. The Journal of Burn Care and Rehabilitation 24: 1–8
11. Perry S, Heidrich G, Ramos E 1981 Assessment of pain by burn patients. Journal of Burn Care Rehabilitation 2: 322–327
12. Choinere M, Melzack R, Rondeau J et al. 1989 The pain burns: characteristics and correlates. Journal of Trauma 29: 1531–1539
13. Melzack R 1990 The tragedy of needless pain. Scientific American 262: 27–33
14. Patterson DR, Everett JJ, Burns GL et al. 1992 Hypnosis for the treatment of burn pain. Journal of Consulting and Clinical Psychology 60: 713–717
15. Patterson DR, Questad KA, Boltwood MD 1987 Hypnotherapy as a treatment in patients with burns: research and clinical considerations. Journal of Burn Care Rehabilitation 8: 263–268
16. Hoffman HG, Hollander A, Schroder K et al. 1998 Physically touching and tasting virtual objects enhances the realism of virtual experiences. Virtual Reality: Research, Development and Application 3: 226–234
17. Kahneman D 1973 Attention and effort. Prentice-Hall, Englewood Cliffs, NJ
18. Shiffrin RM 1998 Attention. In: Atkinson RC, Hernstein RS, Lindzey G et al. eds. Steven's handbook of experimental psychology, vol. 2. Learning and cognition. Wiley, New York, 739–811
19. Hoffman HG, Prothero J, Wells M et al. 1998 Virtual chess: the role of meaning in the sensation of presence. International Journal of Human-Computer Interaction 10: 251–263
20. Hoffman HG, Doctor JN, Patterson DR et al. 2000 Virtual reality as an adjunctive pain control during burn wound care in adolescent patients. Pain 85: 305–309
21. Gasma A 1994 The role of psychological factors in chronic pain. I. A half century study. Pain 57: 5–15
22. Melzack R, Wall PD 1965 Pain mechanisms: a new theory. Science 150: 971–979
23. Turk DC, Meichenbaum D, Genest M 1983 Pain and behavioral medicine: a cognitive-behavioral perspective. Guilford Press, New York

24. Ward RS 1998 Physical rehabilitation. In: Carrougher GJ ed. Burn care and therapy. Mosby Inc, St Louis, MO, 293–327
25. Ehde DM, Patterson DR, Fordyce WE 1998 The quota system in burn rehabilitation. Journal of Burn Care Rehabilitation 19: 436–440
26. Hoffman HG, Patterson DR, Carrougher GJ 2000 Use of virtual reality for adjunctive treatment of adult burn pain during physical therapy: a controlled study. Clinical Journal of Pain 16(3): 244–250
27. Hoffman HG, Patterson DR, Carrougher GJ et al. 2001 The effectiveness of virtual reality based pain control with multiple treatments. Clinical Journal of Pain 17: 229–235
28. Hoffman HG, Garcia-Palacios A, Patterson DR et al. 2001 The effectiveness of virtual reality for dental pain control: a case study. Cyberpsychology and Behavior 4(4): 527–535

WEBSITES OF INTEREST

Human Interface Technology Lab: www.hitl.washington.edu/

Virtual Reality Pain Control: Harborview Burn Centre: www.vrpain.com

3

Enabling communication: pictures as language

Bodil Jönsson

SUMMARY

A developmental disability often includes a language disorder, the results of which render learning, in part, if not entirely impossible. This has drastic consequences for children and adults, and gradually ends up becoming the primary disability.

With today's technology, thousands of personal digital photographs can become an active language. When someone acquires a first language, even when over the age of 50, it can result in the initiation of a learning process – it can even result in that person learning to speak. By seeing the results presented against this fundamental background, they become comprehensible, encouraging and challenging. Three case studies are presented: a boy with autism and two adult men with cognitive limitations.

The Isaac technology unites the chapter. Ten years ago, 'Isaac' was the latest in high tech. Today, 'Isaac' is more of a framework, the critical technological components of which can be purchased as standard equipment. However, without the original implementation neither the user's experience nor the framework would have come to light. That is why we are now implementing Isaac 2002: software for managing the tremendous number of digital photos that enable simple combinations of pictures to become conveyers of meaningful language elements in many situations.

CASE STUDY 1

Abdulkader Faraax is a 10-year-old boy and his story has been written in close cooperation with his teacher, Agneta Dyberg-Ek. Abdulkader was born in Sweden in 1991 after his parents emigrated from Somalia at the end of the 1980s. They have a loving relationship with their son and a close physical one with lots of hugging and kissing.

Abdulkader did not develop like other children. He was extremely active and restless from an early age and he was diagnosed with autism at the age of three. He had already started at day care (at 2½) and continued there with different personal assistants until the autumn of 1997. He and his assistants had a room of their own and worked with a variety of social interaction games, colors and other activities. They used sign language in combination with pictograms and small photographs. The most fun he had was when he was swinging – something he could do for hours in the gym or outside. He also liked to be chased and to run around and around. He had, for the most part, no spoken language.

When Abdulkader started school at 6 years of age with Agneta as his teacher, he could dress and undress himself, eat on his own and manage his toilet needs. He only had a few words: names of those closest to him and single words, such as 'eat' and 'water'. The family wanted him to learn Swedish, but had always spoken Somali with him even though they had been educated in Sweden, having completed upper secondary school.

Agneta had, and still has, close contact with Certec and started participating in the Isaac project as early as 1995/96. The Isaac project involves the use of a large number of personal digital photographs as a means of communication for children and adults with developmental disabilities, autism and aphasia. The colored pictures are viewed, sorted and stored on a computer. They can then be printed, mounted in booklets, on the wall, on posters or on large rollers for easy access. The variety of ways in which the project has developed is a product of the creativity and ingenuity of the teachers, caregivers and family members involved. As a teacher, Agneta has consistently tried, with the aid of personal digital photos, to understand how Abdulkader and other pupils interpret their (our) world and what they wonder about. This means that she has photographed extensively in order to use pictures as language. Pictures now fill the following functions for Abdulkader:

1. Provide awareness that what is invisible at that moment still exists

It made a big difference when Agneta understood that for Abdulkader it was as if his parents had disappeared when he was in school. Correspondingly, Agneta disappeared out of his mind when he was not in school. If she turned up at his home or in a shop, the situation was entirely wrong. She was supposed to be in school and his mother was supposed to be at home. It was first by using photos of people, which they *moved* between photos of different buildings, that he gradually began to realize that people do not disappear just because they can no longer be seen.

All such insight needs to be continually reinforced. One autumn, a classmate of Abdulkader changed classes. He was still in the same building and came by at times, but was no longer a part of Abdulkader's world. Talking about it with him was not enough. Agneta thought that Abdulkader understood, so she had not photographed the event. It wasn't until all the classes were on an outing and Abdulkader started pushing his former classmate that she realized something was wrong. Back at school, she and Abdulkader immediately went to the old classmate in his new classroom, photographed him there and that was enough to satisfy Abdulkader. He stopped picking on his former classmate. Now he knows.

2. Provide confirmation

Closely connected with this is that Abdulkader often *wonders*, wonders intensively about things and people, and that is when he needs to see a *picture* as confirmation that the listener understands what and who he means. If there is no picture, such confirmation is impossible. In his own classroom everything is turned upside down for him if his teacher forgets to photograph something new in the environment or if he does not have access to pictures of those people who are usually there. Not until he is able to see the person in question in a picture and is able to confirm for himself that it is the one he was thinking about, can he settle down.

Example 1: the first few weeks of the 1997 school year were extremely turbulent, but after a month things improved. A letter about this from Agneta has been published.[1] It tells how things did not start to calm down until pictures were taken of almost everything. Suddenly one day, though, all reverted to as it had been before – Abdulkader was tremendously restless all day long, unable to concentrate or to quieten down. When it was time to go home by taxi, and Agneta accompanied him out to the car, she saw that the driver was new. 'Is that what you were trying to tell me all day, Abdulkader? That there was a new taxi driver?' He did not respond. 'Shall I go in and get the camera and take a picture of him?' No response. But Agneta fetched the camera anyway, took the photo, and then, not until then, when Abdulkader could see the photo himself and see that the new driver was also in the picture, did he collapse, totally exhausted in the back seat of the taxi. A whole day of considerable stress and strain was over.

It is worth mentioning that the taxi had dropped Abdulkader off at the wrong address three times in less than 6 months. The last thing he does in school everyday now, before going out to the taxi, is to confirm for the staff with pictures where he is going and with whom he will be spending the afternoon and evening. Then he feels secure. If he is dropped off at the wrong place, though, he quickly loses all the trust that has been built up. So now the staff has established the *routine* that Abdulkader will always have pictures with him of the building to which he is going. The driver gets out of the taxi, opens the door and before they take off asks Abdulkader: 'Where are you going?' When Abdulkader shows the driver his picture, he knows that he has control over the situation and that he will be dropped off at the right place. In this case he is using the picture to answer a *question*.

Example 2: a new question word after the summer of 2001 was, 'Truck?' 'What do you mean by "truck"?' Agneta wondered. She checked to see if he wanted to read about trucks. No, that's not what he meant. He continued calling out, 'truck, truck', and was obviously upset. Was he afraid of trucks? Had something happened involving a truck? She didn't understand. The staff at his after school program said that he was also yelling out 'truck' there.

Days went by. One Monday he shouted 'truck' several times in the morning. Then a big red truck drove up to the school, the one that comes every Monday with supplies, and that Abdulkader had seen through the window for several years. Agneta wondered: 'Is that what he wanted confirmed, so that we would understand what he was thinking of? Or perhaps he was wondering when the truck was going to come?' She photographed the truck immediately, printed it out and Abdulkader calmed down. Now he has a picture of a truck on his Monday schedule. And since then he hasn't called out 'Truck?'.

3. Seeing people

Abdulkader finds it difficult to perceive people even if he is looking right at them. It is not due to a visual impairment or fear of making eye contact, but stems from something else. It seems that with the help of a digital camera, it is possible to make people visible so that he can see them. We do not know why awareness of a person arises through observing a picture but not through observing the real person, however, we have a number of suggestions. One is that it may be because pictures are two dimensional, that they are framed, that they do not move and change, the way human faces do all the time, etc.[2]

On one occasion, we found out by chance something quite surprising. When one of Abdulkader's aides said: 'It's time for us to go and eat, Abdulkader', the child did not react. But one day when the aide had a *photo* of himself on the lapel of his jacket and happened to point at the *photo*, not at himself when he said: 'It's time for us to go and eat, Abdulkader', the boy stood up right away and accompanied him.

4. Asking questions

Abdulkader's path to being able to ask questions has been long and slow. It has mostly consisted of one word or two-word sentences. He has been able to ask for things that he has seen. He has also been able to choose when presented with two pictures and use the words.

Agneta has avoided using pictures to give instructions of the type: 'Now we are going to do this.' She displays a photo and tries to get Abdulkader to orally express or in some other way indicate what he is *thinking* when he sees it. She does this by showing him the picture and saying: 'What shall we do?' If Abdulkader says what Agneta thinks he is going to, they do it. But if he says something totally different, she tries to figure out exactly what he means, shows him other pictures, adds information, and seeks out his confirmation.

5. Showing how things are related

What does, 'Put on your cap!' mean? Abdulkader did not understand, even if Agneta put the cap on him. It wasn't until he saw the picture of himself wearing the cap that he could accept and understand and then put on the cap.

6. Preparing

It would be unimaginable to visit a new place with Abdulkader without preparing him. Agneta has even been able to travel with him and his classmates to Denmark's Aquarium when everything has been photographed in advance, enabling him to obtain confirmation the entire time from the pictures he has with him.

7. Giving instructions

There are situations in which instructions need to be given. If you are on a class outing, you can't just say to Abdulkader: 'Sit down. This is where we are going to eat,' and point at a stone or bench. But it works quite well to take a *picture* of a stone or bench and say: 'This is where you can sit.'

One autumn day after school it was time to make preparations for winter. The table at which Abdulkader usually sat and drew needed to be moved in from a room with no heating. The situation turned chaotic – as expected. But the solution was obvious: show him a picture of the table in its new position with drawing paper and crayons on it and say: 'This is where you can sit and draw.' And that solved the problem.

8. To make apparent through variation – to make the world real

To make *words* visible has meant a lot and has created trust. *Many* visits in *many* different shops were needed before Abdulkader understood what 'shopping' meant. But now he does and he likes to go along. Agneta thinks that it is the multiplicity of his own experiences of reality *remaining* in the pictures that make his world, thoughts and words real for him.

9. Regaining Swedish after the summer of 2001

During the summer of 2001, Abdulkader spent 8 weeks in a totally Swedish-speaking environment without his parents. Nevertheless, it was as though all the Swedish words had disappeared by the time he returned to school in the autumn. The jumping, running around and anxiety that existed with Abdulkader when he started school 4 years earlier were there again, and Agneta was trying to understand what had happened and felt as though she would have to start from the beginning. But when he was able to see his pictures again, his own through the years, he was able to answer in Swedish.

Size of Abdulkader's vocabulary in words and pictures

At the most, Abdulkader has used a total of 300 to 400 words actively, primarily in combination with pictures or objects. A day when he is most talkative, he will produce perhaps 20–30 words. Most are question words (like 'Truck?' in the previous example) or words that he uses to give confirmation. He has spontaneously spoken on a few occasions. One time when he was sitting at the window and the first snow was falling he suddenly said: 'Go sledding'. And on another occasion when he had just had his hair cut, he came up to Agneta and said: 'Cut hair'. His parents have related many similar examples of spontaneous speech.

In his first year in school (1997/1998) he had 400 pictures, in the second an additional 700, in the third he had another 2000, and in his fourth another 1500. He now has a total of 5000 pictures. During an ordinary week at school, though, he does not use more than perhaps 50 to 60 of these actively. Abdulkader does not take any of the photos himself.

The results for Abdulkader should not be measured primarily through the size of his vocabulary, but rather through the decrease in desperation

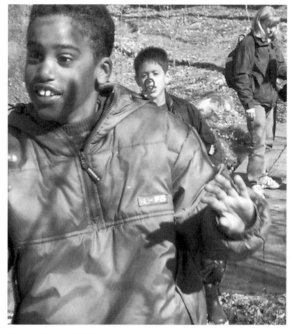

Figure 3.1   Abdulkader at play.

and outbursts of agony and rage. It could be that oral language is more harmful than useful. There is some evidence that if Abdulkader is *not* exposed to sounds, words, noise or music – just to pictures – then his existence becomes less frustrating and more productive.

The situations described here are the ones which Agneta and I have discussed in detail and which we are able to describe even though we do not completely understand them. But there is so much more that has happened and is happening with Abdulkader that we do not understand and find hard to express. His case offers an excellent illustration of the need to strive for better explanatory models and better concepts concerning language and visualization (Fig. 3.1).

INTRODUCTION AND BACKGROUND

Originally, the long-term project called Isaac was based on a personal digital assistant (PDA) for differently abled people. The idea evolved in 1993 through the close cooperation between Professor Lars Philipson, Department of Information Technology, Lund University, and Bodil Jönsson, Professor of Rehabilitation Engineering at Certec, Department of Design Sciences, Lund University, Sweden.

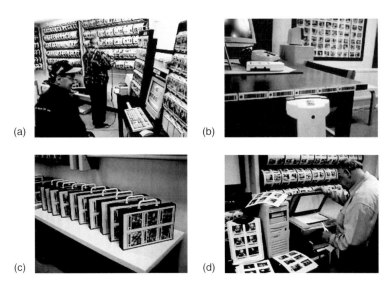

Figure 3.2   Stig and Thomas working with their digital pictures at the Pictorium.

Designed to be used as an aid for individuals with cognitive limitations, Isaac combined in one unit a pen-based computer, a digital camera, a global positioning system (GPS) satellite navigation receiver, and cellular phone channels for voice and data. A number of such mobile units could be in wireless contact with a support center providing assistance over the phone based on pictures, position data and other kinds of information managed by the system.

Although targeted for a special application, Isaac had the potential for much wider use. The emphasis on multimedia and communication put Isaac in the forefront of PDA technology as an example of future personal computing. Information about the original Isaac is available at: http://www. english.certec.lth.se/isaac/isaac1.html. Furthermore, an overview of the project is available at: http://www.english.certec.lth.se/isaac/.

We have seen many generations of Isaac users over the years. Eventually, it became obvious that the key function of Isaac was neither its mobility nor its GPS function. Instead, it was the managing of *many* pictures (with sound) and the bar code interface to the computer that made the difference, and that led to astonishing personal development.

Figure 3.2 shows Stig and Thomas, the two people in the next case study, interacting with the technology. The digital photos can be viewed on the computer screen or printed and mounted on rollers, on the wall, on furniture and other objects. Specially designed software enables those using the program to sort and retrieve stored images. They can then print pictures of their choice, arrange them and photocopy them on their own. Bar codes are added to the photos.

People with developmental disabilities can not only find the picture that they are looking for among thousands of others; what is more important is that they can make *sequences* of pictures (using a bar code scanner), thus giving other people they interact with insights into their world, which were previously completely unknown. This is the beginning of a fruitful spiral; the people using the technology gain a new kind of feedback. As they become more and more used to their ability to make themselves understood, they try harder and harder. Or to state it in two words: they *learn,* as never before. And all that is needed for this to happen are the *elements* (the pictures) that are relevant to them and that they can combine.

Certec has continually developed the Isaac technological/educational concept. Isaac has primarily been used by people with developmental disabilities and limited or non-existent oral language, along with their families, friends and personnel. It has also been applied to and produced significant results for people with aphasia and psychiatric disorders.[3–7] There are now a number of case studies of the interplay between people with different types of language disabilities and a multiplicity of personal digital photographs (over 1000 and often well over 10 000).[8] As demonstrated in the case study at the start of the chapter, there is also a growing and increasingly widespread use of digital photos in the daily activities of special educational facilities and care-giving organizations for the disabled.

WAS THERE A NEED FOR ISAAC? WHAT DIFFERENCE DOES ISAAC MAKE?

Isaac was created entirely at the initiative of engineers and scientists. No user had expressed a 'need' for an Isaac nor had parents, staff or even researchers in cognition, rehabilitation, or education. A possible precursor to Isaac was found in an article by Gregg Vanderheiden of the Trace Center, USA, describing 'The Companion'.[9] This was a somewhat science-fiction-inspired tale of the support that a technological 'companion' might provide to a differently abled person in the future. The account did not play an active role in the creation of Isaac, but to some of us who were involved it was a stimulating background story.

I was the one who at the time of the Isaac technology creation lobbied for the inclusion of a built-in, digital camera, something quite exotic in 1993. It was obviously a 'solution', but to what and why? I was not sure, but the main question was: How do you go about talking to others if you do not have the words? If you want to tell me something about a car, it is most often something about a *special* car: my car, a blue car, the neighbor's van, etc. – not just any car, not just the concept 'car'. Generalized pictures (pictograms, etc.) can never fulfill the task of stimulating communication that is specific and yet varied.

The most striking effect of the picture-as-language concept has been its ability to produce drastic and long-lasting effects on the learning acquisition of people with cognitive limitations/developmental disabilities/learning disabilities/autism. Though there are many groups for which the 'picture-as-language' concept is helpful, none of them suggest why the modern-day availability of a multiplicity of digital photos can be as effective as it is. However, without denying the existence of corresponding motor problems (in walking, hygiene, ability to hold one's head up, etc.), contact avoidance, attention disturbances, compulsive behaviors, etc., if one narrows it down to the *language disorder* as being a significant, often the most significant aspect of the disability, there is value in pursuing the following thought:

What exactly is it in the life of a cognitively limited person that has to do with his/her language disability, and how can the language disability be tackled?

The dramatic effects of the digital pictures appear logical if the following line of reasoning is true: If you are unable to acquire a language you will be unable to *learn* to any great extent. If the effects of this have been accumulating since early childhood, it can result in the developmentally disabled adult being very different from others in the areas of feelings, knowledge, behavior and relationships. But it is never too late. In fact, the introduction of pictures as language to people in their 50s or over can result in a strong, positive change and a constructive process for all involved.[8]

It has been difficult to find explanations for the effects of Isaac. Established research in the fields concerned constitutes a mixture of efforts on different levels. They are so difficult to structure and publish as a literature review that I refrain from even attempting. What is striking is that the research areas involved have different purposes and varying concepts. Furthermore, what is relevant is the *cross section* between:

- the rapidly evolving information and communication technology (ICT), especially its potential for pictures as language;
- language research in its deepest sense;
- research on language difficulties caused by cognitive limitations.

In what follows, I develop more fully our experiences from The Pictorium, a day activity center for adults with cognitive limitations.

The difference Isaac makes for people with cognitive limitations

Changes in the learning acquisition of two adults with cognitive limitations (now in their 50s) over an 8-year period are described. These people appear in the text under their own names – they and their relatives want it that way.

Stig Nilsson and Thomas Åkesson have participated in The Pictorium, a day center for adults with developmental disabilities, for many years. One of its unique aspects is that the supervisor, Göran Plato, with his artistic talents has been able to establish a creative environment. To this he has incorporated advances in information technology to enhance and improve the communication and cognitive capabilities of the adults in his care. He knows them well after all his years of working together with them, but makes every effort to encourage them in their own decision making by finding new ways of enabling them to express themselves. This is why I refer to him as their 'mental companion'. It is difficult to describe The Pictorium in words; it needs to be *seen* and *experienced*. In lieu of that, the following can be of assistance: http://www.english.certec.lth.se/isaac/intro.html, the Swedish TV documentary film,[10] as well as the most recent material published about The Pictorium: *Art and Science – A Different Convergence.*[8]

What has happened to Stig and Thomas during the years has been continuously documented.[1,8,10–18] They are both upper-middle-aged and have developed in a way that has, perhaps, never before been reported – both have gained in stature, in self-respect and have improved their thinking and communication abilities. Thomas has acquired an extensive oral language and Stig has greatly strengthened his ability to express himself, primarily through pictures. After 9 years there is no sign of the development leveling off; if anything, the opposite.

CASE STUDY 2

Stig Nilsson is an extremely communicative person although he has very limited spoken language and only a few signs. He is impatient for everybody in his surroundings to understand what he wants to express. The misunderstandings and total lack of understanding have caused frustration and anger over the years. Even for those working closely with Stig, it was often impossible to comprehend his intentions, not to mention his wishes and dreams.

For Stig to gain access to this multitude of pictures made a significant difference and initiated from the very beginning a rapid development process. He has so many thoughts that he has never been able to communicate. As he has received more feedback, he has been able to proceed through long chains of events and associations. The following is an example that shows how his communication abilities had grown 5 years ago.

Alan Alda visited The Pictorium on 18 August 1997 as the host of the popular TV series 'Scientific American Frontiers', which airs once a month on the American public television network PBS.

The theme of the program in January 1998 was major research breakthroughs in Scandinavia in recent years. After an extensive search, the producers chose Isaac and its users as one of the two Swedish contributions to the program. The day of filming arrived, and Alan Alda whirled into The Pictorium.

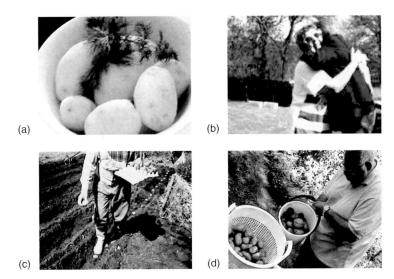

Figure 3.3 The potato growing process.

He was unprepared for the huge number of pictures, the bar coding, the bar code scanner and the computers (his not knowing what to expect is part of the program concept). He tried talking to the users and after a while he realized that he could communicate with them by referring to their own pictures. First, he tried to show them what kind of food he liked. He chose boiled potatoes. When this picture appeared on the screen, Stig, one of the users, turned immediately and pointed to another picture of an older lady, not once, but several times and with great emphasis!

What was Stig trying to tell Alan Alda? What would Alan have understood if he had known more about Stig? Simply that the users at The Pictorium grow their own potatoes, that they grow them in the lady's garden and that the next day they were going to harvest their potatoes (Fig. 3.3)! Not a bad chain of thought for a person who has a developmental disability, who lacks a spoken and written language, and who has very limited sign language. As this example illustrates, Stig had grown tremendously through the use of Isaac. He was able to handle a visit from an English-speaking actor and could tell him about one of his many new perceptions of how things are related. Before Isaac, this would have been completely impossible. Stig was unable to show those around him what he wanted to say and they were unable to guess. With about 10 000 digital photos of his own, however, he has turned the pictures not only into words but also into a language (Fig. 3.4).

Can you actually be certain that you understand what Stig means? Well, it depends on who 'you' are. The advantage of digital pictures for strangers who meet Stig, is that they can immediately carry on a

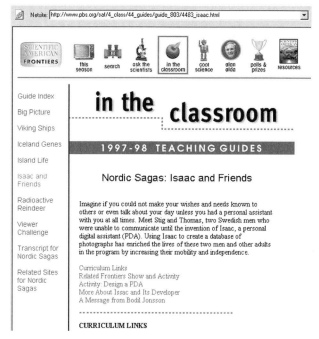

Figure 3.4   Bodil Jönsson answered questions under 'Ask the scientists' at www.pbs.org/saf, the Scientific American Frontiers' site, here featuring 'Isaac and Friends'.

superficial conversation with the aid of the pictures. But for those who already know him, the pictures constitute a different kind of progress, as can be seen in the example above. Stig was telling us that the instant he sees the potatoes, he thinks of them growing in the soil, of the garden where they are growing, of who owns the garden and of when the potatoes will be harvested. Accordingly, we were able to discover complex internal conceptions of how things are related in a way that outsiders cannot. We can ask him questions, and carry on a completely new kind of conversation with Stig. There is no magic in this – the difference between communication with strangers and with confidants is of a similar nature whether you communicate with pictures or with words. In our opinion, the risk of misunderstanding Stig when communicating via pictures is actually smaller than the risk of misunderstanding other people when communicating with words. The reason is that he is not satisfied until he knows that we have understood.

Now, Stig still does not speak a lot, but he expresses so much with photos that it is easy to occasionally forget that he does not talk. Before he had only 'Iiiig' (Stig) and 'Jaaa' (Yes). New word-like sounds from Stig (from Göran Plato's e-mail 2001): ' "Oooooja; Ja; Va, va, va; Na-na-na;

Mu, mu, mu". This happens when he is the one controlling the bar code scanner and picture rollers. Stig usually sits at the computer, looks at his pictures and tries to imitate the sounds I make. He's using many new words that I find difficult to understand.'[8]

CASE STUDY 3

Thomas Åkesson has gained not only in pictorial but to an astonishing extent in oral language as well. Actually, his language development should be measured day by day. Before Isaac, he was a person of extremely few words, having only a couple hundred in his vocabulary, the pronunciation of which was difficult to understand.

The only evaluation carried out by a speech and language pathologist is from the spring of 1998.[18] It revealed the level of Thomas' (and two other persons') oral language in different situations. Or rather the *levels*, because Thomas' oral language differed quite a lot between those situations in which personnel and relatives willingly interacted with him in his picture-filled world and others in which they did not meet Thomas on these terms.

Three years later, in the spring of 2001, Göran Plato wrote to me in an e-mail:

Thomas is using many new word and sentences. I have never heard these before: 'I have to have.' 'Don't you want?' 'Come over, sit here.' 'What are we gonna do now, today?' 'Am better now.' 'That's not right, it's wrong.' 'I wanna go home.' 'Good, you're nice, you coming tomorrow?' 'Will you get me tomorrow?' 'Who's driving tomorrow?' 'Damn it, stop fighting!' 'We need to shop, we're out of a lot' 'I wanna call someone.' 'Shall we work?' 'Don't wanna, do it yourself!' 'What does this say?'[8] (Fig. 3.5).

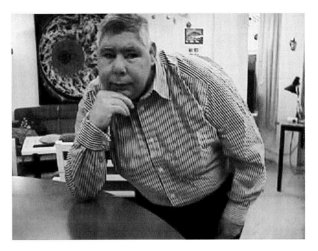

Figure 3.5   Thomas.

Pictures and taking the initiative

One thing is for certain, Göran does not want to make decisions for Stig and Thomas more than is absolutely necessary. It has resulted in Göran signaling them with a wave of the hand about things they can do on their own, at times even waiting them out. But all the new possibilities have resulted in Stig and Thomas starting to take the initiative entirely on their own. Some examples from Göran:

Thomas asked me: 'Plato, you don't happen to have a bag at home that I could borrow?' It's as if the more information pictures we make and the more we produce, the greater the new initiatives they start taking themselves.[8]

Thomas has started taking the initiative to send picture e-mails. One of them was to Arne Svensk at Certec. It was three pictures with the title: Do you want a knuckle sandwich? Arne was urged on by the challenge to provide feedback. He decided to send pictures of the effect Thomas' had on him. Arne added his to the originals so that they could be 'read' in order like a comic book (Fig. 3.6). Thomas' spontaneous reaction was: 'Damn, did I hit him that hard?'

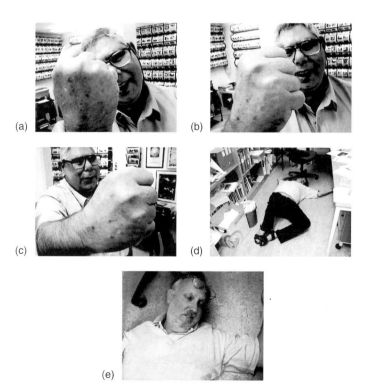

Figure 3.6   Thomas sends a picture e-mail to Arne.

An explosion in the ability to observe and in the perceptual development of how things are related

Closely related to taking the initiative is one's own attention, judgment, and desire to try something new. An example from Göran:

We drive the same route from the area where Thomas lives every day. Thomas has seen a motorcycle there that he likes. One day when we drove by he said: 'Plato, the motorcycle isn't there today.' I hadn't really noticed myself so I had to turn and look and sure enough, there was no motorcycle![8]

All the participants have made tremendous gains in their abilities to make new connections. The habit of using pictures (today between 35 000 and 50 000) has improved their ability to observe the world around them. It is most evident with Thomas since he has become so much more verbal at the same time. Just take the following examples (from Göran's e-mail, 2001):

We often watch the video we took on our Stockholm trip. There is one sequence I find particularly interesting. Thomas was sitting by a window and looking at a building. 'Plato,' he said, 'look at all the window-pictures there are in that building.' He pointed back and forth at the building. I asked what he meant by 'there is a picture in each window'. We videotaped it and I helped Thomas to get a close-up by zooming in on the windows, so he could see what they were doing inside. There was someone sitting at a computer, someone making a phone call, someone drinking coffee, etc. He sat for a long time and looked at it.[8]

This last example shows how we have in a way come full circle. One of the things we discovered a long time ago was that Thomas could not clearly see a picture if it did not have a frame. So we started to frame all the pictures. That gave Agneta Dyberg-Ek, Abdulkader's teacher, a sudden insight: That is the reason why sitting by a window has such a positive effect on some students. It is as though the window gives them a frame through which to see the world. And in that way, one and the same slice of real life becomes easier to handle than the complex, three-dimensional, constantly changing world.[8]

Thomas now saw the windows from the outside as pictures. He even said so: 'there is a picture in each window'. That Göran then had the opportunity to zoom in and show what was actually in the pictures – that was fantastic.

A final example of perceptual development is when Arne sent an e-mail to Thomas with the mere intention of expressing different feelings. Thomas became so fascinated with the pictures that he decided to imitate Arne's body language and he did it with noticeable precision (Fig. 3.7).

Pictures as help when catastrophe strikes

Like the rest of us, people with developmental disabilities have accidents, and like the rest of us things usually work out for them in the end. But the

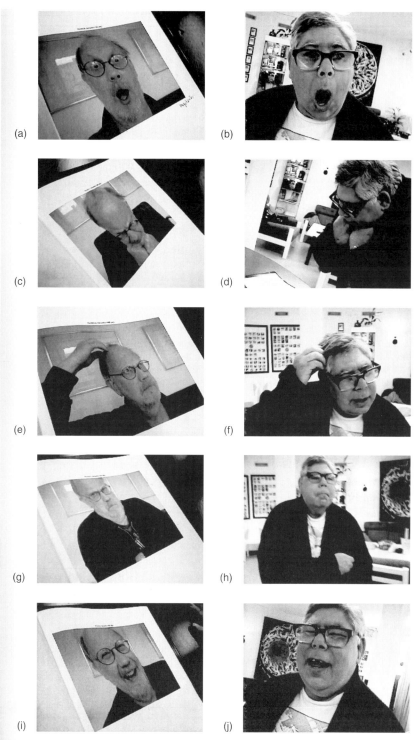

Figure 3.7 Thomas imitates Arne's body language from the pictures Arne sent.

connection isn't always obvious and they lack the ability to generalize to the next difficult situation. Göran has developed a fascinating, effective concept with empty pictures to be filled in step-by-step:

Thomas dropped his glasses and they broke. As if that wasn't enough, the handle on his briefcase was loose. As a result, the briefcase got caught between his legs; he fell on the pavement, cut his elbow, hand and knee. His hand was so swollen that he had to go to the clinic.

And Stig had just had his cast removed when he was going to show a group of visitors a picture. He fell – and his arm swelled up again. What an unfortunate set of accidents the guys have been through.

My recipe: I recreate the events through *pictures*. Build up how they happened. What we are going to do. And see to it that they end with a *positive event*, when everything is fine again.

I've started with pictures of the actual injuries. When the fellows saw them they started laughing, started talking about them with everybody and explaining or trying to explain. In that way they started to *recreate* what had happened and you better believe that they were very good at doing it all over again in pictures, so that they could see for themselves what had happened and tell others on their own. The more they are able to picture-talk about it, the less of a problem it is. Just imagine how little is needed to increase quality of life for them!

To document a negative event in pictures has changed it to a positive, healing one. It has been a kind of first aid. As soon as Stig has a pain or thinks about it, he takes out the pictures and explains how it happened. What we have done. How it will turn out: 'I will be fine!'

They have managed their problems on their own. Fantastic! They have laughed over their accidents. It's terrific that pictures can heal.[8]

Pictures and weight watching

Thomas is overweight. For many years others have tried to get him to lose weight. They have reduced the portion sizes, given him fewer portions, healthier food – and in between a lot of food to comfort, especially from inexperienced staff. The results have been that Thomas has grown heavier and heavier. He finds it hard to walk, cannot bend over to tie his shoes, etc.

It took a while for Göran to understand that the road to success would be through pictures: pictures to display attractive dishes and to show Thomas how to go about losing weight. One day Göran sent the following e-mail:

Thomas wants to send some new pictures of himself. His new weight is 87.5 kilos. He was up to 102. He has really gone all out for this and wants to have pictures of appetizing food. Some of your co-workers from Certec were here yesterday and we invited them to stay for coffee. But when it was Thomas's turn to take a piece of cake, he said he didn't eat it anymore. 'I have my own.'

He can now put on his socks again. And today he picked out a picture of food he had eaten before and asked if he could have it again tomorrow. What progress he has made! I am really touched by it all.

I forgot to tell you about Thomas's morning coffee break. He was able to choose between a baguette with marmalade and a cracker with lettuce, tomato, cucumber and a little slice of low fat cheese. Thomas chose the cracker. 'That one looks really appetizing. I'll take it. Mmmmmmm good,' he said and laughed.

I've started planning a diet for him consisting of 1,500 calories a day. In pictures, of course.[8]

WHAT IS NEEDED FOR ISAAC TO MAKE A DIFFERENCE?

That the Isaac Project found a home at The Pictorium and was further developed there was no coincidence – the environment was already creative and communicative. Human support alone, though, is not enough. Neither Göran Plato nor anyone else could manage by themselves to give Stig and Thomas what they required to develop their thinking skills. What they needed in addition to their already communicative environment were *tools and artifacts to think with*.[19]

The necessity of a multitude of pictures

Many pictures, illustrating the same thing or event, are needed for communication to occur inside or between individuals. It is impossible to know which picture tells a user the most from the beginning. But, even if one picture turns out to be better for a certain user in a certain situation, it is as if the other pictures are needed too, perhaps precisely because they generate perceptions of internal relationships and concepts.

Pictures during and after learning versus pictures as instructions

As it turned out, the digital camera represented a means that was infinitely more successful than we ever could have imagined. For we had only understood the half of it (if even that). From the beginning, we believed that the right kind of *instructions*, created through the use of personal photos, were central. But it turned out to be *not* the chains of correctly constructed instructional photos that resulted in success; it was the chains of photos that were built up *while* learning, as a *support* in learning that made the difference. The pictures help Stig and Thomas while they are in the process and afterwards they are a confirmation that, 'Now I know that.' A happy memory in other words, rather than a set of instructions for future use (Fig. 3.8).

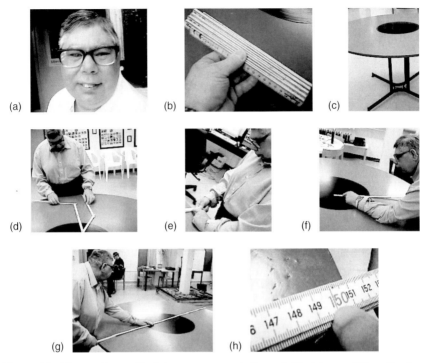

Figure 3.8 Thomas learned to take measurements through 30 pictures of himself using the yardstick. Learning by doing and seeing a multitude of pictures.

The picture and the question versus the picture and the answer

A decisive factor in the success of Isaac at The Pictorium was, most likely, Göran Plato's artistry. Art and science share many points in common. One of these is that both raise new *questions*. But there is a basic difference in how the questions are used. While science immediately throws itself into finding the answers and then making them public, art takes on the role of finding questions, accentuating them and 'hanging' the *questions* up for people to see. So that people can answer themselves – or continue living with the questions.

This has been quite evident in our different ways of working. At first, The Pictorium and Certec are united in the joy of *discovering* the new questions and asking one another: 'Do you think that it can actually be like this?!' But then Certec tries to find the answers, come up with the technical solutions while Göran makes use of our answers by making them over into questions, as it were, that are similar to the original questions and then holds them up in front of Stig and Thomas. It has resulted in a personal development among the participants of The Pictorium closely connected to their interaction with

Göran and with his consistent refusal to live life for anyone else, to decide for anyone else.[10]

If ever there was a group of people who have been more exposed to training in following directions and repetitive practice than others, it is people with cognitive limitations: learning by transfer; an expressed stimuli-response situation, an expressed belief in learning through repetition, combined with assuming guardianship, that is, others doing things and making decisions for the person involved. This approach has dominated and dominates still. The pattern is deeply ingrained even today, in spite of all the good talk of individual development and the right to self-determination that we have heard for a long time.

Perhaps the pattern will not be broken until one understands the difference between elevating the questions versus furnishing the answers. There is no doubt that the people we are involved with need support, lots of it, in order to see structure and context. Read about Henrik Person's black Wednesday.[19] He needs help in many different situations that he does not grasp. But is it preaching, nagging, reproaching and repetition that he needs? Or a more restricted set of values in society saying that people like Henrik really shouldn't be allowed to live on their own, shouldn't be allowed to work, shouldn't …?

There is a polarization in the focus on questions versus answers in different approaches to education. On the one hand, we find constructivism, which with its view of learning as a searching and creative process, places the main emphasis on questions. The supposition is that people learn by asking questions, searching, creating and finding support in the world and inside themselves, all in order to achieve learning, i.e. internal change. On the other hand, there is the psychology of learning, programmed learning, teaching technology and similar approaches, in which learning is studied as if it were independent of content and environment, and as if it could be primarily controlled through situations and instructions arranged in the right manner by the external world.

DISCUSSION AND CONCLUSIONS

Our experience of the effects of the introduction of personal digital photographs as language stretches over a 10-year period. Our reasoning has progressively moved in the direction that all higher mental activity *is* language related (in its broadest sense). According to this line of reasoning, a reduction of the language disability would most likely result in just the developments that we have seen.

But the models we use to explain these effects have never been analyzed by linguists or other researchers in the language sciences. They can be briefly stated as follows:

1. It is essentially the direct and indirect effects of the reduction in *language disability* that we see.

2. The most important effect of pictures-as-language is that it is a means for some people to gain their first user worthy language and in that way drastically improve their ability to *learn*.

3. The prerequisite for all learning is some form of a *relation* between a person and his/her surroundings: the material, the natural and (particularly) the human. *Language* in its broadest sense can be said to constitute this relationship, to be the mental means of conveyance. Many of those we are writing about have previously had weak and monotonous relationships to their surroundings.

4. It seems as though the personal digital photographs are often *more real* for the users than reality itself, i.e. it is easier for them to establish a relationship to the phenomenon through the picture than in direct contact with it. This can be due to a number of factors: that the picture is a still life and immutable, that it is bright, that it has a frame, that it makes it possible for the viewer to look at the situation from different angles, etc.[2]

5. If you examine what a relationship to another person can signify for learning, the most important function of the picture is that it allows an exchange in initiative taking between the differently abled person and his/her surroundings; that it enables conversation based on a common focus and – perhaps most of all – that it enables *variation*.

6. Language is hardly a uniform 'something' that arises and develops in a predetermined manner, neither on the individual level nor collectively. Verbal expression arises in specific contexts, is used for a specific purpose, differentiates successively and gradually develops into an enormous collection of concepts that are interwoven in all that we do; with an emphasis on '*do*'. It is crucial that *action* is coupled to language. This is most likely the same for people with cognitive disabilities.

7. Rich action and rich language presuppose variation.[20,21] It is variation rather than repetition that is the mother of all learning.[16] But the world around us tends to be more repetitive, the greater the dominance it has intellectually, power- or age-wise. In language there are, however, small shifts of already existing meaning, which gradually build up a whole world of internal perceptions. The strength of digital photos in this context is that they can easily become so *many* that they provide a *variation* that offsets what is static and at times meager.

We can go no further than these seven points on our own. In spite of years of intensive work on the project, we have not been able to find more penetrating, applicable explanatory models for the effects, nor relevant, basic theories that we can rely on. Indeed, the digital picture concept is less than a decade old, and on the basis of that it is not unreasonable that theory building hasn't yet caught up. But what we have discovered appears to be so powerful, perhaps even primitive, that it has in all likelihood been studied in the language field. Language has always been shaped and changed through interplay between people. Our language is something that reflects our way of thinking, our relations to other people, our culture, and our identity.[22] We are asking, in other words, for help.

We are eager to *identify* relevant existing theories (along with researchers from different branches) or to come up with new, user worthy theoretical foundations, the effects of which would be at least twofold:

1. To better understand and utilize the results achieved so far
2. To make even more effective implementation than what we have hitherto accomplished.

FUTURE PROSPECTS

Today, you can easily buy over the counter the two essential pieces of hardware that make up Isaac: the digital camera and the computer; the bar coding can also be included. What is missing is a *user worthy and user-friendly Windows application for managing large personal collections of images and sounds, with or without bar coding, with or without frames, etc.* This Windows application will be the Isaac of 2002.

Inspired by many years' experience from the different Isaac generations, Professor Lars Philipson, the original Isaac inventor, has now designed such an application in cooperation with Certec. On 15 August 2002 the beta testing of the first parts of this application began. When development is completed, it will be available free of charge from www.isaac.certec.lth.se. Our sincere hope is that the application will turn out to be valuable, both for the original target group (differently abled people, their relatives and personnel) and in wider circles.

The Isaac project as a whole is a remarkable example of the evolutionary possibilities of contemporary technology. The original Isaac was an exclusive and expensive combination of hardware and software, produced as a prototype in only a few copies and for a special purpose and a special user group. The *years of Isaac user experiences* have been continually discussed, questioned, penetrated, and followed up. The key question has been: How can all this experience be implemented? My answer has been: TTT, thoughts take time.[15] This is paraphrased from the title of a poem 'Things Take Time'[23] by the well know Danish poet and artist, Piet Hein. Later on, 'TTT' took on the meaning 'things that think' at MIT Media Lab. There are two different time aspects:

1. The Isaac *thought* per se has needed its time to develop from thought to implementation to thought to implementation to ... Today, 'Isaac' is more or less a *framework*. Originally, it *was* a specialized combination of hardware and software. But now, it is more an *idea* that can be implemented in many different ways. The technical development has made the basic parts of Isaac (except the above-mentioned software for an easy and adapted managing of *many* pictures) available over the counter: digital cameras, computers and different interfaces. Thus, it is impossible to know

how to count the 'Isaac' users. Nor is it possible to estimate what percentage of use is successful. In Sweden, there are all those hundreds of people (personnel and relatives) who are involved in Certec's courses and discussion groups and who work with 'Isaac' implementations at work or at home. They are all successful, year after year, and they contribute to each other and us all the time. At the same time, there are many failures as well. *If* the people around the people with language difficulties are not genuinely *interested* enough in picture communication, then failure is inevitable. There is also a second TTT aspect here.

2. *Using* Isaac takes *time*. *If* the people around are not prepared to invest a lot of time in the handling of pictures, then failure is also foreseeable. This is no quick fix, nothing that you can just imitate. It is a revolution of the same kind that the Internet brought about in the teaching-and-learning process. The traditional view of the teacher as the possessor of knowledge whose job it was to transmit it to the student in the most appropriate way dramatically changed with the advent of all the information freely available on the Internet. Students have become searchers of knowledge on their own with teachers providing structure, feedback, guidance and help in evaluating the information. Instead of students being told what they have to learn, they are searching for the answers to the questions they have themselves. The information that is gained as a result of answering these questions has a much greater chance than general information of being transformed into knowledge within the person asking the question. This revolution in the teaching-and-learning process brought by the Internet is akin to putting the digital picture taking, storage and sorting capabilities of Isaac into the hands of Stig, Thomas and all the others. But more than just the technology is needed for this to happen and this is where someone like Göran Plato comes in as the one providing the structure, feedback and guidance. We can see no way around this difficulty – you have to accept that the picture language still demands more time than does oral language. But the handling of the wealth of pictures that is needed can be facilitated through an easier interface and faster storage and searching. It is these last thoughts that now form the basis for the new Isaac: a Windows application for many at no cost.

REFERENCES

It is hoped that it is not seen as an act of omnipotence that this reference list, with few exceptions, is as closely related to Certec as it is. It is only meant to express a need for additional help.

1. Jönsson B, Philipson L, Svensk A 1998 What Isaac taught us. Certec, Lund, Sweden, Available online: http://www.certec.lth.se/doc/whatisaac
2. Jönsson B 1996 Datorns attraktionskraft (*The computer's power of attraction*) Report 7. Certec, Lund, Sweden, Available online: http://www.certec.lth.se/dok/datornsattraktionskraft/
3. Andersson G, Knall G 1994 Gun Andersson och hennes väg framåt – om rehabilitering efter en hjärnskada (*Gun Anderson and her road forward*). Certec, Lund, Sweden, Available online: www.certec.lth.se/dok/gunandersson/

4. Andersson G 1997 Min dagbok med digitala bilder (*My diary with digital photos*). Certec, Lund, Sweden, Available online: www.certec.lth.se/ord/dagbok.html
5. Andersson G 1998 Ord som kommer tillbaka men också en del nya ord (*The return of words*). Certec, Lund, Sweden, Available online: www.certec.lth.se/ord/nya_ord.html
6. Andersson G 1999 Det tar aldrig slut (*It never ends*). Certec, Lund, Sweden, Available online: www.certec.lth.se/dok/dettaraldrigslut/
7. Mandre E 2002 Vårdmiljö eller Lärandemiljö? Om personer med autism inom vuxenpsykiatrin (*From medication to education: people with autism in adult psychiatry*). Certec, Lund, Sweden, Available online: http://www.certec.lth.se/doc/frommedicationto/
8. Plato G, Jönsson B 2001 Art and science – a different convergence. Certec, Lund, Sweden, Available online: http://www.certec.lth.se/doc/artandscience/, pp. 20, 28, 36, 38, 40, 42
9. Vanderheiden G, Cress C 1992 Applications of artificial intelligence to the needs of persons with cognitive impairments, the companion aid. In: Resna International '92 Conference. Resna Press, 380–390.
10. Dahlöf A, Iverus M, Dauberübchel et al. 1999 Ovanlig vänskap (*Uncommon friendship*). Documentary film. Uppsala Publishing House, Uppsala, Sweden
11. Bauth R, Jönsson B, Svensk A 1995 Just give us the tools. Sweden: Natur och Kultur, Available online: http://www.certec.lth.se/doc/justgive/
12. Dahlöf A, Larsson S 1999 Växtbok för annorlunda människor (*Growth book for differently abled people*). Uppsala Publishing House, Uppsala, Sweden
13. Danielsson H 2000 Bildpraktik – Om digitala bilders betydelse för personer med kognitiva funktionshinder (*Picture practice – the significance of digital photos for people with cognitive disabilities*). Certec, Lund, Sweden, Available online: http://www.certec.lth.se/dok/bildpraktik
14. Jönsson B, Svensk A 1994 Technology and differently abled people. Natur och Kultur, Sweden, Available online: http://www.certec.lth.se/doc/technologyand
15. Jönsson B 2001 Unwinding the clock: ten thoughts on our relationship to time. Harcourt, New York
16. Jönsson B, Rehman K 2000 Den obändiga söklusten (*The unyielding desire to search*). Brombergs, Sweden, Available online: http://www.certec.lth.se/dok/denobandigasoklusten/
17. Jönsson B 2001 Tankekraft (*Thinking power*). Brombergs, Sweden
18. Sporre M 2000 Digitala bilders kommunikativa funktion för människor med kommunikationshandikapp (*The communicative function of digital photos for people with cognitive disabilities*). Department of Logopedics, Phoniatrics and Audiology: Lund, Sweden, Available online: http://www.certec.lth.se/dok/digitalabilders
19. Svensk A 2001 Design av kognitiv assistans (*Design for cognitive assistance*). Licentiate thesis, Certec, Lund, Sweden, Available online: http://www.certec.lth.se/doc/designforcognitive
20. Emanuelsson J 2001 A question about questions. Acta Universitatis Gothoburgensis, Sweden
21. Marton F, Booth S 1997 Learning and awareness. Lauwrence Erlbaum, Mahwah, NJ
22. Strömqvist S ed. 2002 The diversity of languages and language learning. University of Lund Press, Lund, Sweden
23. Hein P 1998 Collected Grooks 1. Borgens Forlag, Copenhagen, Denmark

WEBSITES OF INTEREST

Art and Science – A different convergence. CERTEC INTERNAL REPORT, LTH, N0 1: 2001. Göran Plato, Bodil Jönsson: http://www.certec.lth.se/doc/artandscience/

Design for Cognitive Assistance. Licentiate Thesis. Arne Svensk. http:// www.certec.lth.se/doc/designforcognitive

Just Give Us the Tools. Bauth R, Jönsson B, Svensk A: http://www. certec.lth.se/doc/justgive/

Isaac – A compilation of information about Isaac: http://www.english.certec.lth.se/isaac/

Isaac – A Personal Digital Assistant for the Differently Abled: http://www. english.certec.lth.se/isaac/isaac1.html

Isaac – The Pictorium, FAQ: http://www.english.certec.lth.se/isaac/intro.html

Moving sound

Phil Ellis

SUMMARY

This chapter describes the results of using an approach called sound therapy with children with profound and multiple learning difficulties and also with the elderly mentally infirm in a long-term care home. Sound therapy was developed by Phil Ellis during the 1990s and uses three examples of sound technology, most importantly the Soundbeam, together with some vibroacoustic techniques. Although the technology is vital, it is the placing of these within a carefully controlled aesthetic environment that is important. Aims of research for both groups are described together with the qualitative research methodology. A range of results mainly from video observation and external validation show in what way sound therapy can be effective. Finally, requirements for sound therapists are drawn from the personal experience of two practitioners: Phil Ellis, the project director and Katy Atak, one of two research assistants employed on the project who authors the second case study below.

CASE STUDY 1

Mary is a severely disabled girl who was 8 years old at the start of the research. She has cerebral palsy, epilepsy, diabetes, has almost no speech – apart from being able to say a kind of 'hello' – has no communication skills, cannot walk, has no self-help skills and generally has an attention span of only a few seconds. Over a period of 5 years Mary regularly attended sound therapy sessions during school term times, usually for about 20 minutes each week.

As with all children with this type of condition, I use a Soundbeam as the most important aspect of technology. This device emits an ultrasonic beam, which will trigger sound if any physical movement is made within the beam itself (a fuller description occurs later in the chapter). The Soundbeam is positioned so that the ultrasonic beam is directed to the top, rear of the head from above. This results in sound being made by the slightest head movement, forwards and backwards or lateral. At first, although there was movement in the beam, and sound caused, there was a time delay between Mary causing a sound and showing a response. Progressively Mary would show more awareness of having some control, and over time the delay in response became shorter, until there was instant response to the sounds caused by her movements.

There were occasions where she would change her behavior completely in these sessions. For example, on one occasion she hadn't vocalized all day, including registration in the afternoon. She apparently wouldn't even say 'hello'. When she came to sound therapy she wouldn't stop saying 'hello'! The stimulation and enjoyment was clear. On arriving in the room she would often look around carefully and watch closely as the beam was being set up. Normally she looks down at her wheel-chair table in a listless fashion.

Often she would have quite stiff and tense muscles, but in the beam she would make lots of physical movements during the session, move her arms, torso, head, and occasionally make a whole body movement, responding to her inner needs, not moving to external commands. Although normally she wears straps over her shoulders, these were often removed and she would show great physical control in moving her head, arms and torso. Sometimes she would make loud and prolonged laughs as she moved in the beam, showing happy emotion and expression.

The head teacher of the school commented: 'Her hearing is great and her vision is great, but she can't verbally express anything except 'hello'. She has got from the unintentional (movement) through to the intentional movement and selection of particular sounds that she has chosen, she enjoys; and it's that innerness – she'll laugh and she'll chuckle and there are more sounds coming now, and I firmly believe that it is as a result of Soundbeam. Because for years she's been in school with speech therapists and physiotherapists and teachers, but there has been no way for her to express herself.'

There are many benefits from this for Mary. She has developed almost instant response to sound and her muscular control has developed significantly. She would anticipate a session and her behavior would change as she was being wheeled to the sound therapy room. Her attention span greatly increased and she would often be fully and actively involved in a session for several minutes, whereas in other situations she would become uninvolved after a few seconds if left on her own. Perhaps most important, as the head teacher remarks, was the ability to express herself. By moving in her chair she could control a whole range of sounds and 'play' them in many different ways. Her classroom assistant remarked that she would 'come alive' during these sessions and her mother observed a significant increase in her physical movements and control. The increased amount of laughter and interactivity is also significant here.

There are numerous examples of children, from 2 to 19 years of age, with a range of profound disabilities responding in similar ways to the sound therapy environment. As with the elderly, it seems that the technology – when used in particular ways – can open doors which either have never been open before, or that have closed through deterioration of some kind or another.

CASE STUDY 2

Linda is 80 years old, the sole survivor of 11 brothers and sisters born and raised in Lancashire, England. Her father was a barber and it was Linda's job to lather up the customers and then fetch him (invariably from the pub!) to shave and groom them. She went on to marry and have five children of her own – three boys and two girls. Her son Colin, who visits her regularly with his own family, told me of his memories of Linda as a loving and caring person, and quite simply, despite having had a hard life, a perfect mother.

Colin and his brother had looked after Linda themselves for 5 years when she suffered ill health through having a number of strokes, but it was after the fifth stroke, 6½ years ago that she started to deteriorate with the onset of senile dementia, and they finally, with reluctance, had to hand over permanent care to a nursing home. Colin feels that she is still the same loveable person that she always was, despite her difficulties, but his sadness is that Linda never mentions his father and that she sometimes uses bad language, unheard of when she was well.

I first met Linda in January 2002. She had been going to sound therapy sessions since May 2000. These sessions had been run by another researcher involved in the project. Pat, the nurse manager of the home said she had enjoyed these very much. Unfortunately, since autumn 2001, my predecessor had been unable to continue her work, therefore Linda had not been able to have any more sessions for a number of months. During this time, Pat had seen a general decline in Linda's health and well-being and was very keen that she should attend sound therapy again with myself.

My first impression of Linda on meeting her in the lounge downstairs was of a quiet, gentle, rather withdrawn lady who did not seem terribly well. She did lift her head to look at me briefly and said 'hello', but did not appear to be communicative. A week later, when she arrived at the sound therapy room, she had no memory of me and the impression I had of her from our first meeting would seem to have been correct. However, within minutes of beginning our first session, I realized that there was far more to Linda than meets the eye. When I greeted her and offered her a microphone, she blew into it and asked what we were doing. I told her that we were going to have some fun and we went on to make various 'daft' vocal sounds together. When I switched on the Soundbeam and moved her hand up and down in it, she seemed quite surprised, exclaiming, 'heavens above!', but she was very receptive to me and after a while moved her hand herself. During this time she gave me some beaming smiles that transformed her from the sad old lady I had met a week ago into a bright, alert and interested Linda. At the end of the session whilst listening to the tape, she asked, 'will this be my music?' and gave me another lovely smile when I assured her that this was indeed her music and her special time. When she had gone I had to admit to myself that I had totally misjudged Linda from our introduction – she clearly had character and opinions and, I felt certain, some memory of previous sound therapy sessions hidden some where in her mind.

I was eagerly awaiting Linda's arrival the following week, expecting to build on the promising start we had made. However, Pat had warned me that Linda had not been well for a few days and had not been eating properly. Earlier on in the day she had said that she had 'given up'. When she arrived at the sound therapy room she had reverted to the Linda I had first perceived – her expression was sad and she seemed to physically droop.

I tentatively tried the beam with her – I programmed in the 'vibes' sound and gently moved her hand up and down to create a rising and falling tinkly sound. I was pleased to see that she smiled and briefly seemed to cheer up, although it only lasted a minute or so before she pulled her hand away. I persevered and programmed in the 'voice' sound, gently moving her hand again to create a soothing 'OOH', undulating between a few notes. Out of the blue she smiled again and raised her eyes to mine, before withdrawing into her self once more. For the remainder of that session, whilst listening to music in the chair, she escaped into her own far away thoughts to a place where I was not needed.

Although I found it upsetting to witness at the time, I feel, on reflection, that I did in fact connect with her through the Soundbeam, albeit briefly, and I learnt a valuable lesson for myself. Linda was a lady with a host of emotions and a great capacity for response, despite her difficulties due to the stroke damage. Like any other person she would have good days and bad days, and I would have to respect whatever mood she arrived in and go at her pace.

Happily, Linda's mood was brighter the following week and during our third session together I felt that we really connected through our Soundbeam work. She was very receptive to me and allowed me to move her hands quite rapidly to stimulate the 'voice' sound, stopping on three occasions to kiss my hand and smile at me. At one point she copied a wiggling motion with the fingers on her left hand – the hand that she generally does not move very much due to the stroke she has suffered – and then went on to move my hand with her right one. She quickly became confident in doing this and initiated a variety of movements before suddenly choosing to stop, leave go of my hand and place her own hands in her lap.

In the next few sessions I discovered some of Linda's likes and dislikes through our Soundbeam work. She is not too keen on singular sounds and she definitely does not like loud, sudden sounds. In one sound setting she stimulates its soothing, resonating sounds with gentle circular hand movements, preferring the lower pitched tones. In another she will sometimes make graceful side sweeping movements, although she finds this more tiring. In recent sessions she demonstrates that she recognizes me and sometimes stimulates the beam independently without having been reminded how to do it, always stopping to give me a beaming smile and often a kiss on my hand.

During our last session I saw that she has quite a sense of humor as she kept her hand up high and wiggled it vigorously to stimulate a disco drum at high speed, again with a cheeky smile. She has started to speak recently of how she likes the 'Sunbeam' – I actually think that her name for it is more pleasant than our own! – and when I ask her how she feels after sessions she will invariably use words such as 'marvelous' and 'I enjoyed it very very much'. Of course, there are moments of confusion and sometimes she thinks that the sounds are coming from the church nearby, but does that really matter? All I know is that through our Soundbeam work, I have discovered a vibrant, affectionate lady with a mind of her own and a range of emotions, and I am glad to say that Pat, who obviously knows Linda intimately, has seen a great improvement in her spirit and health since returning to sound therapy.

AIMS OF SOUND THERAPY

Sound therapy with special needs children

When visiting a school to advise about the purchase of music technology in 1986 I first encountered children with profound and multiple learning difficulties (PMLD). An arrangement was subsequently made to visit the school on a regular basis to explore the possibilities of developing communi-cation skills and physical control for a group of children who had no self-help skills, nor any independent behavior. I experimented with various items of music technology and gradually focused on three, which seemed to have great potential for this group of children. We aimed at the following changes in children's behavior:

- from involuntary to voluntary
- from accidental to intended
- from indifference to interest
- from confined to expressive
- from random to purposeful
- from gross to fine
- from exploratory to preconceived
- from isolated to integrated
- from solitary to individual.

Sound therapy with the elderly mentally infirm

In 1997 I was invited into a home for the long-term care of the elderly mentally infirm (EMI). The aim in this environment was to see if exploiting similar techniques and using the same technology would provide any benefits for people with stroke, dementia and other conditions associated mainly with people in the 'third age'.

The second case study drew on the experience of Katy Atak, one of the researchers involved in this study. The research was sited in three homes for the long-term care of the elderly, and 18 residents were involved during the 2-year programme. There are a number of aims in applying the technology through sound therapy to this group:

- Interactive communication skills. Sound processor and microphone to (re)develop and/or improve:
  - vocal inflection (expression)
  - enunciation
  - range of phonemes (vowels, consonants, etc.)
  - expressive use of voice
  - listening skills
- Independent physical movement and control. Soundbeam and sound module to:
  - (re)develop physical control (typically hand/arm or head, possibly leg)
  - extend/re-energize listening range (quiet/loud, high/low)
  - awaken curiosity through exploration
  - enable self-expression

- Relaxation
  - encourage relaxation
  - promote a general feeling of physical and mental well-being
  - possible trigger for recollection and reminiscence.

When working with PMLD children rather than the elderly the aims of sound therapy are slightly different, particularly in the area of recollection and reminiscence, as these children do not have a rich life experience to draw upon. The emphasis for the children is placed mainly in the first two areas above, but occasionally also for relaxation when appropriate. The vibro-acoustic effects are present throughout sessions, and so provide additional stimulation and feedback when working at developing communication skills and physical movement and control.

TECHNOLOGY USED FOR SOUND THERAPY

Sound processor and microphone

The first piece of technology was a standard sound processor and microphone, encouraging use of the voice for communication through vocal interaction, and the development of enunciation and expression. The effects available through use of the sound processor – including reverberation, echo patterns and pitch-shifting – are highly motivating and intriguing, and encourage vocal interaction and development. The focus given here is not on language and vocabulary as such, but more on expressive communication through changes in pitch, volume and vocal timbre – non-verbal communication.[1-3] It seems possible that some people who have lost the power of speech are able to (re)develop vocal expressiveness by focusing on these elements. The aim is not of learning word sequences, as in melodic intonation therapy,[4] instead the focus is placed on the development of interactive communication through vocal inflection. However, some re-learning of vocal control, including the development of an increased range of sounds, has been observed in the elderly.

Soundbeam

The second piece of technology, called a Soundbeam, became central to the research with both children and the elderly. This piece of technology generates sound from physical movement and works through the use of an ultrasonic beam. A sensor, which looks a little like a microphone, emits an invisible ultrasonic beam. By directing this at a part of the body – the head, an arm or leg, even an eyelid – the smallest movement will result in a sound being heard. The Soundbeam converts physical movement into code and then sends this to a digital sound generator. Effectively you can move your head and play, for example, an electronically generated 'saxophone', 'piano', or any sound you choose. The Soundbeam inventor Edward Williams says: 'this device was the result of my search for ways of enabling dancers to generate and control musical analogies of their own movements in space – at a distance and without any physical contact with the (electronic) musical instrument concerned.'

The most telling use of the Soundbeam since its introduction has been with the disabled, however, and not in the general dance community.

Vibroacoustic devices

The third piece of technology, which is used in therapy, is a vibroacoustic chair or a Soundbox, both developed by the Soundbeam Project. The Soundbox is used with profound and multiply handicapped children, as a wheelchair can be placed on the box. All sounds made in the session are converted into vibration, which is transferred from the surface of the box to the wheelchair and so to the child. The Soundchair is a vibroacoustic chair, which looks rather like a sun-lounger, and is used with the elderly. When sitting or lying on this chair, vibrations can be felt in the chest, abdomen and legs.

Over a number of years in special schools for PMLD children and in homes for the long-term care of the elderly, I have developed sound therapy, an approach which utilizes the technology described.

RESEARCH METHODOLOGY

Evidence for the effectiveness of this approach comes mainly from qualitative methodologies. As each person involved in sound therapy sessions is so individual, all responses tend to reflect this, although there are some common reactions and responses from people with different backgrounds and conditions. In order to bring as much clarity and objectivity into the observation and evaluation process a video-based qualitative research tool was developed which is called layered analysis.[5] This methodology involves using video recordings, which are made of every session of sound therapy, and subsequently disassembling these and reassembling them to build up a comprehensive and detailed series of pictures for each individual. The video processing is in four stages:

1. *Source tape*: A complete recording of each sound therapy session is made. This is not kept from week to week, but initially provides a full record of each session. Its function is to provide temporary storage of data, allowing relevant sequences and events to be identified and archived.

2. *Master tape*: Significant examples of behavior during a session are identified and copied from the source tape. The master tape recording thus gradually increases in length from week to week. This provides a detailed, chronological account of behavior from every session of sound therapy.

3. *Layers tape*: Particular responses from each of the three sections of sound therapy sessions are selected and recorded separately. This provides the most detailed set of sequences revealing particular patterns of behavior, development and progression.

4. *Summary tape*: This is limited to approximately 10 minutes in length for any individual and provides a visual summary of development from the start of a programme of sound therapy, but may not include examples from every month. It is illustrative of an individual's development and is useful in situations where time is at a premium.

From this rich source of data, a list of behavior changes has been developed against which progression and development can be charted for each individual. These lists are different for the children and the elderly.

THE EFFECTIVENESS OF SOUND THERAPY

Over a period of 16 years working with special needs children and 5 years with elderly people, data were collected providing descriptive evidence for the effectiveness of sound therapy.

Special needs children

Starting in 1992 I worked for a 6-year period in a school for children with PMLD, gradually developing the techniques of sound therapy.[6-8] Case study 1 is representative of more than ten children with whom I worked during this period, and of many more who have subsequently been involved in follow-up work. One-to-one sessions with 45 children were performed weekly over periods between 2 and 8 years.

As a result of our video analysis, the following changes can be seen as indicative of development and progression over time:

- developing a number of individual ways of performing expressively with sound
- clearly listening with care and enjoyment to the sounds they articulate
- showing a developing discrimination in the selection and rejection of particular sounds
- often making some vocal response as they move in the Soundbeam
- developing structures in sound which repeat and grow from week to week
- showing aesthetic resonance through most telling facial expressions and body movements
- being actively involved for extended periods of time, far in excess of normal activity
- developing a greatly increased level of concentration

- beginning to discover, explore, give expression to and communicate their own feelings
- making significant physical responses – movements and gestures which have not been seen before, or which have not previously been made independently
- showing satisfaction and pleasure from their own achievements in structuring sound.

The single feature which all children revealed is their active involvement for extended periods of time. Focused activity for minutes at a time was often observed in children whose attention span in other situations could often be measured in seconds.

Elderly mentally infirm

Weekly one-to-one sessions were performed with 25 elderly and mentally infirm over periods of 1–2 years. For this group we have seen improvements in:

- mood
- level of distress
- level of depression
- level of aggression
- level of anxiety
- level of relaxation.

After sound therapy sessions, all those involved would seem happier and would smile more, with greater awareness of other people. This could last overnight and sometimes for days.

The effects of the sound therapy experience for many elderly people seems to:

- encourage eye-to-eye contact
- develop vocal communication, both verbal and through inflection
- improve hearing ability, sometimes beyond the immediate sound therapy environment
- develop listening skills
- encourage and develop physical movement
- provide opportunities for individual exploration and control
- enable deep relaxation and pleasure
- provide opportunities for recollection and happy reminiscence
- promote a general feeling of physical and mental well-being
- re energize and motivate
- develop positive self-esteem
- produce smiles, happiness and a positive outlook, which can permeate other aspects of experience.

External validation

A recent short study of five residents over a 10-week period was conducted by Steven Dennett of STB Consultancy Ltd. The residents were nearing the end of the 2-year project referred to earlier and had all been receiving therapy during the past 6 months. This study was based on the Well and Ill Being Scales (WAIBS) devised by the Bradford Dementia Group, and only the well-being scores were included, as the ill-being scores were deemed unsafe due to participant dropout. Although only a very small-scale research project, and, therefore, necessitating caution in interpretation, it revealed some interesting findings.

From Table 4.1 and Figure 4.1 it can be seen that there was an overall increase in well-being in the hour after the sessions for all participants. There was also an unexpected indication of expectation, with residents apparently

Table 4.1   Summarized WAIBS well- and ill-being scores for five participants (average age 82) over 10 weeks in which sound therapy was provided once a week

		Stage ONE (sessions running) Well-being scores summary table				
	Participant number	Period 1 Monday	Period 2 Wed pre session	Period 3 Wed post session	Period 4 Wed end	Period 5 Friday
	1	51	59	64	38	68
	2	30	53	81	82	69
	3	21	15	25	26	27
	4	29	38	71	72	66
	5	17	24	68	72	59
Total		**148**	**189**	**309**	**290**	**289**

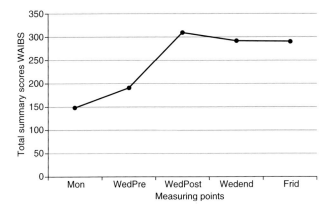

Figure 4.1   Total of summarized well- and ill-being scores for five participants (average age 82) over 10 weeks in which sound therapy was provided.

showing small improvement leading up to the session. A reading of the total scores over the 10 weeks reveals that this positive change effect remained high and only dropped off over the following days.

For the future, a research programme set in residential settings with a control group designed to assess the psychological, psychosocial and illness factors that might be affected by sound therapy is required. Such a programme would validate the value of this approach from a quantitative research perspective. Using the Soundbeam to control visual in addition to aural feedback is an area of growing interest. This might have significance for both PMLD children and the elderly. The technology can already provide this facility and long-term study would be needed to evaluate the potential benefits.

It seems that the use of technology in very controlled ways can affect psychosocial aspects of patients' functioning in many ways. However, the technology itself cannot achieve anything, it is the way in which it is used that is crucial, and this is at the heart of sound therapy. The *aesthetic resonation*, which results from this approach, is its power.

DISCUSSION

The techniques of sound therapy have gradually developed over a number of years, and are still evolving. It brings together aspects of different worlds that have a connection with music but without being dependent on traditional musical skills or thought processes. I have deliberately avoided use of the word 'music' in describing this approach as it is distinct from the approach known as 'music therapy'. In this 'the music therapist is a skilled musician',[9] and their training can reflect the formal thinking, which lies behind many traditionally based approaches. There is clear benefit from the work of Orff or Nordoff and Robbins for example,[10,11] but these demand considerable training of already traditionally trained musicians. In sound therapy a broader view of music itself is taken, and we move away from particular ways of organizing sound towards the view of sound itself as the most important element.[12] Therefore, although practitioners of sound therapy will need to have 'open' ears,[13,14] traditional musical skills, such as the ability to read music notation or play an instrument, are not prerequisites.

Sound itself is the medium of interchange, and in sound therapy this is used in a particular way and in a particular environment. Before discussing this it is useful to refer to some other approaches, which use sound and/or music as a medium of therapeutic intervention.

Tomatis' sound therapy approach[15] has alleviated many physical conditions, including voice/speech disorders, tinnitus, learning disabilities, and autism by correcting hearing deficiencies. To do this a number of carefully produced recordings of music have to be listened to over a period of time, during which the frequency deficiencies noted in a client are 'revitalized' and a more normal audiogram should result at the end of a period of treatment.

The work of Guy Berard[16] is similarly impressive, with direct connections being made between an individual's audiogram and a variety of conditions, including autism, dyslexia, hyperactivity and depression. By progressively 'retraining' a person's hearing and gradually normalizing the audiogram, these conditions can apparently be ameliorated, sometimes cured. In the field of neuro-developmental psychology the importance of sound is given a high profile: 'the significance of sound for learning is immeasurable'.[17] The work of Colin Lane of the Arrow Trust seems to resonate with this, and he has achieved impressive results in the improvement of children's literacy ability.[18] 'Signature sounds' is another approach, devised by Sharry Edwards, in which tones particular to any individual are used in a treatment program, with many physical and psychological benefits apparently accruing from this treatment.[19,20]

A common feature of all these techniques, and of other approaches to music therapy, is that of 'treatment', of direct intervention and imposition of external stimuli determined by an outside agent. Even where a music therapist may claim to be 'responding' to a patient's music, this is a personal response on the part of the therapist. The 'patient' or 'client' is viewed in a clinical way, with a condition, which needs to be treated or ameliorated. There are clearly defined goals with these treatments, and success is measured according to how effective the treatment has been in terms of the clinical or medical condition. The modus operandi of these approaches is essentially from the outside-in.

In sound therapy a different approach is taken. The therapy is essentially non-invasive, with an emphasis placed on the creation of a highly controlled environment in which individuals are able and choose to (re)develop a range of skills through *aesthetic* interaction with sound. Whilst progression and development remain a key focus, the essence lies in the internal motivation of the individual; in working from the inside-out. At all times the individual is given the opportunity to take control of the situation as far as possible. Certain aspects are controlled externally – notably the sonic environment – but the essence lies in allowing the individual the freedom to act as she or he chooses within available parameters, which remain as open as possible. In this way, 'learning' occurs incidentally. As a result we can see progression and development in a variety of ways across a range of disabilities.

The power and effectiveness of sound and music in enabling people to come to terms with, sometimes even overcome, disabilities has been noted by many authors.[21–25] Compelling cases have been made for the holistic treatment of patients across a variety of disorders, rather than treatment focused exclusively on chemical or medical interventions:

We now know, and can demonstrate with the most rigorous modern science, that the perceived separation between mind and body is, in fact, an illusion, and that we as whole persons function like eco-systems, responding to every stimulus in global ways.[26]

And such approaches can even affect the survival chances of the terminally ill:

Psychologically motivated endeavours can significantly affect the *quality* of life, sometimes even the survival chances, of patients with terminal illnesses.[27]

Another important aspect of sound therapy, which is used with both the children and the elderly, is that of vibroacoustics. Much work is being done in this area with impressive results published concerning the treatment of patients with a variety of conditions.[28] Mixing low frequency sine tones with music has been found to produce beneficial effects for a variety of conditions.[29,30] Perhaps the most significant conditions relevant to sound therapy through vibroacoustic techniques include anxiety, muscular pain, tension and depression. The psychophysiological effects observed in the elderly appeared to be entirely positive, with residents regularly reporting, at the conclusion of sessions, improved feelings about themselves both physically and mentally. A tape was prepared for this part of the therapy, which combined pulsed sine tones between 40 and 75 Hz, with music, which can be described as slow moving, gentle, peaceful and calming. For the children, this aspect of the therapy can yield remarkable results. For those who for a variety of reasons might become overwrought, totally frustrated or angry, and are almost unreachable, the vibroacoustic tapes can regularly be the means of allowing the individual to calm and regain control, whilst inducing a feeling of well-being.

Also crucial to the success of the approach is the creation of an environment within which the therapy sessions are held. The importance of physical space to the psychological well-being of people has been documented elsewhere,[31] and the creation of particular psychological environments forms an essential element in the potential for many treatments. Hence a very quiet room is needed, with no external distractions – visual or aural. A gentle acoustic is helpful, something which is often not easy to find in schools! A low level of lighting is also a useful touch.

The effectiveness of this approach is closely linked to cause and effect, to the participant being in total control of the sound environment. The perception-action and biofeedback loops created by movement → sound → vibration → movement seems to be a very powerful circle of experience. It has certainly provided a new opening, improved quality of life and developmental experience for many people.

What does it take to become a sound therapist?

What are the qualities needed by a person wishing to practice sound therapy? In conclusion Katy Atak has these thoughts:

It came as quite a shock to be asked this question, because after almost 2 years of working as a research assistant on the sound therapy project, I have become accustomed to focusing on the children and adults I work with and digging deep into their skills, their qualities, not my own. I am extremely reluctant to write a prescriptive list of attributes because this would imply that I believe I have discovered a magic formula that works, and that is simply not the case. Perhaps the most important 'skill' that I have learnt is that every client is an individual and that what works with one will not necessarily work with another. Therefore I will simply reflect on the skills I hope I have been developing whilst working on the project, and in so doing, clarify the personal qualities that can grow from the experience.

As a teacher I am used to working with children in an extremely interactive way. It becomes second nature to impart and tease out knowledge and then comment about the experience, usually within a fairly rigid time structure. In sound therapy I very quickly realized that some of my teaching skills I had to leave at the door. I am not there to teach, to tell, to share my views and knowledge. I am there to create an environment in which children and adults with communication difficulties have the opportunity to express themselves freely in their own personal style and at their chosen pace. So often, people with profound difficulties have power and choice taken away from them and it is usually done with the best intentions by well-meaning carers whose job it is to help that person through essential daily tasks.

Through nobody's fault it is all too easy to deal with the physical problems and somehow forget that underneath the damage there is a human being with emotional and aesthetic needs and a personality that longs to be expressed. Sound therapy, over a period of time, can provide a capsule in which a person's problems and difficulties are put aside and their abilities and preferences are brought to the fore.

Therefore, it is essential for me to provide an environment in which damaged people are empowered. I am there to help them create their own environment in which they choose the sounds and vibrations that express how they are feeling at that time. To do this I have to put my personal preferences and tastes aside. There may be sounds chosen that I do not like or even find unpleasant, but that does not mean they are sounds to be avoided. There may be sounds chosen repeatedly to the point where I am longing for variation, but it is not my tolerance in question. There may be sounds discarded which in my opinion are beautiful and interesting, but it is not my thoughts that are important. There may be a wealth of sounds that I would like to introduce and explore, but I must respect that my ability to listen, feel, digest and choose is different from that of the person with whom I am working.

Life today moves at an incredible pace with time restraints thrust upon us at every turn, yet in sound therapy I can give someone the luxury of having time to express themselves and make choices without the clock ticking away and deadlines having to be met.

There may also be sessions where there is no great response and for a variety of reasons the adult or child may be uncooperative. When this happens I have to accept that all human beings have 'off days' and expression of feelings cannot just be switched on at my convenience. Therefore I must not allow myself to be disheartened by what I perceive as a negative response, but rather view it as one valid step of many on a long journey to communication.

In the recording process of the research I have always felt that it is important to document the negative response alongside the positive, as over a period of time the variety of response builds up a true picture of the person with whom I am working, rather than a fairy tale, idealistic picture which bears little resemblance to reality.

I have always included my own mistakes in the documentation process – not easy for a teacher! – and in doing so it has helped me to learn from them and hopefully change my approach slightly the next time a similar situation arises.

The one element of teaching that is essential in sound therapy is the ability to observe. It is actually a great luxury to have the time to focus all my attention on one other human being and over a period of time become accustomed and tuned in to their mannerisms, facial expressions, vocal sounds and movements. It is only after working with the same group of children as a class music teacher for a number of years, and subsequently on an individual basis in sound therapy that I realize how much more I was able to learn about their inner being by studying them closely and observing their responses within the intimacy of our sessions.

So what skills and qualities does a person require in order to research the benefits of sound therapy?

If I had to summarise them in one phrase I would have to say: 'Learn to keep quiet, watch, listen and leave your own opinions at the door; with patience you will discover a person who is every bit as opinionated as yourself.'

ACKNOWLEDGEMENTS

I am grateful to ExtraCare and the Linbury Trust for financial support, to the pupils and staff of the Lambert School in Warwickshire, to the residents and staff of ExtraCare, West Midlands, Mapleford Home, Lancashire, Eshton Hall, Yorkshire, Leonard House, Sunderland, and to researchers Katy Atak and Helena Moorwood, without whom this work would not have been possible.

REFERENCES

1. Knapp ML, Hall JA 1992 The effects of the face on human communication, in nonverbal communication in human interaction. Harcourt Brace, Fort Worth
2. Izard C 1989 Human emotions. Plenum Press, New York
3. Vargas MJ 1986 Louder than words. An introduction to nonverbal communication. Iowa State University Press, Ames
4. Springer S, Deutsch G 1998 Left brain right brain: perspectives from cognitive neuroscience. WH Freeman and Company, New York
5. Ellis P 1996 Layered analysis: a video-based qualitative research tool to support the development of a new approach for children with special needs. Bulletin for the Council for Research in Music Education 130: 65–74
6. Ellis P 1995 Incidental music. British Journal of Music Education 12: 59–70
7. Ellis P 1996 Incidental music: Sound therapy for children with special educational needs. Video programme and booklet, available from the Soundbeam Project
8. Ellis P 1997 The music of sound: a new approach for children with severe and profound and multiple learning difficulties. BJME 14(2): 173–186
9. Wigram T, Saperston B, West R eds 1995 The art and science of music therapy: a handbook. Harwood Academic Publishers, Chur, Switzerland
10. Nordoff P, Robbins C 1971 Therapy in music for handicapped children. Gallanc, London
11. Aldridge D, Gustoroff G, Neugebauer L 1995 A pilot study of music therapy in the treatment of children with developmental delay. Complementary Therapies in Medicine 3: 197–205
12. Ellis P 1994 Special sounds for special needs; towards the development of a Sound Therapy. In: Heath L, ed. Musical connections: tradition and change. International Society of Musical Education
13. Schafer RM 1979 The rhinoceros in the classroom. Universal Edition, Canada
14. Truax B 1984 Acoustic communication. Ablex Publishing Corporation, Norwood, NJ
15. Steinbach I 1995 Samonas Sound Therapy – background and uses. Hamm, Germany
16. Bérard G 1993 Hearing equals behaviour. Keats Publishing Inc, Connecticut, USA
17. Goddard S 1996 A teacher's window into the child's mind. Fern Ridge Press, Oregon
18. Lane C 1991 Can you hear me? Special Children 10–12
19. Edwards S 1992 Signature sound technologies. Sound Health Inc, Ohio, USA
20. Beaumont R 1994 Breaking the sound barrier. Kindred Spirits 3(5): 28–30.

21. Critchley M, Henson RA eds 1977 Music and the brain. Heinemann Medical Books Ltd, London
22. McClellan R 1991 The healing forces of music: history, theory and practice. Element, Dorset
23. Sacks O 1973 Awakenings. Pan Books Ltd, London
24. Storr A 1992 Music and the mind. Harper Collins, London
25. Wigram T, Saperston B, West R eds 1995 The art and science of music therapy: a handbook. Harwood Academic Publishers, Chur, Switzerland
26. Watkins A ed. 1997 Mind-body medicine: a clinician's guide to psychoneuroimmunology. Churchill Livingstone, London
27. Greer S 1994 Psycho-oncology: its aims, achievements and future tasks. Psycho-oncology 3: 87–101
28. Skille O, Wigram T 1995 The effect of music, vocalisation and vibration on the brain and muscle tissue: studies in vibroacoustic therapy. In: Wigram T, Saperston B, West R eds. The art and science of music therapy: a handbook. Harwood Academic Publishers, Chur, Switzerland
29. Wigram T, Dileo C eds 1997 Music vibration. Jeffrey Books, New Jersey
30. Williams E 1997 An introduction to vibroacoustic therapy. The Soundbeam project, Bristol
31. Senior P, Croall J 1993 Helping to heal. Calouste Gulbenkian Foundation

WEBSITES OF INTEREST

Soundbeam: www.soundbeam.co.uk

CARESS: Creating Aesthetically Resonant Environments in Sound: www.bris.ac.uk/caress

5

Robotics and rehabilitation: the role of robot-mediated therapy post stroke

Emma K. Stokes

SUMMARY

Physiotherapy rehabilitation following stroke began as an intuitive and heuristic approach and for many years, the strategies employed were retained because of familiarity and an absence of alternatives. Recent evidence in support of physiotherapy in stroke rehabilitation advocates exercise-based interventions that enable the patient to carry out repetitive and meaningful movements. In order to relearn movement following brain injury, considerable repetition is necessary. In theory, technology provides a means to deliver this type of therapy in a manner that is designed by a physiotherapist but mediated or delivered by a robot. To syllogistically apply this thesis, without research, in an era of evidence-based practice is not possible. This chapter reviews the research work to date in the potentially exciting area of physiotherapy for people with stroke that is delivered by using robotics. In particular, this chapter emphasizes the current development of a European system designed to deliver robot-mediated therapy to the upper limb – GENTLE/s.

CASE STUDY

Mr G. was the first participant in the GENTLE/s study on the effects of robot-mediated therapy (RMT) for the upper extremity post stroke. The methodology for this study employed a series of single case studies, with a baseline phase 'A', a 'B' phase, which employed robot-mediated therapy and a control phase 'C', which comprised sling suspension for the upper extremity. The latter is a simple form of limb suspension employing slings and pulleys, which enables the affected limb to be supported fully for movement. The ultimate sample size included in the study was 20 and was completed in September 2002. During each phase of 3 weeks, all outcome measures were observed on 8 to 9 occasions.

Table 5.1   Maximum voluntary isometric contraction slopes for phases A, B and C

	Power (lbs)		
	A	B	C
Elbow flexion	0.17	0.72	0.43
Elbow extension	−0.0	0.5	0.31
Shoulder flexion	0.1	0.45	0.32
Shoulder extension	−0.1	0.68	−0.13

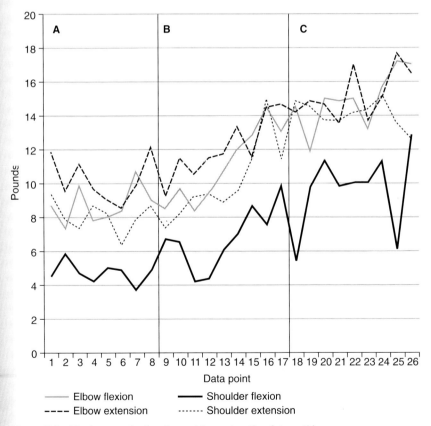

Figure 5.1   Maximum voluntary isometric contraction (strength).

Mr G. was 71 years of age at entry to the study and presented with a left hemiparesis, following a stroke 5 months previously. His CT scan reported the findings of periventricular changes and changes in the right centrum ovale consistent with ischemia. The stroke was classified as a lacunar infarct. He is right-hand dominant. He presented with no deficits in sensation, no unilateral neglect and no visual-field defects. Figures 5.1–5.3 and Tables 5.1–5.3 represent the changes over the three phases in strength, motor activity using the Fugl Meyer Test,[1] and physical performance using the Motor Assessment Scale.[2] The 'A' phase establishes a baseline, which becomes relatively stable and takes on

Table 5.2 Fugl Meyer Test (total score) slopes for phases A, B and C

	A	B	C
Fugl Meyer Test – total	0.57	1.18	0.61

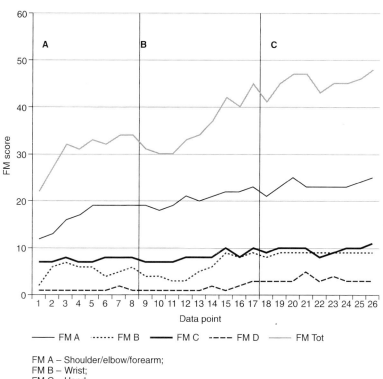

FM A – Shoulder/elbow/forearm;
FM B – Wrist;
FM C – Hand;
FM D – Co-ordination/Speed;
FM Tot – cumulative score of subsections

Figure 5.2 Fugl Meyer Test (motor activity).

board any learning effect of performing the activities required during testing and/or natural recovery. All domains measured demonstrate an upward trend during the robot-mediated therapy 'B' phase, comprising three sessions weekly for 3 weeks. This appears to continue during the 'C' phase, also three times weekly for 3 weeks, albeit at a slower rate, reflected by a smaller slope. Additional small benefits were a decrease in pain and tone at the wrist. There was no change in quality of life as measured by the SF-36.[3] While patient satisfaction was not formally measured in this phase of the study, the anecdotal reports of this participant, indeed all participants, were very positive. Feedback during the robot-mediated therapy was favorable and functional gains, not measured by the methods employed, were reported, for example, simple tasks such as managing to open doors more easily.

Table 5.3   Motor Assessment Scale (total score) slopes for phases A, B and C

	A	B	C
Motor Assessment Scale – total	−0.09	0.3	0.2

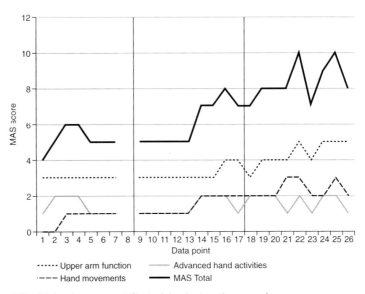

Figure 5.3   Motor Assessment Scale (physical performance).

INTRODUCTION

The word robot derives from the Czech for forced labor and was first penned by Karel Capek in the 1930s. While the role of the robot in Hollywood has developed from the simple R2D2 of 'Star Wars' to the very human representation in 'Artificial Intelligence', their role in the real world of industry and service provision has also changed and developed, albeit in a more pragmatic manner.[4] While industrial robots are larger and have little human interaction, the development of smaller robotic systems saw their emergence into service provision areas – surveillance, product assembly, laboratory and medical/rehabilitation applications.[5] The initial uses of robotic systems in the field of rehabilitation were as aides for activities. Depending on the nature of the control mechanisms, they fall into two categories – 'robot as assistant' or 'robot as extension'. In the case of the former, the robotic system carries out the task, whereas in the latter the tasks are directly linked to the physical input of the user.[4]

In the 1990s, the use of robotics in rehabilitation underwent a paradigm shift, a move towards intervention rather than simply assistance. Erlandson[5] describes the emerging applications of robotic and mechatronic systems in special education, vocational training and rehabilitation training. A wide variety of potential applications have been reported,[6–10] however, only a small number have reached the stage of full clinical trials.[11–13] This shift towards the provision of therapy by robotic systems addresses, for the most part, the rehabilitation of the upper extremity. Indeed, 75% of the output of the 'Therapy' section of the 7th International Conference on Rehabilitation Robotics (ICORR),[14] deals with the use of robotics for treatment or assessment of the upper extremity. Nonetheless, there is also some emerging work on their use in the lower extremity in combination with unweighted treadmill systems.[15]

Stroke rehabilitation, with a particular emphasis on the upper extremity, has become the focus of attention for robot-assisted therapy for a number of reasons. Stroke is one of the most common causes of acquired disability in many countries in Europe and in the USA, with an incidence ranging between 100 and 180 per 100 000 of the population.[16–18] Approximately 80% of people with stroke present with impairments of the upper extremity, with only half regaining functional use during the rehabilitation process.[19–21] Even though many people manage to perform activities of daily living competently with one functioning upper extremity, residual loss of upper extremity function is reported as being a significant contributory factor to decreased well-being.[22]

Currently, physiotherapy rehabilitation is very 'hands-on'. Interventions are often guided and informed by the principles described by Bobath,[23] Brunnstrom,[24] Rood,[25] Johnston,[26] and Carr and Shepherd.[2] A recent systematic review confirmed there is actually little evidence to guide therapists in their choice of intervention.[27] What is known is that more therapy is better and in the 'black box' of rehabilitation interventions, those that are task-oriented and repetitive will optimize cortical reorganization as part of guided recovery.[28] During a physiotherapy session, only approximately 17% of time is spent on the upper extremity (UE).[29] Active participation in rehabilitation comprises only a small part of any given day in the rehabilitation setting. Hence, it is desirable to augment current rehabilitation strategies with those that enable a patient to continue activities and exercises, in the absence of direct physical contact with a therapist. It is envisaged that robot-mediated therapies (RMTs) are a novel way of addressing this aspiration.

A number of clinical trials are ongoing and in the USA a number of research groups have reported the results of randomized-controlled trials. Their work will be considered in detail and the results discussed below. Emerging European work – GENTLE/s – is discussed in the context of preliminary data.

MIME – Mirror-Image Motion Enabler

A decade ago the developers of MIME (Fig. 5.4), the Veteran Affairs Palo Alto Rehabilitation Research and Development Center, explored the concept of using a robotic system for mediating exercise of the upper extremity with therapists, engineers and physicians who simulated hemiplegia. Despite not achieving clinically acceptable performance of their system in this early stage, they drew on other sources,[30–32] and with further developmental work, on normals and men with hemiplegia, created a system which provides full support to the hemiplegic upper extremity and has four modes of therapeutic movement – three unilateral and one bilateral.

The participant in the therapy sits in a wheelchair. In the unilateral modes, the affected upper extremity is attached to the robot via a customized orthosis for the forearm. The robot exerts forces, as required, on the upper extremity, which can move in one of 12 individualized, pre-programmed trajectories of movement. The modes of movement are passive, active assisted and active constrained. Passive requires no volitional movement from the participant, active assisted requires initiation of movement and

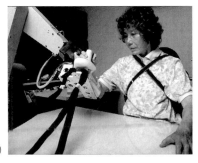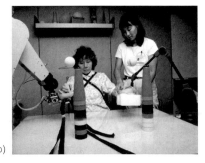

(a)   (b)

Figure 5.4   Mirror Image Motion Enabler (MIME). (a) depicts 'MIME-bimanual'. (b) depicts 'MIME-unilateral'.

active constrained requires the generation of force against a velocity-sensitive resistance. In the bilateral mode, the unaffected upper extremity acts as the mediator of movement. As it passes through movement patterns, a position digitizer incorporated in the system results in the affected upper extremity moving through a mirror-image movement pattern. The robot-mediated movement enables the patient to move through therapeutic movements, comprising tabletop tracing of circles and polygons and 3-D reaching movements.

Preliminary results of clinical trials were published in 1999 and 2000.[13,33,34] Twenty-three subjects were recruited for a randomized, controlled trial. Data are available on 21 subjects, a further stroke and hip fracture accounted for the attrition. Subjects were randomized into either robot therapy (RT) or a control group (CT). Both groups were approximately 26 months post stroke, and they continued their usual medical treatments and home intervention. The subjects attended 24 treatment sessions, each of 1-hour duration, over a 2-month period. The treatment sessions were similar to the extent that they employed stretching, exercises and tracking tasks, and they were supervised by the same therapist. In the RT group, the robot, and not the therapist, assisted the movements in the exercise component. To diminish the potential confounding effect of exposure to a novel device in the RT group, the CT group was exposed to the robot for 5 minutes, when it placed the targets for a tracking task.

The outcome measures employed by an independent, blinded, metrologist were:

- Functional Independence Measure (FIM)[35]
- Barthel Index (BI)[34]
- Fugl-Meyer (FM) Scale,[1] which is a clinical measure of motor activity of the shoulder, elbow, wrist and hand
- isometric strength of eight shoulder and elbow movements
- free-reach kinematics – as measured by the MIME system
- electromyography of the shoulder and elbow muscle groups.

No significant changes were noted in the functional measures – BI or FIM. The overall upper extremity FM scores were not significantly different for either group; however, a trend favored the RT group. When consideration was given to the shoulder/elbow components of the FM, those actually exercised during the robot-mediated therapy, the RT group showed a significantly greater improvement than the CT group.

Statistically significant improvements in all strength measures occurred between pre- and post-intervention measures in the RT group. There were significant differences between the RT and CT groups only in adduction and shoulder flexion strength, with a trend towards greater strength improvements in other movements. In reviewing the kinematic data, both groups demonstrated improvements in the ability to voluntarily move towards a target (free reach/EMG), the RT group demonstrating a trend towards greater improvements. Further results of an extended sample[37] ($n = 27$) suggest that, although the RT group had statistically larger improvements in proximal motor function as measured by the FM at 1 and 2 months of treatment, this difference was not present at follow-up 6 months later. Neither were significant differences in the passive range of motion and pain noted between RT and CT. The RT group did have a clinically moderate, but a statistically significant, greater increase in the FIM.[38] Further work with MIME discussing the mechanisms of these improvements is in press.[39] For example, a 4-year study is ongoing, investigating the relative contributions of the unilateral and bilateral movements in subjects in a sub-acute period post stroke. Furthermore, a multi-center trial is investigating the effects in an acute stroke population. These data should be available in 2004 or 2005.[39]

MIT-Manus

In the past 7 years, the group of researchers involved with MIT-Manus has used back-drivable robots (that is, robots that have low mechanical impedance) as the 'key enabling technology' for developing objective and sensitive measures to monitor changes that occur in the upper extremity as a result of brain reorganization in the rehabilitation process and for a practical and economically feasible 'clinician-supervised, robot-administered therapy'. The results of their clinical trials[12,40–43] are presented in Table 5.4.

With the MIT-Manus system (Fig. 5.5) the patient sits in a chair, with the shoulders strapped, facing a support board. On this support board are a series of round targets over which the robot arm and handle are suspended. The affected upper extremity is supported at the elbow by a low friction pad. The participant faces a video screen, and this provides visual feedback of the actual targets beneath the arm and forearm. Auditory feedback is provided for correct movements, which focus on the shoulder and elbow. Initially, 20 participants were recruited for study.[40,41] The subjects were approximately 3 weeks post stroke. The method of randomization to either CT or RT was designed in such a way that no more than three patients were in the RT at any given time. If the RT group had three participants when a further subject was recruited, they were automatically assigned to the CT and vice versa. A further 56 subjects were recruited and their outcomes reported separately and summatively with the first 20 subjects.[42] A 3-year follow-up of the first 20 patients is also reported.[43] All participants received their conventional therapy. In addition, the RT group had 4–5 hours per week of RMT as outlined above. The CT group was exposed to the robot for 1 hour per week, but it did not move their upper extremity, that is, they performed free-reaching movements. The robot moved the target to which they reached.

Table 5.4 Results of clinical trials: MIT-Manus

	Preliminary 20 subjects[40,41] (Mean ± SD)	56 subjects[42] (Mean ± SD)	3-year follow-up preliminary 20 subjects[43] (Mean ± SEM)	76 participants[12] (Composite results of 20 subjects ± 56 subjects, whether SD or SEM is presented is not clear)
Age (years)	RT 58.5 ± 8.3, CT 63.3 ± 10.6	RT 62 ± 2, CT 67 ± 2	RT 54 ± 3, CT 66 ± 2	
Gender (M/F)	RT 5F/5M, CT 4F/6M	RT 14F/16M, CT 12F/14M	RT 2F/4M, CT 3F/3M	RT 19F/21M, CT 16F/20F
FIM total	RT 25.7 ± 12.25, CT 25.6 ± 7.23		RT 41.3 ± 3.6, CT 39.7 ± 4.3	
FIM motor		***RT 25.0 ± 3.5, CT 19.5 ± 3.5***		
FIM cognitive		RT 6.0 ± 2.0, CT 5.5 ± 2.5		
FM total	RT 14.10 ± 9.7, CT 10.10 ± 11.63		RT 12.2 ± 4.6, CT 12.8 ± 5.0	RT 9.25 ± 1.36, CT 7.1 ± 1.20
FM SE		RT 5.0 ± 2.5, CT 4.0 ± 2.0	RT 8.0 ± 3.7, CT 8.0 ± 4.0	
FM WH		RT 1.0 ± 1.0, CT 0.0 ± 0.0		
Muscle strength	RT 3.88 ± 2.45, CT 2.30 ± 2.89	***RT 4.1 ± 1.4, CT 1.7 ± 1.7***	***RT 9.1 ± 2.0, CT 5.1 ± 1.6***	***RT 3.99 ± 0.43, CT 2.0 ± 0.32***
MSS SE	RT 9.44 ± 5.90, CT 1.8 ± 3.34	***RT 8.3 ± 2.5, CT 4.4 ± 2.0***	RT 21.4 ± 4.6, CT 9.2 ± 4.2	***RT 8.15 ± 0.79, CT 3.42 ± 0.62***
MSS WH total	>degree of improvement in RT	RT 0.8 ± 0.8, CT 0.0 ± 0.0	RT 17.0 ± 7.7, CT 11.7 ± 6.6	RT 4.16 ± 1.16, CT 2.64 ± 0.78

RT: robot therapy; CT: control therapy; FIM: Functional Independence Measure; FM: Fugl Meyer; SE: shoulder/elbow section; WH: wrist/hand section; MSS: Motor Status Scale.
Figures in italics and bold represent a statistically significant difference between robot and control group.

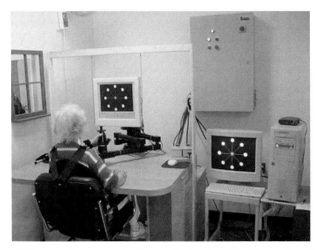

Figure 5.5 MIT-Manus. Reproduced with permission from the Massachusetts Institute of Technology, Newman Laboratory for Biomechanics and Human Rehabilitation.

The outcome measures employed by an independent, blinded metrologist were:

- Functional Independence Measure[35] (FIM) as a total score (FIM total) and as subsections. The motor subsection (FIM Motor) includes sections on locomotion, self-care and mobility. The cognitive subsection (FIM Cognitive) includes social cognition and communication.
- Fugl-Meyer[1] (FM) a clinical scale used to quantify motor impairment. FM total includes all the upper extremity components. In this study, the authors subdivided it into shoulder/elbow (FM SE) and wrist/hand (FM WH).
- Strength of the muscle groups of the upper extremity using the grading system, where 0 is no contraction and 5 is normal strength, similar to the Oxford scale.[44]
- Motor Status Scale (MSS), a scale designed by the researchers that considers control of movement. The total score (MSS Total) is the sum of all the movement scores from 10 shoulder movements/4 elbow movements (MSS SE) and 3 wrist/12 hand movements (MSS WH). Scoring is from 0 to 2, with the anchors representing no movement and normal controlled movement respectively.

The figures represented in italics in Table 5.4 are those measures that demonstrated a statistically significant improvement in the RT group compared with the CT group. The MIT-Manus trial results are not dissimilar to the MIME system. Improvements in function were only noted to be statistically greater in the RT group than the CT group in one trial. This difference in the improvement in function is represented by a 5.5 point difference between the RT and CT groups, out of a possible score of 77. The motor subsection of the FIM represents self-care, locomotion and mobility, and since it is not explicitly stated in the results, it is possible that the improvement does not constitute increased upper-extremity function. The FIM and the BI reflect general ability in activities of daily living and it is possible that they may not be sensitive enough to identify subtle upper-extremity functional improvements. It is possible to complete the Barthel Index with one hand. The total score for the FM scale – considering motor performance – demonstrated a trend towards greater improvement in the RT group. When specific consideration was given to the components of this scale, which measure activity at the shoulder and elbow, the parts of the upper extremity targeted by RMT, this improvement reached statistical significance. Improvements in muscle strength were noted to be statistically significant in most trials. This was also the case with measures that considered control of movement.

In the MIT-Manus and MIME systems, improvements are noted at the level of body structures/functions[45] and less at the level of participation or functional activity, for the most part. This may be simply a product of the outcome measure used, or possibly insufficient sample sizes. Since these are the first sources of clinical research on RMT, it is too early to draw unequivocal conclusions.

ARM Guide

While traditional clinical outcome measures have been employed by both the MIME and MIT-Manus research groups, both have also considered robot-generated or system measures and have completed mathematical modeling and small clinical trials with a view to ascertaining their potential benefits in affording deeper insights into the process of recovery[34] and motor control.[46] It was the aspiration to create an improved diagnostic tool to evaluate impairment of the upper extremity after brain injury that led to the development of the ARM Guide (Assisted Rehabilitation and Measurement Guide).[11] The ARM Guide is a device that provides mechanical assistance to reaching movements. It is capable of measuring hand position and the forces generated during reaching movements of the upper extremity.[47] It allows the seated participant to reach in a linear path, at different workspace angles. The initial pilot work on the ARM Guide addressed its potential to assess impairments of movement in hemiparetic upper extremities[48] and the relative contribution of such impairments to decreased active range of motion.[47] Recent research has evaluated the effect of the ARM Guide in delivering therapy post stroke.[49] In attempting to answer the question, 'is the robotic component of RMT necessary or is it simply the repetitive nature of the activity which might cause improvement in the upper extremity?', 10 subjects with chronic arm impairment following stroke were randomized into two groups. One group used the ARM Guide to perform repetitive reaching movements (RT) and a control group (CT) performed a matched number of free-reaching arm movements, i.e. without robotic assistance. No significant differences were noted in either functional or bio-mechanical evaluations between the groups, both of whom demonstrated improvements. However, the authors suggest that these data must be interpreted with caution due to the small sample size and the baseline differences that existed between the two participant groups.[49]

Other emerging technologies

Other developing robotic technologies with upper-extremity applications include Driver's SEAT[6,50] and Java Therapy.[51] Java Therapy is web-based robotic rehabilitation, and represents the concept of telerehabilitation, using a joystick to assist or resist exercises. A web page provides the interactive forum with the patient and software has been developed to assess status, deliver therapy games and produce therapy reports. The assessment component can measure speed, coordination, strength and finger speed. The therapy games include a blackjack game and a checkers-type game. Preliminary work has focused on development, initial and ongoing user testing.

The Driver's Simulation Environment for Arm Therapy (SEAT)[6,50] is a rehabilitation device, which is designed to improve upper-extremity activity following stroke, by employing a steering wheel as the basis of bimanual movement of the upper extremities. It employs steering tasks, in passive-assisted and active-assisted modes to deliver a 'meaningful and purposeful task' for people with stroke and resultant hemiparesis of the upper extremity. The authors suggest that by employing a bimanual task, such as steering, there is a potentially strong motivating reason for use of the affected upper extremity. The technology is designed such that overuse of the unaffected side results in a negative consequence for the user, hence forcing the affected upper extremity to engage in the activity. Preliminary testing on a small sample of eight participants, to investigate if this therapy will increase force production in the affected upper extremity, has yielded positive results.

THE EUROPEAN DIMENSION – GENTLE/S

GENTLE/s is an inter-disciplinary research consortium, funded as part of the 5th Framework Programme of the European Commission. The project is pan-European in nature; the author of this chapter is the principal investigator at Trinity College, Dublin, one of the eight partners in the consortium. The project aims to design, build and evaluate a system that delivers RMT to the upper limb.[52] The first prototype (Fig. 5.6) comprises a three-degree of freedom haptic interface arm (Haptic Master) with a wrist attachment mechanism, two embedded computers, a large monitor and speakers, seating for the patient, and an overhead arm support system.

The patient is seated at the work surface with their arm in an elbow orthosis (Fig. 5.7), which is attached to the overhead frame via a constant

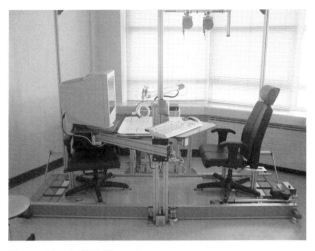

Figure 5.6   GENTLE/s system.

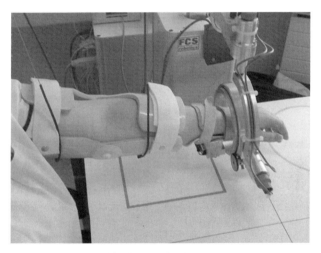

Figure 5.7   GENTLE/s elbow orthosis.

force spring. This allows the de-weighting of the arm, eliminating the effects of gravity and minimizing the risk of subluxation of the gleno-humeral joint. The patient is connected to the robot arm via a magnetic wrist attachment mechanism. This incorporates a quick-release safety mechanism, under patient control, which disconnects the patient from the robot at the touch of a button and a breakaway mechanism, which detaches the patient from the robot if there is a distraction force on the arm. In this system, RMT is provided as repetitive movement – three different modes are possible, namely passive movement (no patient effort), assisted active (patient and robot) or

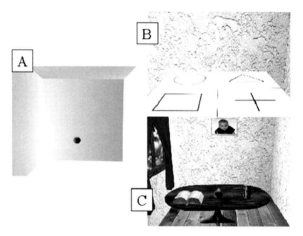

Figure 5.8   Virtual rooms in the GENTLE/s system.

active (patient). This enables people with all levels of upper-extremity movement to take part in therapy. Movement occurs in patterns, individually tailored and set up in the GENTLE/s system by the therapist. Movement can be set between a series of points in space, or along an arc of movement defined by setting points in close sequence (Fig. 5.8). The movement patterns are represented on screen in a 3-D environment. As the GENTLE/s system develops, these have become more relevant to daily activities and incorporate, for the second prototype, activities related to shopping (moving items from a shelf into a basket) and functional activities (moving items around a workspace). These 'rooms' are presented graphically on a monitor of a computer screen, and actual movement of the upper extremity corresponds to the movement of the objects on the screen. This unique aspect grounds the repetitive activity in tasks that relate to daily living. Similar to other systems discussed, it also provides motivation for movement. Feedback regarding the correct movement pattern is provided by the robot's haptic interface.[53,54] The amount of force used to bring the arm back to the pre-set movement pattern can be varied to suit the needs of the individual.

The first clinical trials commenced in September 2001 and were ongoing until September 2002. A series of single case studies, employing a multiple baseline period and randomization into ABC or ACB is the methodology of choice. 'A' represents the baseline measurement period and 'B' is RMT, which takes place three times weekly for 3 weeks. 'C' represents the same period of time spent with the upper extremity deweighted, when movement occurs in slings. This dimension is examined to enable more directed consideration of the 'robotic' components of RMT, as opposed to simply the increased therapy, which is established as producing results. The outcome measures utilized in this study are similar to those employed in the previously discussed studies – upper-extremity strength, upper-extremity range of motion, and the Fugl Meyer Scale.[1] The inclusion of the Motor Assessment Scale[2] – a scale designed specifically to measure movement and function post stroke, may allow more sensitivity in changes in this domain to be observed. Measurements are taken during baseline and repeatedly during the 'B' and 'C' phases. A total series of 20 subjects were completed by September 2002. The case study presented at the beginning of this chapter provides a brief insight into the data generated by the first participant in this study.[55] In addition to examining the therapeutic implication of RMT, internally generated measures, such as force production and error correction along a path of movement,[56,57] are also being examined with a view to improving measurement and informing clinical practice and intervention in the areas of movement analysis. The GENTLE/s system also incorporates an existing test to enable movement analysis – a labyrinth. Movement analysis, e.g. consideration of force generated and speed of movement, may provide additional information on the performance of particular movements, inform changes over time and aid in designing interventions. Performance on this maze, through which a curser is moved, has been analyzed in healthy adults and people with movement disorders.[58]

USERS AND CLINICAL APPLICATION

The use of robotics in rehabilitation post stroke is in its infancy. Many questions remain unanswered about physiotherapy rehabilitation post stroke, both in the context of traditional interventions as well as more novel approaches. It would not be acceptable to introduce another item to the 'black box' of physiotherapy strategies without fully investigating the evidence. Indeed, a recent commentary[59] by de Weert and Feys has suggested that the appropriate application of research to physiotherapy in stroke rehabilitation is to consider individual therapies, and in establishing what are effective interventions, thereafter considering the package of therapy in its entirety. Therein lie the challenges, but also the exciting phase of physiotherapy development.[60] Happily, the development and design of RMT, while driven by technologists, has involved clinicians. The theoretical framework in support of RMT exists, i.e. dose-dependent, task-oriented, repetitive movements. RMT is not being developed to replace the therapist, but to augment rehabilitation in a clinical and cost-effective manner.

The question still remains, if the clinical evidence is produced, will the results influence clinical practice? Will therapists and patients accept the notion of RMT? Erlandson[5] suggests that one of the forces that will shape the use of robotics as mediators of therapy, rather than aides to activities, is the traditionally slow diffusion of information about technology across professional boundaries. De Weert and Feys[59] consider that the adherence to established schools of thought might be one explanation for the tardiness in employing evidence-based practice in physiotherapy.

Research addressing user attitudes has been explored for RMT. In the early 1990s Dijkers et al.[61] reported on patient and staff acceptance of robotic technology to deliver therapy in occupational therapy. The patients were positively disposed to the therapy, found it helpful, interesting and not confusing. Ninety percent of participating occupational therapists indicated that their overall response was positive, but 63% were hesitant about using the system due to lack of familiarity with computers. In the preliminary development of the MIT-Manus system,[40] attitudinal disposition of patients towards various aspects of the system was documented using scoring on a Likert scale, from 0 to 7, with the anchors representing strongly disagree and strongly agree to positive statements respectively. In this case a mean score for all patient responses of 3.5 would represent a theoretical neutral. Participants found the therapy comfortable (mean score 5.92), enjoyable (mean score 5.71), and beneficial (mean score 5.67). They were less positive about the unique benefits of working with the robot (mean score 4.82) and most certainly would not wish the robot to replace the therapist (mean score 2.58). The attitudinal disposition of therapists was not considered by the previous authors, but has been documented by Coote and Stokes,[62] with both patients and therapists reporting positive attitudes to the GENTLE/s system. While therapists are positive towards RMT, it has been noted that exercise equipment, available in many physiotherapy departments, is not used very frequently in rehabilitation post stroke.[63] This may reflect the fact that therapists use the approach that was most prevalent during their training as the rationale for choice of treatment in stroke rehabilitation.[64,65] In the future, if RMT is deemed to be successful, and financial constraints notwithstanding, education will be fundamental to its widespread use. The term 'robot' is relatively unfamiliar to therapists. In a recent survey,[66] 61.5% of therapists reported that robots could be used for rehabilitation of the upper-extremity post stroke, while 72.7% of the same respondents agreed that a machine, controlled by a computer that could guide a patient's arm through a movement (a description of the essentials of a rehabilitation robot) could be usefully employed. The 11.2% difference suggests that careful explanation of the role of robotics in rehabilitation is required. Even a small amount of exposure to RMT, for example, a poster presentation at a national conference, has a positive effect on the understanding of therapists.[66]

CONCLUSION

Integrating technology into rehabilitation is challenging and exciting. The role of robotics in rehabilitation is potentially vast, RMT in stroke rehabilitation representing only one facet of the multifarious applications. Clinical trials are ongoing to establish which, if any, of the components of RMT most contribute to effective and functionally relevant motor recovery post stroke. In the absence of this evidence, RMT should not become part of recognized rehabilitation strategies. The evidence of clinical and cost effectiveness will be insufficient if the therapy is not made accessible to both the therapy and client users. The future of RMT rests in the hands of engineers, computer scientists, therapists, neuroscientists, and the people who require rehabilitation following stroke, all of whom have a role to play in driving its transfer from the design and testing stage to appropriate routine use in the clinical, and perhaps, the home setting.

REFERENCES

1. Fugl-Meyer AR, Jaasko L, Leyman I et al. 1975 The post-stroke hemiplegic patient: a method for evaluation of physical performance. Scandinavian Journal of Rehabilitation Medicine 7: 13–31
2. Carr JH, Shepherd RB 1982 A motor relearning programme for stroke. Heinemann, London
3. Ware JJ, Sherbourne CD 1992 The MOS 36-item short-form health survey (SF-36). I. Conceptual framework and item selection. Medical Care 30: 473–483
4. Mahoney RM 1996 Editorial. Technology and Disability 5: 121–123
5. Erlandson RF 1995 Applications of robotic/mechatronic systems in special education, rehabilitation therapy and vocational training: a paradigm shift. IEEE Transactions on Rehabilitation Engineering 3(1): 22–34
6. Johnson MJ, Van der Loos HFM, Burgar CG et al. 1999 Driver's SEAT: simulation environment for arm therapy. Proceedings Sixth International Conference on Rehabilitation Robotics 227–234
7. Takahasi Y, Kobayashi T 1999 Upper limb motion assist robot. Proceedings Sixth International Conference on Rehabilitation Robotics 216–226
8. Rao R, Agrawil SK, Scholz J 1999 A robot test-bed for assistance and assessment in physical therapy. Proceedings Sixth International Conference on Rehabilitation Robotics 187–200
9. Richardson R, Austin ME, Plummer AR 1999 Development of a physiotherapy robot. Proceedings International Biomechatronics Workshop 116–120
10. Nagai K, Nakanishi I, Kishida T 1999 Design of robotic orthosis assisting human motion in production engineering and human care. Proceedings Sixth International Conference on Rehabilitation Robotics 270–275
11. Reinkensmeyer DJ, Kahn LE, Averbuch M et al. 2000 Understanding and treating arm movement after chronic brain injury: progress with the ARM Guide. Journal of Rehabilitation Research and Development 37(6): 653–662. Available online: http://www.vard.org/jour/00/37/6/reink376.htm
12. Krebs HI, Volpe BT, Aisen M et al. 2000 Increasing productivity and quality of care: robot-aided neuro-rehabilitation. Journal of Rehabilitation Research and Development 37(6): 639–652. Available online: http://www.vard.org/jour/00/37/6/krebs.htm
13. Burgar CG, Lum PS, Shor PC et al. 2000 Development of robots for rehabilitation therapy: the Palo Alto VS/Stanford experience. Journal of Rehabilitation Research and Development 37(6): 663–673. Available online: http://www.vard.org/jour/00/37/6/ burga376.htm
14. Mokhtari M ed. 2001 Integration of assistive technology in the information age. Proceedings Seventh International Conference on Rehabilitation Robotics. IOS Press, Amsterdam, 39–134
15. Reinkensmeyer D, Lum P, Winters J 2002 Emerging technologies for improving access to movement therapy following neurologic injury. In: Winters J, Robinson C, Simpson R

et al. eds. Emerging and accessible telecommunications, information and healthcare technologies: engineering challenges in enabling universal access. IEEE Press

16. American Heart Association 2001 Heart and stroke statistical update. American Heart Association, Dallas, TX

17. Irish Heart Foundation Council on Stroke 2000 Towards excellence in stroke care in Ireland. Eireann Healthcare Publications, Dublin

18. The Stroke Association 2002 Stroke facts. Available online: http://www.stroke.org.uk

19. Parker VM, Wade DT, Langton-Hewer R 1986 Loss of arm function after stroke: measurement, frequency, and recovery. International Rehabilitation Medicine 8: 69–73

20. Wade DT, Langton-Hewer R, Wood VA et al. 1983 The hemiplegic arm after stroke: measurement and recovery. Journal of Neurology, Neurosurgery and Psychiatry 46(6): 521–524

21. Heller A, Wade DT, Wood VA et al. 1987 Arm function after stroke: measurement and recovery after the first three months. Journal of Neurology, Neurosurgery and Psychiatry 50(6): 714–718

22. Wyeller TB, Sveen U, Sodring KM et al. 1997 Subjective well-being one year after stroke. Clinical Rehabilitation 11(2): 139–144

23. Bobath B 1978 Adult hemiplegia: evaluation and treatment. Heinemann, London

24. Brunnstrom S 1979 Movement therapy in hemiplegia: a neurophysiological approach. Harpers and Row, Hagerstown

25. Rood M 1954 Neuropsychological reactions as a basis for physical therapy. Physical Therapy Review 34: 344–449

26. Johnstone M 1983 Restoration of motor function in the stroke patient. A physiotherapists approach. Churchill Livingstone, Edinburgh

27. Pomeroy VM, Tallis RC 2000 Physical therapy to improve movement performance and functional ability post stroke. Reviews in Clinical Gerontology 10: 261–290

28. Robertson IH, Murre JMJ 1999 Rehabilitation of brain damage: brain plasticity and principles of guided recovery. Psychological Bulletin 125(5): 544–575

29. Ballinger C, Ashburn A, Low J et al. 1999 Unpacking the 'black box of therapy – a pilot study to describe occupational therapy and physical therapy interventions for people with stroke. Clinical Rehabilitation 13: 301–309

30. Lum PS, Reinkensmeyer DJ, Lehman SL 1993 Robotic assist devices for bimanual physical therapy: preliminary experiments. IEEE Transactions on Rehabilitation Engineering 1(3): 185–191

31. Lum PS, Lehman SL, Reinkensmeyer DJ 1995 The bimanual lifting rehabilitator: an adaptive machine for therapy of stroke patients. IEEE Transactions on Rehabilitation Engineering 3(1): 22–34

32. Hogan N, Krebs H, Chamnarong J et al. 1992 MIT MANUS: a workstation for manual therapy and training II. Proceedings of Telemanip Tech-SPIE: International Society for Optical Engineering, 1833, Nov

33. Burgar CG, Lum PS, Shor M et al. 1999 Rehabilitation of upper limb dysfunction in chronic hemiplegia: robot-assisted movement versus conventional therapy. Archives of Physical Medicine and Rehabilitation 80(9): 1121

34. Lum PS, Burgar CG, Kenney DE et al. 1999 Quantification of force abnormalities during passive and active-assisted upper-limb reaching movements in post-stroke hemiparesis. IEEE Transactions on Biomedical Engineering 46(6): 652–662

35. Hamilton BB, Granger CV, Sherwin FS et al. 1987 A uniform national data system for medical rehabilitation. In: Furher MJ ed. Rehabilitation outcomes: analysis and measurement. Brookes, Baltimore, 37–147

36. Mahoney FI, Wood OH, Barthel DW 1958 Rehabilitation of chronically ill patients: the influence of complications on the final goal. Southern Medical Journal 51: 605–609

37. Shor PC, Lum PS, Burgar CG et al. 2001 The effect of robot-aided therapy on upper extremity joint passive range of motion. Integration of assistive technology in the information age. Proceedings Seventh International Conference on Rehabilitation Robotics. IOS Press, Amsterdam, 79–83

38. Lum PS, Burgar CG, Shor M et al. 2002 Robot-assisted movement training compared with conventional therapy techniques for the rehabilitation of upper limb motor function after stroke. Archives of Physical Medicine and Rehabilitation 83(7): 952–959

39. Burgar CG 2002 Personal communication
40. Krebs H, Hogan N, Aisen ML et al. 1998 Robot-aided neurorehabilitation. IEEE Transactions on Rehabilitation Engineering 6(1): 75–87
41. Aisen ML, Krebs H, Hogan N et al. 1997 The effect of robot-assisted therapy and rehabilitative training on motor recovery following stroke. Archives of Neurology 54: 443–446
42. Volpe BT, Krebs HI, Hogan N et al. 2000 A novel approach to stroke rehabilitation. Robot-aided sensorimotor stimulation. Neurology 54: 1938–1944
43. Volpe BT, Krebs HI, Hogan N et al. 1999 Robot training enhanced motor outcome in patients with stroke maintained over three years. Neurology 53: 1874–1876
44. Wade DT 1992 Measurement in neurological rehabilitation. Oxford University Press, Oxford
45. World Health Organization 2001 International Classification of Functioning. Available online: http://www3.who.int/icf
46. Krebs HI, Aisen ML, Volpe BT et al. 1999 Quantization of continuous arm movements in humans with brain injury. Proceedings of the National Academy of Science USA 96: 4645–4649
47. Reinkensmeyer DJ, Schmidt BD, Rymer WZ 1999 Mechatronic assessment of arm impairment after chronic brain injury. Technology and Health Care 7: 431–435
48. Reinkensmeyer DJ, Dewald JPA, Rymer WZ 1999 Guidance-based quantification or arm impairment following brain injury: a pilot study. IEEE Transactions on Rehabilitation Engineering 7(1): 1–11
49. Kahn LE, Averbuch M, Rymer WZ et al. 2001 Effect of robot-assisted and unassisted exercise on functional reaching in chronic hemiparesis. Proceedings 23rd Annual IEEE Engineering in Medicine and Biology Conference, Istanbul, Turkey, October 25–28.
50. Johnson MJ, Van der Loos HFM, Burgar CG et al. 2001 Designing a robotic stroke therapy device to motivate use of the impaired limb. Integration of assistive technology in the information age. Proceedings Seventh International Conference on Rehabilitation Robotics. IOS Press, Amsterdam, 123–134
51. Reinkensmeyer DJ, Pang CT, Nessler JA et al. 2001 Java Therapy: web-based robotic rehabilitation. Integration of assistive technology in the information age. Proceedings Seventh International Conference on Rehabilitation Robotics. IOS Press, Amsterdam, 66–71
52. Harwin W, Loureiro R, Amirabdollahian F et al. 2001 The GENTLE/s project: a new method of delivering neuro-rehabilitation. In: Andrich R ed. Assistive Technology-Added value to the quality of life. IOS Press, Ljubljana, 10: 36–41
53. Amirabdollahian F, Loureiro R, Harwin WA. Case study on the effects of a haptic interface on human arm movements with implications for rehabilitation robotics. 1st Cambridge Workshop on Universal Access and Assistive Technology (CWUAAT) (incorporating 4th Cambridge Workshop on Rehabilitation Robotics). University of Cambridge, Cambridge, UK, March 25–27
54. Loureiro R, Amirabdollahian F, Coote S et al. 2001 Using haptics technology to deliver motivational therapies in stroke patients: concepts and initial pilot studies. In: EuroHaptics, Birmingham, UK, July 1–4, pp. 1–6
55. Cootes S, Stokes EK eds. Unpublished data
56. Amirabdollahian F, Loureiro R, Harwin W 2002 Minimum jerk trajectory control for rehabilitation and haptic applications. International Conference on Robotics and Automation, Washington DC, USA, May 11–15, 4: 3380–3385
57. Amirabdollahian F, Loureiro R, Driessen B et al. Error correction movement for machine assisted stroke rehabilitation. In: Mokhtari M ed. Integration of assistive technology in the information age. IOS Press, Vol. 9, 60–65
58. Bardofer A, Munih M, Zupan A et al. 2001 Upper limb motion analysis using haptic interface. IEEE/ASME Transactions on Mechatronics 6(3): 253–260
59. De Weert W, Feys H 2002 Assessment of physiotherapy for patients with stroke. Commentary. Lancet 359: 182–183
60. Pomeroy VM, Tallis RC 2002 Restoring movement and functional ability after stroke. Now and the future. Physiotherapy 88(1): 3–17

61. Dijkers MP, deBear PC, Erlandson RF et al. 1991 Patient and staff acceptance of robotic technology in occupational therapy: a pilot study. Journal of Rehabilitation Research and Development 28(2): 33–44
62. Coote S, Stokes EK. Robot mediated therapy: attitudes of patients and therapists towards the first prototype of the GENTLE/s system. Technology and Disability. In press
63. Coote S, Stokes EK. Current practice in physiotherapy post stroke: challenges to incorporating non-traditional treatment methods. Submitted
64. Nilsson LM, Nordhlom LA 1992 Physical therapy in stroke rehabilitation: basis for Swedish physiotherapists choice of treatment. Physiotherapy Theory and Practice 8: 49–55
65. Carr JH, Mungovan SF, Shepherd RB et al. 1992 Physiotherapy in stroke rehabilitation: basis for Australian physiotherapists choice of treatment. Physiotherapy Theory and Practice 8: 49–55
66. Coote S, Stokes EK. Moving robot-mediated therapy from research into clinical practice, an exploration of potential barriers to its implementation. Proceedings 8th International Conference on Rehabilitation Robotics. In press

WEBSITES OF INTEREST

GENTLE/S: Robotic assistance in neuro and motor rehabilitation:
http://www.gentle.rdg.ac.uk

MIME: Mirror-Image Movement Enabler: http://guide.stanford.edu/ICORR2001/shor.pdf

MIT-Manus: http://web.mit.edu/newsoffice/nr/2000.manus.html

ARM Guide: http://sulu.smpp.northwestern.edu/arm_guide/

Listening to the body

PART CONTENTS

6

Psychophysiological recording and biofeedback: tools enabling people to control their own physiology

Richard A. Sherman

SUMMARY

Real-time recordings of the body's physiological levels of functioning are used to help people become aware of what their bodies are doing and when they are not performing, as they should. Biofeedback is simply showing these recordings to the person being recorded so that the person can learn to control the physiological system being observed. The chapter follows a typical patient as he participates in diagnostic procedures enhanced by psychophysiological recordings, learns to recognize how his body is malfunctioning to cause his problems and uses the biofeedback devices to help him control the systems, and finally participates in desensitization training whose progress is guided by psychophysiological recordings. Recent advances in the field are also discussed.

CASE STUDY

Howard (a pseudonym) was referred for treatment of headaches, non-cardiac chest pain, and anxiety by his family practitioner after unsuccessful management attempts by a psychotherapist, a neurologist, and a physical therapist. He was a 34-year-old computer technician who had held his job for 7 years. He was a quiet, private person who liked to work alone. His headaches began about 5 years previously for no apparent reason and had gradually become more frequent and intense so that he now had headaches nearly every day. His chest pain started at about the same time and had followed the same course. Howard reported a life-long history of being uncomfortably anxious, but his anxiety became so difficult to deal with over the last year that he sought professional help. The sharp increase in anxiety coincided with a change in his work environment when his work location was shifted from a private office to a large open area containing dozens of workers performing diverse tasks.

The psychophysiological portion of Howard's assessment began with his filling in a very detailed body diagram on which he indicated the exact locations, descriptions, and intensities of his pain problems. The diagram showed that his headaches were a tight band around the top of his head. He also reported pain in his shoulders, neck, and across his chest. The shoulder and neck pain usually began before the pain in his head, while the pain in his chest changed independently of the other painful areas. He did not know what made his pain better or worse. His posture was normal, the physical therapist had not been able to help his pain, and he did not have any trigger points. Thus, the odds were that he was experiencing stress-related tension headaches.

The next step involved performing a psychophysiological profile of Howard's responses to stressful and relaxing images. Sensors were placed on him as a means of recording tension in his jaw, trapezius, and forehead muscles, respiration patterns from his chest and abdomen, and heart rate, sweating, and skin temperature (caused by near-surface blood flow) from his hands. Heart rate, sweating, and near-surface blood flow are all very sensitive indicators of stress responses.

While Howard was sitting quietly (if a bit nervously after being coated with all those sensors), his breathing was relatively fast (about 20 breaths per minute) and shallow with almost no abdominal breathing, and his muscles were tenser than would be expected of a slightly nervous person. The other systems were about normal. After about 5 minutes of recording, Howard was asked to imagine a very stressful scene in great detail. He indicated that he did not understand what we wanted so we guided him through the harrowing details of driving along an ice-coated highway at night during a sleet storm with huge trucks and four-wheel-drive vehicles whizzing by in the fast lane. He was asked to notice how tense his hands were on the wheel, his breathing, etc. As soon as he had a clear image of the situation, we told him that a colossal double trailer was roaring past, spraying his windshield to opacity with sleet, suddenly cutting in front of him, and then slamming on its breaks. There was a very clear change in his respiration pattern and his muscle tension increased to highly abnormal levels, while the other systems showed minimal changes indicative of normal stress responses. His jaw was especially reactive and remained clamped shut for several minutes after the exercise. After giving him a few minutes to recover, he was guided through a quietly relaxing walk at the end of which he mixed with a group of people having a quiet party. While imagining the quiet walk, his breathing slowed slightly and his muscles relaxed but, again, there were no significant changes in the other parameters. When we got to the part of the scene where he was mixing with people at the party, he showed nearly as bad a stress response as he showed while imagining the truck cutting him off, with the addition of a very significant increase in sweating. After a few minutes for a final baseline, we removed the sensors and discussed the changes in muscle tension and respiration with him.

The profile confirmed our initial view that:

1. His headaches were due to stress-induced muscle tension in the masseter (jaw muscles) and upper trapezius (shoulder muscles), as they were sufficiently tense at baseline to cause pain. Muscles only have to be sustained at about 5% tenser than normal to cause pain.[1]

2. His usual feelings of anxiety and non-cardiac chest pain were probably due to habitual, rapid, shallow chest breathing with the pattern being intensified by stress. This was made more likely by his psychotherapist failing to find any particular reason for his being anxious and both the breathing pattern, the anxiety, and the chest pain being exacerbated by stress. Shallow rapid breathing from the chest causes too much carbon dioxide to be released, which, in turn, causes the blood to become too basic. This sets off a cascade of events leading to initiating and sustaining feelings of very mild suffocation and anxiety. This condition frequently results in both non-cardiac chest pain and chronic anxiety. Gevirtz's team[2] and many others have now shown that as many as half of the patients carrying a diagnosis of chronic anxiety actually have a breathing disorder, and that when it is corrected, this results in the anxiety going away without further intervention.

3. The recent intensifying of his anxiety coincident with the change in work environment seemed to be a somewhat phobic response to having to be around a crowd of people. The likelihood of this being correct was increased by the stress response elicited during the profile when he imagined being around a group.

On the basis of our interviews and the physiological profile, we decided to perform a three-step intervention. First, we would treat his headaches with a combination of muscle tension biofeedback from his shoulders, jaws, and forehead in the clinic,[3] in conjunction with home practice of progressive muscle relaxation exercises[4] to sensitize him to how tense his muscle were and to help him learn to relax. Second, after he had gained control of his muscles and confidence in his ability to control his body's reactions to stressful situations, we would treat his general anxiety and non-cardiac chest pain with respiration retraining, consisting of a combination of biofeedback of his breathing patterns in the clinic, in conjunction with home practice of breathing exercises. Third, after the team's clinical psychologist had done a further evaluation of Howard's reaction to crowds and determined that he was having a phobic reaction, we would use a standard desensitization intervention with his physiological stress responses being used as a marker to objectively determine whether he was still responding to the stressor at each stage in desensitization. He was given a log to keep on a daily basis of his headache intensity, duration, and frequency, as well as his chest pain and anxiety, so that the progress of the treatment could be tracked.

The biofeedback training progressed very quickly. As illustrated in Figure 6.1, we placed sEMG (muscle tension) sensors on his face, forehead, and shoulders.

At the first session, it turned out that he was unable to recognize how tense his jaw and shoulder muscles actually were. If somebody without musculoskeletal pain is asked to tense any muscle to 100% of its maximum, then any other percentage, such as 50, 25, 75, etc., he or she will be able to do so very accurately. The person's sensations are accurately calibrated with actual tension. However, people with musculoskeletal pain in a particular muscle, such as the jaw or low back, can almost never perform this task accurately for that muscle – their sensation to muscle-tension level is out of calibration.[5] Our first task was to help him recalibrate his sensation to the muscle-tension system. This was accomplished easily by showing him the levels of his jaw muscle tension on the monitor and having him practice tensing and relaxing, while associating sensations with actual levels of tension. After several sessions, he was able to close his eyes and still match muscle tension levels to any requested percent of maximum.

Our next task was to teach him to relax his muscles when he wished to. The relaxation training he was doing at home had helped sensitize

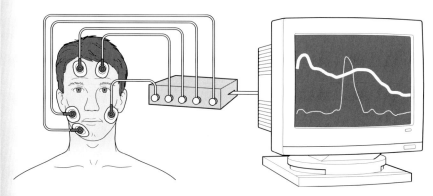

Figure 6.1 Illustration of averaged signals recorded from the forehead and jaw areas. The active sensors are over the frontal (forehead) and right masseter (jaw muscle) regions with the reference over the left masseter. The display shows the signals from the frontal area as a thin white line and the masseter as a thicker line. The signals have been averaged over time (root mean square – RMS), so appear as smooth lines which go up and down with changes in muscle tension.

him to when he was becoming tenser than he should for longer than he should, but he could not relax his muscles quickly upon demand. We helped him accomplish this by showing him a display of the signals from his jaw muscles and having him work toward specific goals of sequentially reducing his tension by lowering the signal in a series of graduated steps during which he reduced his signal slightly to a threshold line set just below the lowest level he could reach voluntarily. This 'shaping' process speeds muscle-control training considerably and is illustrated in Figure 6.2. He succeeded in learning the required tasks, and his headaches gradually decreased sufficiently in intensity, duration, and frequency over a period of about 5 weeks that we felt it was time to proceed to the next step in training.

The next stage in his training was to help him become aware of, and correct his pattern of relatively rapid, shallow, chest breathing so that he would form a habit of breathing more slowly using his diaphragm/abdomen to a greater extent. Our intention was to help him change his breathing patterns to decrease the abnormally low level of carbon dioxide resulting in feelings of anxiety with concomitant anxiety-based chest pain. Pneumatic respiration sensors were placed over his chest and abdomen to pick up expansion and contraction as he breathed. This is illustrated in Figure 6.3. He quickly learned to recognize incorrect patterns of breathing and to correct them while watching the display, but it took over a month of practice at home before he was able to habitually change his breathing patterns in his real life. According to his log, his feelings of general anxiety and his chest pain gradually subsided as his

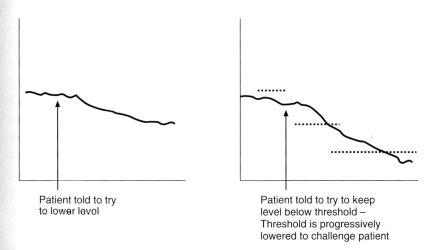

Patient told to try
to lower level

Patient told to try to keep
level below threshold –
Threshold is progressively
lowered to challenge patient

Figure 6.2   Demonstration of using threshold changes to shape learning. The display shows the averaged signal (solid line) being successively lowered to meet ever lower dashed threshold lines.

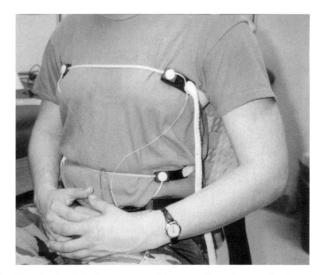

Figure 6.3   Respiration is being measured by recording changes in chest and abdominal circumference during inhalation and exhalation using belts placed around both the chest and abdomen (a pneumograph). This gives measures, which change nearly in proportion to volume.

breathing patterns normalized. However, he became very aware that his breathing was out of control when he had to perform tasks such as presentations in front of his colleagues and when the crowd in his office environment became particularly 'agitated'.

The third phase of the treatment was initiated in order to help Howard reduce his stress responses to being around groups of people. During the physiological profile we had noted that his sweating increased markedly when crowds were discussed. Changes in sweating are a great marker of sympathetic reactions to stress and this is recorded by sending a tiny current between two sensors held firmly against two nearby parts of the body, such as two fingers. Sweat is, of course, salt water, which conducts electricity. As sweating increases, the increased amount of salt water on the skin reduces resistance to the current flowing from sensor to sensor. These changes in resistance are used to mark changes in the underlying sympathetically mediated stress response. Figure 6.4 shows a recording of this galvanic skin response (GSR).

Our clinical psychologist performed a standard progressive desensitization protocol. He began by having Howard describe his feelings about being with groups of people. Both watched the monitor to see if his skin resistance changed – and it did. They worked until Howard no longer showed stress responses to just talking about crowds. Then they proceeded to his imagining being in a crowd and continued until he was able to actually be in a group of people without becoming too upset. They knew when it was appropriate to proceed to

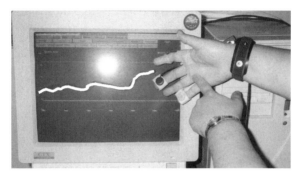

Figure 6.4 Illustration of a recording of the galvanic skin response (GSR), otherwise known as skin conductance level (SCL), skin resistance level (SRL), etc. The sensors are over the palmar surfaces of two fingers. The response is being elicited by stroking the palm.

the next step when he no longer showed changes in sweating. Having an objective marker available to determine when it was time to proceed speeded up the process enormously.

We followed Howard for nearly a year. He continued to practice his relaxation and breathing skills and was very aware of when his physiology was responding to stressors. His headaches were very rare and, when they did occur, were minor (low intensity and brief duration). His anxiety was minimal and clearly related to specific incidents when he did experience it. His chest pain was gone and he was much more comfortable in his work environment.

When Howard began working with us he expressed considerable doubt about the ideas that his body's reactions to stress were causing his pain and that he could learn to control his body sufficiently to avoid and manage his problems. He found the profile's results both startling and thought provoking. They convinced him of the relationship between his responses and his problems. He was quite surprised when he could not tense and relax his muscles to the percents of maximum on demand, and was even more surprised when he learned to perform the task quickly and accurately by watching the biofeedback display. He finally became convinced that the treatment was not just wand-waving when he began to gain control of his headaches. By the time he was ready to learn respiration-control techniques, he had become a real believer in his ability to control his body and virtually led the way through the rest of the treatment.

INTRODUCTION

Psychophysiology is the study of how the mind and physiology continuously interact to produce the levels of physiological functioning which govern how the body functions. This long-established field has gradually made the transition from a basic science into the realms of education, sports enhancement, and clinical practice. Psychophysiological recordings are commonly made of muscle tension, heart rate, brain waves, blood pressure, sweating in response to stress, and skin-temperature representations of near-surface blood flow to assess their patterns and levels of function. For example, these recordings are used in hospital sleep laboratories to assess stages of sleep and physiological sleep disorders as well as in respiration function laboratories to objectively assess breathing patterns. Figure 6.5 shows a recording being made of tension in the biceps and triceps muscles as the arm is successively bent and straightened at the elbow.

Muscles make electricity. They produce proportionately more electricity with increasing tension. The signal coming out of the muscles is transmitted to the skin's surface where it can be recorded using sensors taped to the skin over the muscles of interest. This is called a surface electromyographic (sEMG) recording. In the figure, you can see the sensors taped over the biceps. A similar set is taped over the triceps. When muscle tension is recorded, the sensors are placed parallel to the length of the muscle and on top of it as accurately as possible to minimize confusing the signal from the muscle with other electrical signals generated throughout the body including nearby muscles.

The signals are tiny – a few millionths of a volt – so need to be amplified as close to the sensors as possible in order to avoid confusing them with similarly sized signals from the body and air, from the lights, radio transmissions, etc. The signals reaching the sensors travel to the recording device via wires, light, or radio waves. Once there, they are enlarged enough to be used by an

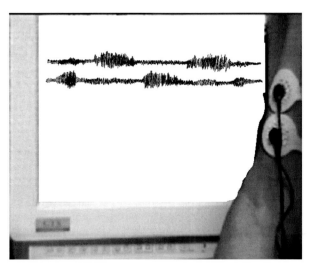

Figure 6.5 Typical display of tension in the bicep and triceps showing the 'raw' signals changing over time as the arm is consecutively bent and straightened at the elbow (pen tracing of an actual recording for clarity).

amplifier in very much the same way a radio amplifies the tiny radio signals traveling through the air. The figure depicts three sensors mounted over the biceps. Only the outer two actively pick up the signal from the muscle. The third is a reference sensor, which picks up signals from the whole body. The amplifier compares signals coming from the active sensors with the reference sensor to sort out the part of the signal generated by the muscle. If the sensors are put in the wrong place, it is impossible to tell what the muscle is doing. As long as the sensors are placed correctly, there is a good correlation between how tense the muscle is and the signal picked up by the amplifier. After the signal is amplified, it is filtered to get rid of noise and then converted to a form that can be shown on the screen or heard as a sound.

In figure 6.5, the display on the monitor shows how tension in the biceps and triceps changes as the patient is alternately tensing and relaxing them to control bending the arm at the elbow. The 'raw' muscle tension signals look like waves: the higher the waves, the stronger the tension. Figure 6.6 shows what the signals are supposed to look like when a patient can control the muscles correctly and what happens when things go wrong – such as too little tension applied to move the arm or the muscles not relaxing when they are supposed to after a movement.

Virtually all of the signals recorded for a psychophysiological assessment go through the same process of carefully placing the sensors so they can

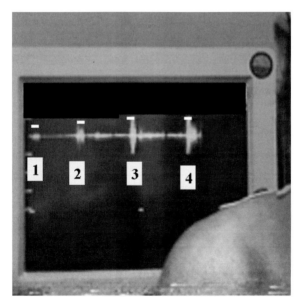

Figure 6.6 Simulated problems during a shoulder shrug. 1) Too little force to produce required motion. 2) Normal contraction. 3) Good but relaxation followed by spasm. 4) Muscle does not quiet at end of shrug. The bars above the raw signal show the approximate period of motion.

pick up the correct signal, amplifying the signal, and then displaying it so the therapist and patient can make an objective judgment as to what the body is doing. Examples of a variety of the signals typically recorded will be discussed throughout the chapter.

BIOFEEDBACK

The newest branch of psychophysiology is biofeedback. Biofeedback is the process of showing patients their psychophysiological recordings in real time, just as they are made, so patients can learn to associate sensations with the levels shown on the recording and see the effects of thoughts and control strategies on physiological functioning immediately. For example, if a person sits typing at a computer monitor for hours at a stretch without taking any breaks and has the arms and head slightly in the wrong positions so that the muscles are just 5% tenser than they should be, the person will probably develop wrist, arm, and head pain. The person probably would not be aware of holding him or herself slightly incorrectly and remaining so tense for so long that pain begins. As part of assessing why a patient hurts, a therapist might record muscle tension in the shoulders and arms while the patient simulates working, and then have the patient watch the recordings as they are being made (biofeedback) so the patient learns to recognize when he is tensing more than necessary for so long that pain begins. The patient would learn to recognize what muscles feel like at different levels of tension so he recognizes when they are tenser than they have to be. The patient would also learn to be very aware of changes in muscle tension in his normal environment, so that he can correct it as needed to avoid remaining so tense that pain begins.

People sometimes have urinary incontinence because their pelvic floor muscles are too weak to prevent urine from squirting out when the abdomen tenses up or after a cough, and because they have stopped tensing up when they should to keep from leaking.[6] Figure 6.7 shows a recording of the average of muscle tension in both the abdomen and pelvic floor before and after biofeedback training. The 'raw' signals have been averaged so they appear as lines instead of waves. The higher the line appears on the monitor, the tenser the muscle. In the figure, the left side shows muscle tension patterns in the abdomen and pelvic floor before biofeedback training and the right side shows them afterwards. At first, when the patient is told to tense up the pelvic floor without tensing the abdomen then keep it tense for a few seconds, she is unable to keep the abdominal muscles relaxed and the pelvic floor muscles only gradually tense up slightly, cannot maintain whatever little tension they do achieve, and then are too weak to remain tense long enough to do anything. As can be seen on the right side of the figure, after a few sessions of watching tension on the monitor and practicing tensing the muscles at home, the patient becomes really good at controlling both the pelvic floor and abdominal muscles so they perform as they are supposed to.

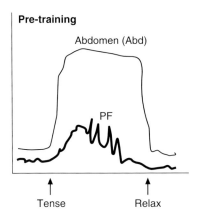
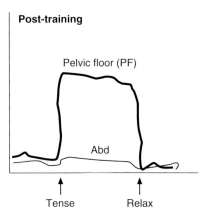

Figure 6.7 Illustration of patterns of relative muscle tension in the lower abdomen (thin line) and pelvic floor (thick line) before and after biofeedback training when only the pelvic floor muscle is to be tensed. Before training the pelvic floor has poor strength and control while the abdomen is tensed inappropriately.

Biofeedback got its start in the late 1940s when rehabilitation medicine professionals such as Basmajian[7] began showing their patients signals from their muscles being recorded on oscilloscopes as part of the muscle-function evaluation process. It quickly became apparent that patients could rapidly achieve more control of their muscles by watching the display than they could by being told how to change their muscle tension by the therapist. Some years later, other scientists began showing patients recordings of their brain waves in an effort to train them to control anxiety and epilepsy. Still others recorded patterns of respiration to help their patients recognize incorrect patterns of breathing leading to anxiety. Recordings of forehead muscle tension were shown to patients so they could learn to avoid tension headaches by keeping their muscles relaxed. Eventually, just about any aspect of the body's functioning, which could be recorded from the outside, was 'fed-back' to patients so they could learn to control inappropriate patterns of functioning.

In those early days, the displays were wavy lines on an oscilloscope, arrows moving across a meter's dial, a few lights glowing on a bar, or even just a series of beeping noises. Patients frequently had a lot of trouble telling what was going on and therapists did not have much control of the displays. Today, therapists can display just about whatever they want to on computer monitors and through highly flexible audio feedback systems. The therapist has nearly unlimited control of the display through controlling the computer's software. Therefore, displays which provide the information patients really need to rapidly learn to control their physiology can be generated on demand. In fact, there have been lots of other changes in biofeedback systems over the years. Muscle-tension and brain-wave sensors used to be very difficult to attach correctly because the skin had to be carefully scrubbed in order to get a good signal. Now, changes in amplifier technology mean that just a brief wash with soapy water or a rub with an alcohol pad does it. Lots of artifacts used to be introduced into the signals as wires swayed and sensors moved around. Now, the signals can be amplified right at the sensor and sent to the biofeedback device through fiber-optic cables, light, and radio waves largely impervious to noise.

Virtually all of the multichannel biofeedback devices in use today are controlled by software, which can be run on laptop computers. The computer's screen and sound systems provide highly flexible feedback displays, which are easily controlled throughout the session. Because the programs run on laptops, biofeedback is applied wherever the patients are – be it in factories, offices, or clinics. Many high-quality, pocket-size biofeedback devices have been developed that can be used to make longitudinal recordings of physiological functioning in the patients' normal environments to help determine what is causing problems. These devices can also be used as home trainers, so patients can not only monitor their physiological status, but also can practice self-control strategies virtually anywhere.

Today biofeedback is incorporated into standard treatments intended to help patients cure themselves of such problems as migraine and tension headaches,[8,9] muscle-related orofacial pain,[10] musculoskeletal low back pain,[5,11] cramping and burning phantom-limb pain,[12] posture-related pain,[1] muscle-tension-related urinary and fecal incontinence,[13] stress labile hypertension,[14] ADHD,[15] non-cardiac chest pain,[2] irritable bowel syndrome,[16] Raynaud's syndrome,[17,18] epilepsy,[19] anxiety,[2] and many more. More recently, a combination of electroencephalographic (EEG) biofeedback, respiration and temperature training is being shown effective for control of drug and alcohol addiction.[20]

Biofeedback is well accepted by the traditional medical community for the treatment of anxiety and headaches, and is now recommended by several national medical organizations, such as the College of Pediatrics and the College of Neurology, as initial approaches to treatment of headache. The use of biofeedback for urinary incontinence is spreading rapidly and is gaining popularity in the traditional medical community. Biofeedback systems for urinary incontinence are now common in the urology departments of large teaching hospitals and the American government has recently decided to authorize insurance reimbursement for the technique. As innovative uses for biofeedback, such as treatment of addiction and ADHD, spread and prove themselves, people's abilities to work with technology to increase their own abilities to control difficult medical problems is growing rapidly. Two of the most exciting innovations in biofeedback involve teaching pain patients to control their brain's reactions to pain signals coming from the body. When a pain signal comes into the brain from the body, the brain shows a characteristic change in brain waves about 100 ms after the pain begins. Flor[21] and others have used biofeedback to teach people to lower the amplitude of the responding brain wave. When patients reduce the size of the response, the magnitude of the reported pain goes down proportionately. Another innovation is the use of biofeedback techniques to train pain patients to actually reduce the representation of painful areas in the brain's sensory homunculus. The size of a painful body part, such as the left low back, has a greater volume of representation in the homunculus than in patients without pain or the corresponding pain-free area on the other side of the body (the right low back in this example). When the patient learns to reduce the painful area's representation on the homunculus, perceived pain intensity decreases.[21]

Research supporting the efficacy of several biofeedback techniques is quite impressive. For example, biofeedback treatments for both migraine and tension headaches are effective for about 80% of patients and the reductions in pain were still there after 15 years among those people who continued to practice their skills.[8,22] The author[23] recently reviewed the strength of evidence supporting biofeedback's efficacy when incorporated into treatment of these and many other problems, so that publication may be of interest to readers interested in further details on the topic.

Biofeedback does have its disadvantages relative to taking medications to ameliorate disorders. The most significant of these is that the patient must be willing to take responsibility for doing the work necessary to learn the required skills, and then practicing them sufficiently and consistently enough for the disorder to be affected and then to remain ameliorated. If the patient does not learn the skills, the disorder will not be affected. If the patient does not continue to practice newly learned skills, the disorder will return, so this may be a life-long commitment. Many people are not interested in doing the work required to learn the skills nor in continuing to apply them for years. Some people cannot learn the required skills for any of a variety of reasons. The case study at the beginning of the chapter provides a flavor of the psychophysiologically guided assessment and biofeedback-enhanced treatment process. The literature leads us to believe that 'Howard' will maintain his gains for as long as he continues to keep his skills sharp and in use.[8,24]

FUTURE PROSPECTS

Biofeedback is changing rapidly both in machinery and the uses it is being put to. Of greatest importance from the author's perspective is the fact that the devices are becoming far easier to use and give increasingly more information to the therapist about how well the device is functioning. All too many therapists have a very limited background in physiology and do not really know how to recognize bad recordings. The best of the newer devices guide therapists through checking the sensors and then warn them if a signal goes bad during the recording because a sensor becomes loose or a myriad of other problems occur. These advances permit the therapist to concentrate more on the therapy and less on technical aspects of biofeedback. Of course, no instrument can guarantee that the therapist places the sensors in the correct location or is applying the techniques in a rational manner. The Association for Applied Psychophysiology and Biofeedback is the major organization representing the field. Their newsmagazine 'Biofeedback' recently devoted an entire issue[25] to innovators' ideas on new techniques coming into practice or just over the horizon. Interested readers can view this issue on the organization's website www.aapb.org

CONCLUSION

Psychophysiological assessment and biofeedback have matured sufficiently in both the equipment available and the techniques used that they can be incorporated into the clinical armamentarium of virtually any practitioner working with patients willing to expend the effort to ameliorate a wide variety of problems. Recent reviews, such as that by the author,[23] show that biofeedback can be effective for a wide variety of problems including migraine and tension headache, urinary incontinence, phantom-limb pain, jaw-muscle dysfunctions, etc. Readers are encouraged to perform their own literature searches to learn how these techniques can be applied to areas of interest and to contact organizations, such as the AAPB (www.aapb.org), to find out how to get training in the use of biofeedback and psychophysiological recording equipment.

REFERENCES

1. Middaugh S, Kee W, Nicholson J 1994 Muscle overuse and posture as factors in the development and maintenance of chronic musculoskeletal pain. In: Grzesiak R, Cicconie D eds. Psychological vulnerability to chronic pain. Springer, New York, 55–89
2. DeGuire S, Gevirtz R, Hawkinson D et al. 1996 Breathing retraining: a three-year follow-up study of treatment for hyperventilation syndrome and associated functional cardiac symptoms. Biofeedback Self-Regulation 21: 191–198
3. Sherman R 1985 Relationships between jaw pain and jaw muscle contraction level: underlying factors and treatment effectiveness. The Journal of Prosthetic Dentistry 54: 114–118
4. Jacobson E 1970 Modern treatment of tense patients. Charles C. Thomas, Springfield
5. Flor H, Birbaumer N 1994 Psychophysiological methods in the assessment and treatment of chronic musculoskeletal pain. In: Carlson J, Seifert R, Birbaumer N eds. Clinical applied psychophysiology. Plenum, New York, 171–184
6. Sherman R, Davis G, Wong M 1997 Behavioral treatment of urinary incontinence among female soldiers. Military Medicine 162: 690–694
7. Basmajian JV, Gowland CA, Finlayson MA 1987 Stroke treatment: comparison of integrated behavioral – physical therapy vs traditional physical therapy programs. Archives of Physical Medicine and Rehabilitation 68: 267–272
8. Blanchard EB 1992 Psychological treatment of benign headache disorders. Journal of Consulting and Clinical Psychology 60: 537–551
9. Penzien D, Rains J, Andrasik F 2002 Behavioral management of recurrent headache: three decades of experience and empiricism. Applied Psychophysiology and Biofeedback 27: 163–181

10. Glaros A, Glass E 1993 Temporomandibular disorders. In: Gatchel R, Blanchard E eds. Psychophysiological disorders: research and clinical application. American Psychological Association, Washington DC, 299–356
11. Flor H, Birbaumer N 1993 Comparison of the efficacy of EMG biofeedback, cognitive-behavioral therapy, and conservative medical interventions in the treatment of chronic musculoskeletal pain. Journal of Consulting and Clinical Psychology 61: 653–658
12. Sherman RA, Devor M, Jones D et al. 1996 Phantom pain. Plenum: New York
13. Tries J, Eisman E 1995 Urinary incontinence: evaluation and biofeedback treatment. In: Schwartz M ed. Biofeedback: A practitioner's guide. Guilford, New York, 597–632
14. McGrady A 1996 Good news-bad press: applied psychophysiology in cardiovascular disorders. Biofeedback Self-Regulation 21: 335–346
15. Lubar JF, Swartwood MO, Swartwood JN et al. 1995 Evaluation of the effectiveness of EEG neurofeedback training for ADHD in a clinical setting as measured by changes in T.O.V.A. scores, behavioral ratings, and WISC-R performance. Biofeedback Self-Regulation 20: 83–99
16. Humphreys PA, Gevirtz RN 2000 Treatment of recurrent abdominal pain: components analysis of four treatment protocols. Journal of Pediatric Gastroenterology and Nutrition 31: 47–51
17. Freedman R 1991 Physiological mechanisms of temperature biofeedback. Biofeedback and Self-Regulation 16: 95–115
18. Middaugh S, Haythornthwaite J 2001 The Raynaud's treatment study: biofeedback protocols and acquisition of temperature biofeedback skills. Applied Psychophysiology and Biofeedback 26: 251–278
19. Sterman MB 2000 Basic concepts and clinical findings in the treatment of seizure disorders with EEG operant conditioning. Clinical Electroencephalography 31: 45–55
20. Walters D 1998 EEG neurofeedback treatment for alcoholism. Biofeedback Spring: 18–33
21. Flor H 2002 Modification of cortical reorganization and chronic pain by sensory feedback. Applied Psychophysiology and Biofeedback 27: 215–237
22. Hermann C, Blanchard E 2002 Biofeedback in the treatment of headache and other childhood pain. Applied Psychophysiology and Biofeedback 27: 142–162
23. Sherman R 2002 Biofeedback. In: Leskowitz E ed. Complementary and alternative medicine in rehabilitation. Harcourt (W.B. Saunders), New York, 125–138
24. Blanchard E, Andrasik F 1985 Management of chronic headaches. Pergamon Press, New York
25. Moss D, Sherman R eds. 2002 Biofeedback 30 # 1. Association for Applied Psychophysiology, Colorado

WEBSITES OF INTEREST

Association for Applied Psychophysiology and Biofeedback: www.aapb.org

Behavioral Medicine Research & Training Foundation: www.behavmedfoundation.org

7

Affective feedback

Gary McDarby *James Condron* *Darran Hughes*
Ned Augenblick *John Sharry*

SUMMARY

In this chapter we introduce the concept of affective feedback. This involves augmenting the traditional methods of biofeedback, with sensory immersion, novel signal processing, compelling game play and narrative, and intelligent technology having an active role in the biofeedback loop. Biofeedback is a powerful under-utilized concept that can be used to enable and empower an individual by giving them access to the information only technology can provide. Its usefulness is hampered by inappropriate technology and wild claims about what it can do. Affective feedback is a way of making better use of the power of biofeedback and relies on the integration of available technologies and expertise, which are outlined in this chapter.

CASE STUDY

Peter was a 9-year-old boy who often suffered from anxiety attacks. The anxiety could be provoked by many different things, such as cars skidding, thunder, or news of disasters on the television. In response to these events, he could become fearful that something bad was going to happen (e.g. that the car would crash into him or his family) and the anxiety could build until he became very distressed. His anxiety was quite disabling and he would frequently refuse to go out, as he feared something bad would happen to him. Once his parents had to be called to his school as he became very distressed during a rainstorm and he had to leave the classroom.

Peter was referred for psychotherapy to help him manage his fears. The goal of treatment was to help Peter learn how to relax in the face of his fears. Central to the approach was the use of the affective feedback game 'Relax to Win' (described later in this chapter), which capitalized on Peter's strong interest in video games. It was explained to Peter, that the more he could relax, as measured by galvanic skin response (GSR), the faster his dragon would travel. In the one player version of the game, Peter raced against a 'ghost dragon' that represented his previous best score. In this way, Peter could learn how to progressively relax and to improve this ability over time.

The therapist coached Peter through the process, helping him name and understand the physical changes in his body that occurred when he was agitated and when he was relaxed. At the end of the sessions, they would plan how Peter could use these skills in the face of outside fears. When he gained more control of his arousal, Peter used the game to practice relaxing in the face of fears. At the beginning of the game, Peter would think of a scary situation (and thus agitate himself) and then apply all his relaxation skills (e.g. breathing deeply, imagining more pleasant things). As the speed of the dragons was determined by the difference in physiological arousal, this approach made the dragon go faster and thus allowed Peter to get his best scores. This was a great reward to him. After four sessions, Peter had made great gains in how he could manage his fears. The 'Relax to win' game was an important component of this improvement in providing a fun game that engaged Peter, while helping him understand how he became distressed and to name his relaxation skills.

INTRODUCTION

Throughout each day, a person's mental state can seamlessly change from groggy to aware, relaxed to agitated, or happy to sad. These changes have a profound effect on the way that people interact with themselves and the world, and yet, many people feel that they do not have control over their own internal state. The internal state referred to here is the automatic ability for conscious and subconscious control via the central and peripheral nervous systems, therefore, internal physical as well as mental health. From attention deficit disorder (ADD) patients who cannot focus, depressed people who cannot escape dark moods, to many people who have a difficult time relaxing – the inability to have self-control over internal states is extensive across society. There are many ways for a person to positively affect their mental state, from taking drugs to going to the movies. These are only temporary measures and in the case of drugs often have negative side effects. What if there was a more controlled, predictable, and long-term way to help people reach specific mental states?

AFFECTIVE FEEDBACK

Affective feedback is the process of using technology to help people achieve and maintain specific internal states. Essentially, we are trying to create immersive systems that encourage people to reach a specific state, such as relaxation or concentration, and 'teach' them how to control it. This turns out to have therapeutic use as a significant number of disorders are linked to a person's natural tendency towards certain particular destructive internal states. For example, a child with ADD, who has a tendency towards an unfocused state, can use the system to learn how to maintain a concentrated state. Another example could be a person prone to depression learning how to maintain a more elevated state of mind.

How is this accomplished?

We first need the technology to create sensory immersive environments that engage and captivate the user. We then need ways and means to measure the effect of these sensory immersive environments. If we allow the technology to experiment with different sensory experiences, and to record relevant effect, we have created an affective feedback system. If the goal is to help a person reach and maintain a specific internal state, the first step is to identify the factors that can cause changes in a person's state over time. This is the experimental phase. The second step is to associate particular internal states with sensory experiences. The final step is to identify comparatively positive states of mind according to that user and facilitate the user maintaining these states. This is affective feedback. For example, a person listening to their favorite piece of music whilst relaxing is in an entirely different mental state to when they are subjected to music they do not like. If the environment was intelligent enough to 'know' this state, then it could select appropriate music to relax a person. Another example of this would be an environment reminding a person to stay actively focusing on positive, relaxing thoughts and breathing deeply to cause a more 'relaxed' internal state. These states are brought about by external environmental factors facilitating the changing of internal states.

How could a system 'harness' the natural power of both conscious self-control and the external environment to 'help' the user reach and maintain a specific internal state? First, it has been shown that people's innate ability to control their own internal state can be refined through a process known as biofeedback.[1] However, this process is very tedious. The first part of this chapter will discuss biofeedback and show various ways in which it can be improved. 'Enhanced' biofeedback is the key to unlocking the potential of self-control of one's internal state and is the first step to affective feedback. The second part to affective feedback is using the power of the environment to directly affect a person's internal state. This will be discussed in the latter part of the chapter. In its 'static' form, this simply entails presenting the user with visual and auditory stimuli that invoke the appropriate internal state. The more advanced 'dynamic' form involves a system that actually learns which environmental factors cause different internal states and, therefore, is able to intelligently pick the appropriate stimuli to create a specific state for each unique user.

We have created two immersive video games, which help the user reach and maintain both relaxed and concentrated states. The games are designed with a structure that demonstrates the real-world application of affective feedback, which will be described later in the chapter.

BIOFEEDBACK vs. AFFECTIVE FEEDBACK

The first key to affective feedback is to utilize the user's innate power to consciously control an aspect of their physiological state. This control could be enhanced through the process of biofeedback (see also Sherman in this volume). However, traditional biofeedback can be a long, tedious and uncomfortable process. This section of the chapter discusses traditional biofeedback and the multiple ways we believe it can be improved to make it more effective and efficient.

Suppose that a person is learning how to play darts for the first time. If their first few tosses don't make it to the board or land far left of the target, they will react by throwing the dart faster and more to the right on the next toss. After multiple throws, the person will slowly gain a 'feel' for how the subtleties of their actions influence the final position of the dart on the board. Intuitively, the key part of this process is receiving 'feedback'; evaluating the result in relation to the original goal. For example, if the room were completely dark, the person would never perceive the result of their efforts and would soon give up on trying to learn to play darts. In a basic form, this is referred to as 'operant learning': someone throws the dart, receives feedback from the result, and changes their next throw accordingly. It is important to note that the operant learning model requires some sense of motivation – a person who does not care about darts will not learn as effectively as a person who is passionate about the sport.

Now, imagine a person trying to learn how to control the blood flow to their hand. Generally, people have some innate sense of the state of warmth in their hands, but the gradient of differentiation between levels (cold, normal, hot) is very large. In other words, the quality of feedback is poor. This is similar to playing darts in the dark and only being able to hear if the dart hits the board or the wall. It is possible to learn to hit the board, just as it is possible to learn that focusing thoughts on the hand for an extended period will warm it up. However, as the quality of feedback is directly linked to the level of learning, it is impossible to gain more subtle control without better feedback.

Clearly, feedback is not the only issue. A sense of causation between the action and the system you are trying to affect is necessary: receiving feedback concerning moon cycles will not give a person control of the moon. In fact, for many decades, it was assumed that the autonomic nervous system (ANS), which controls homeostatic control systems in the body such as heartbeat, was not under voluntary control. This has proved to be untrue.[2] Medical science and technology have advanced to provide new methods of displaying biological states (such as real-time blood pressure and body temperature). With more refined feedback, it is clear a person *can* control these previously considered involuntary biological functions.[3–5]

This process is known as biofeedback, and has been used to gain conscious control over many aspects of the ANS. For example, Dewan in 1971[6] showed the possibility of gaining control of brainwaves to send Morse code messages by consciously oscillating certain brainwave frequencies. There are many other examples of conscious control of brainwaves, heart rate, specific sections of muscles, and blood flow, among others.[7–11]

Is there any practical use in learning how to control the ANS, or is it simply a skill like throwing darts? It turns out that biofeedback has significant therapeutic uses and is employed for that purpose in many fields. Controlling blood flow is a method of helping people with Raynaud's disease,[12] which is characterized by poor circulation to the extremities. Gaining muscle control through biofeedback is a preferred therapy for treating incontinence.[9,10,13] Similarly, musculoskeletal biofeedback is consistently used for physical therapy.[14]

However, the most interesting, and perhaps most controversial form of biofeedback is known as neurofeedback and involves learning how to control one's brain state. But how does one 'display' a 'brain state' in order to present a person with accurate real-time feedback? This problem will be discussed in the next section of the chapter. For now, it is only important to note that it *is* possible to provide very limited feedback regarding brain events with an electroencephalogram (EEG). Using this information, people can learn how to increase the relative amplitude of certain frequencies of brainwaves (which, in broad categories, map to brain states such as concentration) in different topical areas of the brain. This is not easy and requires a significant number of training sessions to master[8,15,16] (see also Chapter 8). However, after a sufficient number of training sessions, it is believed that the long-term structure of the brain actually changes in a way that makes this brain state more possible in the future.[2] As multiple disorders, such as epilepsy[16–32] and depression[7,8,15,33] have been linked to time-reliant irregularities in certain frequencies in specific areas of the brain, biofeedback can be used to treat these problems. For example, training children to increase high-frequency brainwaves, which roughly map to a state of concentration, has been shown to be an effective treatment for ADD.[1,3–5,35–43]

While it has been proven that people can use biofeedback to gain control of functions that were previously thought to be out of conscious control, there are serious limitations. In the early stages of biofeedback in the 1970s, the over-excitement and non-scientific claims of many practitioners tarnished the reputation of the discipline to the point that it is only recovering today. The simple lesson is that denying the problems with biofeedback is more dangerous than exposing them. As with the examples of playing darts or controlling heartbeat, the learning process is severely dependent on the quality of feedback. This is not as much of a problem for monitoring a simple, low-noise bio-signal, such as a heartbeat; however, a signal, such as an EEG is weak and plagued with noise that reduces the quality of the feedback. Additionally, measuring bio-signals often involves a large amount of expensive equipment consisting of electrodes and wires, which must be directly applied to the person's body. This reduces the number of people with access to the technology as well as making the process uncomfortable for the user. Motivation is also a huge issue, especially for children, as the training period is long and demanding. If the person is not completely behind the process, effective biofeedback is very difficult. Finally, as with any skill, humans are limited by their own personal capacity. Just as a person can only play darts so well, a person can only gain so much control of their ANS.

While the last problem is inescapable, the first three can be partially solved if the biofeedback system is improved. The first step towards affective feedback is to make multiple enhancements to traditional biofeedback.

As the general idea of feedback is a necessity, the key is to 'house' the feedback in a more effective environment. This section of the chapter will discuss ways to 1) improve traditional biofeedback directly and 2) create a framework that increases motivation in the user.

Improving biofeedback directly

As mentioned earlier, two major issues confronting biofeedback are the relatively poor quality of some bio-signals (and hence the feedback) and the fact that the equipment is not wireless. Improving upon traditional biofeedback has become realistic with the advent of new affordable technologies. Therefore, solving these problems through the use of non-invasive, affordable wireless sensors and advanced signal processing is a necessary, but not sufficient step towards achieving affective feedback. Another important step toward affective feedback is the use of multiple bio-signals, a 'multi-modal approach.'

Affordable wireless sensors

Currently, professional equipment to measure bio-states for research purposes, such as the Biopac© System, cost upwards of $11 000 (2001 pricelist).

Dedicated biofeedback machines designed for a specific training system on a PC, such as the WaveRider Pro, cost about $1500 (2001 pricelist).[44] This is significant expenditure for home use or even for a professional practice. In addition, the equipment is generally not wireless, requires substantial effort to use, and is uncomfortable.

For our last two projects, we have developed custom amplifiers and biosensors to circumvent these problems. Our goal was to design affordable, comfortable, small, systems that produced accurate and clean bio-signals. Some of the problems that we tackled during the design phase included power consumption, weight, and movement artefact. The final product was custom GSR and EEG sensors and amplifiers. We are working to make the system wireless.

Using signal processing

Extracting pertinent information from a bio-signal demands complex signal processing. By their very nature bio-signals are non-stationary and so their frequency characteristics change with time. This means that techniques like Fourier analysis need to be modified to account for issues like drift, noise and information in the signals changing form over time. In addition, to provide effective feedback information, it is necessary to display an accurate representation of the current state of the system being influenced. Therefore, one of the first issues in biofeedback is finding a concrete way of displaying systems that are abstract (like brain state) or directly immeasurable (like sweat gland activity). Quasi real-time feedback is also necessary, because as the time lag gets greater, it is harder to decipher which actions associate with the system's reactions. Novel real-time signal processing is, therefore, an essential part of affective feedback.

Multi-modal approach

If a user is trying to learn how to increase 'alpha' waves in the brain, the feedback information should clearly reflect the level of 'alpha' waves. But, what if one is trying to promote an abstract mental state, such as 'relaxation?' Alpha waves are a useful measure of mental inactivity that can be associated with psychophysiological relaxation, whereas heartbeat variability and GSR can have characteristics associated with motor relaxation. While these signals are correlated, they still contain independent information. Therefore, it is reasonable to assume that they reflect different aspects of 'relaxation'. If this is the case, the measure (and feedback) of 'relaxation' should somehow reflect a combination of these signals. In other words, it is always helpful to gather as much meaningful information as possible.

This is the logic behind a so-called 'multi-modal' approach – the use of multiple bio-signals for feedback. This is an important method for encouraging any abstract mental state, and is crucial to the concept of affective feedback.

Improving motivation

Operant learning relies heavily on the user's desire to determine the relation between their actions and its effect on the outside system. In fact, user motivation is usually one of the key reasons that biofeedback training fails, especially with children. It is not easy to convince anyone, let alone a child, to put full effort into a time-consuming, difficult task with abstract goals. This is where affective feedback comes in – to 'house' the training in an environment that provides the motivation necessary to succeed.

Originally, feedback was simply a dot on a screen, which only moved vertically to demonstrate the level of achievement.[6] Clearly, a person must be very focused on the end goal of controlling their bio-state in order to endure hours of staring at a dot! As it became obvious that this was not compelling enough for children (or most adults), practitioners headed in the direction of affective feedback by housing the biofeedback in a simple game. An example is a commonly used modified Pac-man game, in which the Pac-man gobbles more dots as the desired bio-signals are produced. The problem is that these games are essentially just a graphically enhanced representation of the 'dot,' which soon loses its novelty. Nonetheless, the games are more effective than traditional biofeedback and see widespread use. Affective feedback is the continuation of this trend towards a situation where people are keen to participate in the experience of biofeedback without having to focus on the long-term goals of bio-signal control. There are a few ways this is accomplished.

Augmented reality to immerse

A student who drifts off or loses interest during a lecture will not learn as much as a student who is paying complete attention. Good advertisers, teachers, and preachers keep this in mind when trying to hold the attention of their audience. Two complementary ways to achieve this goal are to make the message itself more interesting and to remove all possible environmental factors that might create a distraction.

When watching a movie in the theater, it is very difficult not to pay attention, even if the movie is terrible. This is due to the fact that the auditory and visual display of the movie overwhelms the senses: the movie is the entire environmental experience and it is nearly impossible to avoid paying attention to it. Therefore, one way to increase the attention of the user (and block distractions) is to completely control their sensory input, 'immersing' them in an augmented world.

Clearly, this is not enough to guarantee interest as the user can always turn their mind inward. The next step is making the environment more intriguing, so that the person has an interest in paying attention to it. While the user will never forget that they are in a 'false' world, the new environment will command more attention and have a greater effect on their internal state as their 'presence' (engagement in the world) increases. How much realism is necessary to completely draw the attention of the user? It turns out that, if a person is completely immersed, very simple scenes can draw significant attention resources.[45]

Gaming environment and storyline

Evolutionary psychologists believe that humans (as well as some other primates) have a natural inclination to play 'games', because they allow for the practice and perfection of skills in a relatively non-threatening environment.[46] Therefore, using a game is an optimal way to teach a skill as it creates natural motivation and interest in the user. Generally, success within the game provides the primary reward, while secondary skills are learned as a bi-product. Note that games can be used to train relatively arbitrary skills: children are physiologically aroused, and learn how to press buttons in a certain order very quickly if connected with success in an interesting computer game. These enhancements make biofeedback more comfortable, enjoyable, and effective. They do not require the user to have an interest in succeeding in the biofeedback process – only that they enjoy playing an immersive game. Over time, the user will be able to control an aspect of their physiological state, which is the first step to affective feedback.

ENVIRONMENTAL CONDITIONS AFFECTING INTERNAL STATE

People are not as consistent as they would like to believe. While every person does have a set of tendencies to act and react in certain ways, personality is somewhat plastic. The same person can be competitive or cooperative, relaxed or stressed, and generous or stingy depending on their environment. Therefore, the immediate environment can play a huge role in the way that a person thinks and who they 'are' in that moment. This suggests that a person's environment can be manipulated to directly affect their internal state. Architects and designers, for example, have known about this for a long time: places where we live and work are specifically designed to elicit a generally positive emotion in the user.

However, while we use this principle every day without recognition, it is an extremely powerful idea when combined with the application of biofeedback. In its 'static' form, this involves using the framework that houses the biofeedback to directly influence the bio-state of the user and, hence, the effectiveness of the training. This type of affective biofeedback is 'static' because the environmental framework does not change for different users. Alternatively, the more advanced 'dynamic' affective feedback involves the

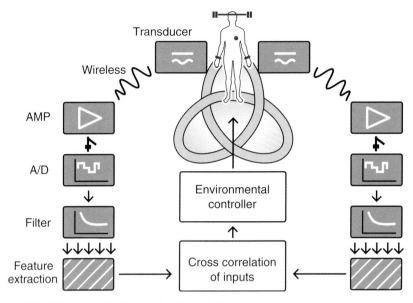

Figure 7.1 Dynamic affective feedback block diagram.

environmental controller actually 'learning' which situations bring out different bio-states in each individual user and uses that knowledge to promote the desired state.

Traditional biofeedback can be seen as an operant learning loop between the user and the computer – the person acts, notices changes in the display based on their bio-signs, and reacts accordingly. Dynamic affective feedback introduces a new loop – the computer acts by manipulating the user's environment, recording the changes in the user, and reacting appropriately (Fig. 7.1).

It is important to note that this new loop can be implemented without biofeedback. If the user does not want to actively participate in the feedback process, the computer can work in the background to subtly change the user's environment and learn its effects on their state. Over time, the computer will have the power to proactively affect the internal state of the user in a predictable way. This technology can help the user reach a chosen internal state without requiring significant effort from the user.

A cloudy and rainy day has a very different effect on a person than a clear and sunny day. In general, simply displaying warm colors instead of cold colors can set different moods. The effect is not solely color based: large and open rooms create a different 'feel' to claustrophobic ones. A simple and uncluttered scene affects people differently than a cluttered, gaudy setting. After analysis, it is clear that virtually everything human made, from homes and products to clothes, is designed to create specific sensations in the user. This power can be captured and used in a constructive way to help people achieve and maintain different beneficial mental states.

Static affective feedback (SAF) is essentially the marriage of biofeedback with multiple technologies shown to affect the user's internal state. While the connections between technologies are original, the individual technologies are not. However, dynamic affective feedback (DAF) is a radical new method that will drastically change the way that computers react to people.

Technology has reached the point that computers can begin to receive information from their users in a more profound way than by using a keyboard. There is, in fact, a new trend in computing to create computers with the ability to recognize and react to the user's emotional state.[47] However, most applications of this concept involve using a simple algorithm to link the computer with the user: the computer determines that the user is in state 'X' and therefore does 'Y.' However, why not enable the computer to be an active participant in the process?

SAF relies on the fact that different scenes create different moods. However, it ignores the fact that a specific scene can have a different effect on each individual person. A simple look at how people decorate their homes suggests that people have unique feelings associated with different environments. Therefore, a way to improve on SAF would be to determine how different environments affect each individual, rather than assuming environments have the same effect on all people. For example, if the computer is trying to 'help' put the user in a concentrated state, what environment should it use? Take a look at where people study; some people feel more focused in an open and busy environment, like a café, while others prefer a quiet and closed setting, like a library. The only way the computer can determine its type of user is by testing out different environments and seeing how the person reacts.

In the traditional biofeedback process, the person receives information about their bio-state from the computer and they slowly learn how to maintain these states, by associating internal changes with external changes. In DAF, the computer receives information about the person's bio-state from the sensors and slowly learns how to affect it, by associating its environmental changes with bio-changes in the person. Although it is convenient to see this as the addition of a new separate feedback loop, it is clear that the loops are not independent.

What parts of the environment can the computer manipulate to learn how to affect the user's internal state? Essentially, most of the components mentioned in the SAF section can be dynamically manipulated with appropriate effort. In theory, it is entirely possible to change the underlying framework, such as the characters and fundamental storyline, dynamically.

INTERFACING TO THE VIRTUAL WORLD

The virtual world has many advantages for creating an immersive environment. One of the greatest advantages is that all visual and auditory parameters can be directly controlled and, more significantly, recorded. The fact that all of the sensory information can be controlled, enables psychologists and psychotherapists alike to produce a sensory state that has a direct influence on the inner state of the person. This can be independent of biofeedback. For example, an extremely simple virtual scenario called 'SpiderWorld' (see Fig. 2.1, Chapter 2, p. 24) is used to treat arachnophobia by helping patients to confront their fear in a safe environment.[48–50] The world consists of a very basic modeled kitchen with a less-than-realistic spider crawling around. Even though it is very basic, subjects are very attentive and respond as if the scene was real.

However, does this increase in attention reduce the effect of outside distractions? Researchers working at the University of Washington found that when burn victims were immersed in a 'Snow World' (see Fig. 2.4, Chapter 2, p. 29), the pain of dressing the wounds was lessened.[51,52] Why? 'Being drawn into another world drains a lot of attentional resources, leaving less attention available to process pain signals' according to Dr Hunter Hoffman of the University of Washington Human Interface Technology Lab.

Controlling the user's entire auditory and visual sensory input focuses their attention to the point of distracting the person from pain. This shows that the use of immersive reality acts not only to captivate the user, but also to reduce possible environmental distractions. It is with this in mind that the Mindgames group has produced two games in particular to examine the validity of this concept: 'Relax to win' and 'Brainchild'.

'RELAX TO WIN'

'Relax to win' is a competitive two player racing game. Each player controls an animated 3-D dragon in a virtual racetrack environment where the goal is to cross the finish line first (Fig. 7.2). While the game itself is quite visually impressive, the main value lies in the fact that the player's stress level, as measured by their GSR, controls the action of the dragon. The dragon has three successively faster 'states': walk, run and fly. If a player relaxes, their skin resistance increases and the dragon will shift up to the next faster state. Conversely, an increase in 'stress' causes the dragon to shift to a slower state. The end result is that the player who 'relaxes the most' over the game will reach the finish line first. The game places users in a competitive environment not only to provide motivation, but to teach them how to relax in a stress-inducing situation.

'BRAINCHILD'

Brainchild is a biometrically controlled modular computer game that teaches the user how to gain control over various bio-signals. The game immerses the player in a compelling fantasy storyline using professional-quality sound and video (Fig. 7.3). The user is taught how to train their

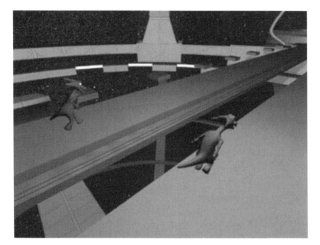

Figure 7.2   Screen shot from 'Relax to win'.

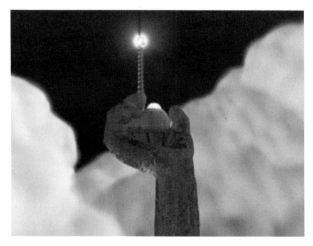

Figure 7.3   Screen shot from 'Brainchild'.

'magic' (biometric) skills by a mentor character who leads the user through the story and process. For example, the player's skill of relaxation is mapped to the 'magical' skill of telekinesis. In the first level of the game, the player is brought to a lock mechanism that they must open with their mind. The mentor 'helps' the user to relax using interactive dialogue that changes in response to perceived levels of relaxation as measured by a combination of GSR and alpha wave content, and the lock begins to open as the person relaxes. Later in the game, if the player requires the power of telekinesis, he must again relax. Note that various elements of the game directly 'help' the user reach their desired bio-state. If the user is learning how to control their relaxation level, the music, video, and dialogue will 'help' put them in this state. Overall, the game provides the perfect structure to explore and experiment with the 'affective feedback' concept.

ACKNOWLEDGEMENTS

The authors would like to acknowledge the contributions of Ned Augenblick who provided the framework for this chapter, and the MindGames group in Media Lab Europe for all the technical details and gaming technologies.

REFERENCES

1. Shouse MN, Lubar JF 1979 Operant conditioning of EEG rhythms and Ritalin in the treatment of hyperkinesis. Biofeedback and Self-Regulation 4(4): 299–312
2. Schwartz MS ed. 1995 Biofeedback: a practitioner's guide. 2nd edn. Guilford Press, New York, 493–524
3. Lubar JO, Lubar JF 1984 Electroencephalographic biofeedback of SMR and beta for treatment of attention deficit disorders in a clinical setting. Biofeedback and Self-Regulation 9(1): 1–23
4. Alhambra MA, Fowler TR, Alhambra AA 1995 EEG biofeedback: a new treatment option for ADD/ADHD. Journal of Neurotherapy 1(2): 39–43
5. Lubar JF, Swartwood MO, Swartwood JN, Timmermann DL 1995 Quantitative EEG and auditory event-related potentials in the evaluation of attention-deficit/hyperactivity disorder: effects of methylphenidate and implications for neurofeedback training. Journal of Psychoeducational Assessment ADHD Special: 143–160
6. Dewan EM 1967 Occipital alpha rhythm, eye position, and lens accommodation. Nature 214: 975–977
7. Othmer S, Othmer S 1995 EEG biofeedback training for bipolar disorder. Presentation at Annual Conference of the Society for the Study of Neuronal Regulation, Scottsdale, Arizona, USA, April 28–May 1, 1995
8. Gruzelier J 2000 Self regulation of electrocortical activity in schizophrenia and schizotypy: a review. Clinical Electroencephalography 31(1): 23–29
9. Burgio K, Whitehead WE, Engel BT 1985 Urinary incontinence in the elderly: bladder-sphincter biofeedback and toileting skills training. Annals of Internal Medicine 104: 507–515
10. Burns PA, Pranikoff K, Nochajski T et al. 1990 Treatment of stress incontinence with pelvic exercises and biofeedback. Journal of the American Geriatrics Society 38(3): 341–343
11. Akkpinar S, Uleft GA, Itil TM 1971 Hypnotizability predicted by computer analysed EEG pattern. Biological Psychiatry 3: 387–392
12. Leshtz A 2002 Biofeedback and Raynaud's phenomenon. Available online: http://members.aol.com/raynauds/biofeed.htm
13. Burton J, Pearce L, Burgio KL et al. 1988 Behavioral training for urinary incontinence in elderly, ambulatory patients. Journal of the American Geriatric Society 36(8): 693–698
14. Holroyd KA, Penzien DB, Hursey KG et al. 1984 Change mechanisms in EMG biofeedback training: cognitive changes underlying improvements in tension headache. Journal of Consulting and Clinical Psychology 52: 1039–1053
15. Saxby E, Peniston EG 1995 Alpha-theta brainwave neurofeedback training: an effective treatment for male and female alcoholics with depressive symptoms. Journal of Clinical Psychology 51(5): 685–693
16. Finley WW, Smith HA, Etherton MD 1975 Reduction of seizures and normalization of the EEG in a severe epileptic following sensorimotor biofeedback training: preliminary study. Biological Psychology 2(3): 189–203

17. Seifert AR, Lubar JF 1975 Reduction of epileptic seizures through EEG biofeedback training. Biological Psychology 3(3): 157–184
18. Finley WW 1976 Effects of sham feedback following successful SMR training in an epileptic: follow-up study. Biofeedback and Self-Regulation 1(2): 227–235
19. Lubar JF, Bahler WW 1976 Behavioral management of epileptic seizures following EEG biofeedback training of the sensorimotor rhythm. Biofeedback and Self-Regulation 1(1): 77–104
20. Finley WW 1977 Operant conditioning of the EEG in two patients with epilepsy: methodologic and clinical considerations. Pavlov Journal of Biological Science 12(2): 93–111
21. Sterman MB, Macdonald LR 1978 Effects of central cortical EEG feedback training on incidence of poorly controlled seizures. Epilepsia 19(3): 207–222
22. Kuhlman WN 1978 EEG feedback training of epileptic patients: clinical and electroen-cephalographic analysis. Electroencephalography and Clinical Neurophysiology 45(6): 699–710
23. Quy RJ, Hutt SJ, Forrest S 1979 Sensorimotor rhythm feedback training and epilepsy: some methodological and conceptual issues. Biological Psychology 9(2): 129–149
24. Sterman MB, Shouse MN 1980 Quantitative analysis of training, sleep EEG and clinical response to EEG operant conditioning in epileptics. Electroencephalography and Clinical Neurophysiology 49(5–6): 558–576
25. Lubar JF, Shabsin HS, Natelson SE et al. 1981 EEG operant conditioning in intractable epileptics. Archives of Neurology 38(11): 700–704
26. Whitsett SF, Lubar JF, Holder GS et al. 1982 A double-blind investigation of the relationship between seizure activity and the sleep EEG following EEG biofeedback training. Biofeedback and Self-Regulation 7(2): 193–209
27. Tansey MA 1985 The response of a case of petit mal epilepsy to EEG sensorimotor rhythm biofeedback training. International Journal of Psychophysiology 3(2): 81–84
28. Lantz DL, Sterman MB 1988 Neuropsychological assessment of subjects with uncontrolled epilepsy: effects of EEG feedback training. Epilepsia 29(2): 163–171
29. Tozzo CA, Elfner LF, May JG Jr 1988 EEG biofeedback and relaxation training in the control of epileptic seizures. International Journal of Psychophysiology 6(3): 185–194
30. Hansen LM, Trudeau DL, Grace DL 1996 Neurotherapy and drug therapy in combination for adult ADHD, personality disorder, and seizure. Journal of Neurotherapy 2(1): 6–14
31. Walker J 1995 Remediation of nocturnal seizures by EEG biofeedback. Presentation at the Annual Conference of the Society for the Study of Neuronal Regulation, Scottsdale, Arizona, USA, April 28–May 1, 1995
32. Sterman MB 2000 Basic concepts and clinical findings in the treatment of seizure disorders with EEG operant conditioning. Clinical Electroencephalography 31(1): 45–55
33. Rosenfeld JP 2000 An EEG biofeedback protocol for affective disorders. Clinical Electroencephalography 31(1): 7–12
34. Duffy FH 2000 The state of EEG biofeedback therapy (EEG operant conditioning) in 2000: an editor's opinion. Clinical Electroencephalography 31(1): V–VII
35. Kaiser DA, Othmer S 1997 Efficacy of EEG biofeedback for attentional processes. Presented at American Psychiatric Electrophysiological Association, San Diego, 1997
36. Lubar JF, Shouse MN 1976 EEG and behavioral changes in a hyperkinetic child concurrent with training of the sensorimotor rhythm (SMR): a preliminary report. Biofeedback and Self-Regulation 1(3): 293–306
37. Tansey MA, Bruner RL 1983 EMG and EEG biofeedback training in the treatment of a 10-year-old hyperactive boy with a developmental reading disorder. Biofeedback and Self-Regulation 8(1): 25–37
38. Lubar JF 1991 Discourse on the development of EEG diagnostics and biofeedback for attention-deficit/hyperactivity disorders. Biofeedback and Self-Regulation 16(3): 201–225
39. Lubar JF, Swartwood MO, Swartwood JN et al. 1995 Evaluation of the effectiveness of EEG neurofeedback training for ADHD in a clinical setting as measured by changes in T.O.V.A. scores, behavioral ratings, and WISC-R performance. Biofeedback and Self-Regulation 20(1): 83–99
40. Linden M, Habib T, Radojevic V 1996 A controlled study of the effects of EEG biofeedback on cognition and behavior of children with attention deficit disorder and learning disabilities. Biofeedback and Self-Regulation 21(1): 35–49

41. Fenger TN 1998 Visual-motor integration and its relation to EEG neurofeedback brain wave patterns, reading, spelling, and arithmetic achievement in attention deficit disorders and learning disabled students. Journal of Neurotherapy 3(1): 9–18

42. Othmer S, Othmer SF 1989 EEG biofeedback training for hyperactivity, attention deficit disorder, specific learning disabilities, and other disorders. Available online: http://www. eegspectrum.com/Applications/ADHD-ADD/Hyper-ADD-OtherIntro/

43. Othmer S, Othmer SF, Marks CS 1991 EEG biofeedback training for attention deficit disorder, specific learning disabilities, and associated conduct problems. Available online: http://members.aol.com/eegspectradhd91/adhd91.htm

44. Elixa Peak Being. WaveRider Pro 4 channel biofeedback. Available online: http://www.elixa.com/mental/wrpro.htm 8 Nov 2002.

45. Mager R, Bullinger AH, Mueller F et al. 2001 Real time monitoring of brain activity in patients with specific phobia during exposure therapy, employing stereoscopic virtual environment. CyberPsychology and Behaviour 4(4): 465–469

46. Handelman D 1990 Models and mirrors: towards an anthropology of public events. Cambridge University Press: New York

47. Picard RW 1997 Affective computing. MIT Press, Cambridge

48. Hoffman HG, Garcia-Palacios A, Carlin C et al. Interfaces that heal: coupling real and virtual objects to cure spider phobia. International Journal of Human–Computer Interaction. In press

49. Garcia-Palacios A, Hoffman HG, Carlin C et al. 2002 Virtual reality in the treatment of spider phobia: a controlled study. Behaviour Research and Therapy 40: 983–993

50. Carlin AS, Hoffman H, Weghorst S 1997 Virtual reality and tactile augmentation in the treatment of spider phobia: a case study. Behavior Research and Therapy 35(2): 153–158

51. Hodges LF, Anderson P, Burdea G et al. 2001 VR as a tool in the treatment of psychological and physical disorders. IEEE Computer Graphics and Applications 21(6): 25–33

52. Garcia-Palacios A, Hoffman HG, Kwong See S et al. 2001 Redefining therapeutic success with VR exposure therapy. CyberPsychology and Behavior 4(3): 341–348

WEBSITES OF INTEREST

Jonathan Walker, MD, Neurologist, Dallas, TX, May, 1995:
http://www.snr-jnt.org/ NFBArch/Abstracts/walkerj1.htm

Media Lab Europe: The European Research Partner of the MIT Media Lab:
http://www.medialabeurope.org

Raynauds disease sufferer's opinion on feedback:
http://members.aol.com/raynauds/biofeed.htm

Virtual reality therapy for burn victims: http://www.hitl.washington.edu/projects/burn/

Virtual reality therapy for spider phobia:
http://www.hitl.washington.edu/projects/exposure/

Waverider feedback hardware and software resources:
http://www.elixa.com/mental/wrpro.htm

8

The Thought Translation Device: communication by means of EEG self-regulation for locked-in patients

Andrea Kübler   Niels Birbaumer

SUMMARY

In this chapter psychophysiological training devices to modify ongoing behavior or to teach a new behavioral response are introduced; such devices are referred to as behavioral neuroprostheses or brain–computer interfaces. The first part of the chapter describes how these devices are used to treat chronic pain, tinnitus, Parkinson's disease, and epilepsy. The second part explains how a brain–computer interface can be used to maintain or reinstall communication in patients with severe motor impairment. The electrical activity of the brain is used as an input signal carrying messages from the user's brain to a computer that translates this electrical activity into an output signal suitable for controlling an application adapted to the individual patient's needs. Patients undergo an extended training procedure to learn how to self-regulate their slow cortical potentials of the brain including operant learning, shaping of behavior and online feedback of the slow cortical potential amplitude of the brain. Self-regulation of the slow cortical potential amplitude is then used to control a cursor on a computer screen with which letters or words can be selected in a language support program.

Das Leben selbst drängt zum Gelingen des Lebens (Life itself pushes for its success – patient HPS)

CASE STUDY

Male patient HPS, a 44-year-old lawyer, has been diagnosed with amyotrophic lateral sclerosis (ALS) for 10 years. ALS is a neurological disorder, which involves steadily progressive degeneration of central and peripheral motoneurons leading to severe or total motor paralysis. In the end-stage patients can only survive with artificial ventilation and tube feeding. HPS worked for the social services of the local state and formerly practiced a number of sporting activities: skiing, tennis, gymnastics and volleyball. His first symptom was a weakness of the right arm after an accident in a volley ball game. For 7 years he has been artificially fed and ventilated. His motor abilities are reduced to two facial muscle movements and weak eye movement. Muscle control is exhausting and unreliable over a longer period of time. Although almost completely paralyzed, HPS is still interested in law and in current affairs, and watching sport events on television keeps him in touch with his former sporting activities. He lives in an apartment on his own, but needs 24-hour care. He organizes his household, and his parents and friends visit him frequently. HPS was intubated in emergency, allowing invasive artificial ventilation, against his previously declared will, but now rates his quality of life and his desire to live highly.[1] The most important issue in maintaining quality of life is the ability to communicate.[2]

HPS was trained to use the Thought Translation Device (TTD, explained in detail below) over several months and has been using the TTD for communication for more than 6 years. For HPS, using the TTD means the regaining of autonomy. He can now write letters to his friends without the aid of caregivers.[1] Concerning the time needed to communicate by means of the TTD, HPS stated that he – as in all other aspects of his life – made 'the discovery of slowness' (quoted from the book *Die Entdeckung der Langsamkeit* by the German author Stan Nadolny). It may be comparable to a beginner who learns to write in primary school, he said.[1,3] HPS is connected to the TTD two to three times a week for 4 hours. His performance varies between 3 to 0.15 letters per minute.[4]

Recently HPS wrote a detailed description of his strategy to control cursor movement (see below) and how he tries to suppress distracting thoughts: to produce a positive slow cortical potential amplitude (explained below) he tries to generate pressure in the brain by, e.g. imagining an athlete starting to run with the starting signal or an arrow shooting up from the bow. In contrast, to produce negative slow cortical potentials, he tries to create a kind of mental void by relaxing the brain. HPS explains that with relaxation he means to let go, to say 'good-bye' to his thoughts. However, it turns out, he says, that almost regularly, new uninvited thoughts disturb the void. He found a visual image for this situation: 'There is a "rear area" free of thoughts against which uninvited thoughts form a "front area" making the rear area disappear'.[5] After 4 weeks of training (two to three times per week) HPS was able to produce negative and positive slow cortical potential amplitudes according to the task requirement (explained below). After 2 months he was able to select letters in a preliminary language support program. Within the following year he succeeded in writing his first message with the TTD by using self-control of his electrical brain activity only. HPS was the first patient who was trained to use the TTD. He has been followed by 15 other paralyzed patients. However, with his aid the TTD, the language support program and the training schedule were further developed.[1] Consequently, other patients needed only about 2–3 months from learning to self-regulate their slow cortical potentials to using this ability to select letters, words or commands from a presented menu.[6,7]

INTRODUCTION

Most of the behavioral neuroprostheses described in the chapter encompass psychophysiological training devices aimed at the learned modification of a physiological process responsible for a particular group of disease symptoms. Physiological and biochemical pathologies are treated as behavioral responses dependent upon the immediate consequences and contingencies. Through contingent reinforcement, punishment or feedback these pathological responses can be changed permanently, sometimes affecting the pathological processes directly, sometimes by suppression of symptoms (such as in epilepsy). The construction of behavioral neuroprostheses often depends on neurobiological models describing cortical and subcortical reorganization in the course of disease processes. Built upon the knowledge of cortical and subcortical reorganization, these neuroplastic alterations are modified by behavioral strategies (e.g. see paragraph on phantom-limb pain). Behavioral neuroplasticity, therefore, involves interdisciplinary action of behavioral psychology, psychophysiology and the cognitive neurosciences.

Chronic pain

The International Association for the Study of Pain (IASP) defines chronic pain as continuous pain lasting more than 3 months. Behavioral responses with such a subjective intensity and significance result in neuroplastic changes at the peripheral and, most likely, also at the level of the central nervous system. The processes associated with such enduring neuroplastic changes have been termed 'pain memory' if they result in chronic pain even after the peripheral pathophysiological causes of the pain symptoms have vanished. For several types of chronic pain syndromes, the neuroplastic changes have been identified, and behavioral and physical treatment modalities were developed to ameliorate 'pain memories'.

Muscular-skeletal pain

Chronic low-back pain, headache (including migraine headaches) and face pain are the most frequent and costly disease conditions. Flor and colleagues[8] have shown that these chronic syndromes can be traced back to three causal factors: classical conditioning of muscular tension, operant reinforcement of pain behavior, and medical/orthopedic determinants. One-third of the patients suffer from an increase in muscle tension in personal stressful situations leading to a sequence of pathological changes in the periphery and the central nervous system.[8] One-third acquire subjective and behavioral pain responses through operant reinforcement, mostly in the family context and by the reinforcing properties of analgesic medication,[9] and the last third of these pain syndromes do have clear medical origins, such as disc problems and traumatic injuries to the skeletal system. We have shown[10] that in all three types of determining factors extensive cortical reorganization of the somatosensory cortex can be observed, leading to an enlargement and hyper-sensitivity of the cortical and subcortical representation of the painful body area (Fig. 8.1).

For both types of learned pain behavior (instrumental and classical conditioning), behavioral neuroprostheses were developed and tested. For those syndromes related to classical conditioning of muscle tension in personally stressful life situations, electromyographic biofeedback of the specific painful area (i.e. low-back muscles) in the presence and in the context of the personally relevant stressful situation is the most effective treatment approach. Portable devices allow the patient to test muscular self-control in the relevant social situations in real life.[11] Patients whose syndromes follow the operant model of chronic pain[12] profit most from a learned change of the contingencies within the family and a change in the timing of pain medication, including increase of socially rewarding physical activities.[13]

Neuropathic pain

Birbaumer et al.[14] and Flor et al.[15] have shown that chronic phantom-limb pain is caused by cortical reorganization in the anatomical representations of the deafferented area. Birbaumer et al.[16] have shown that the relationship between the invasion of the brain area in SI (primary sensory cortex) adjacent to the deafferented area is causally related to the amount of experienced phantom-limb pain. Consequently, treatment strategies aimed at a behavioral modification of the underlying cortical reorganization were developed. One of these strategies consists of asynchronous tactile stimulation of the stump area and the face (both located side by side at the sensory-motor homunculus in SI and MI [primary motor cortex]). The asynchronous stimulation (3 hours per day over several weeks) was aimed at dissociation of pathologically associated synaptic connections. Huse et al.[17] demonstrated that after long-term non-contingent tactile stimulation of peripheral areas represented adjacent at the cortical homunculus, a substantial reduction of chronic phantom-limb pain could be achieved. The development of chronic neuropathic pain can be prevented altogether if formation of associative

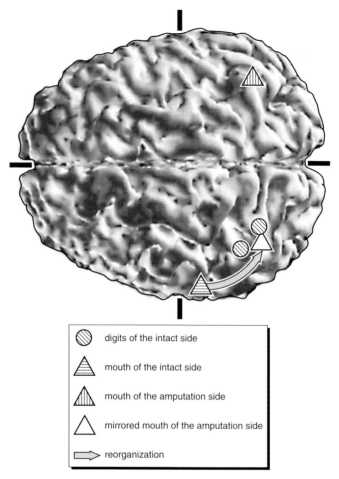

Figure 8.1 Extensive cortical reorganization of the somatosensory cortex in patients with phantom-limb pain (amputation of lower or upper arm) measured with magnetencephalogram. Representation of digits (contralateral to the intact arm) and mouth areas (bilateral). The mouth area of the amputation side is mirrored to the intact side: it does not overlap with the mouth area of the intact side; instead it is represented in the original area of the digits of the amputated hand. The arrow indicates the direction of cortical reorganization, but the reorganization itself occurred in the right hemisphere. The triangle with vertical lines is mirrored to the intact side to show the ultimate location of the mouth representation within the digit representation, because the digit representation cannot be assessed in the right hemisphere (amputated limb).

networks between highly active nociceptive brain areas is blocked by pharmacological substances, such as NMDA-receptor blockers (NMDA = N-methyl-D-aspartate). These prevent the formation of associative (Hebbian) synaptic connections.[18] Again, prevention and treatment of chronic neuro-pathic pain syndromes depend on the understanding of the underlying neurobehavioral mechanisms involved in the formation and maintenance of pain behavior in cortico-subcortical networks.

Parkinson's disease

Parkinson's disease is a chronic progressive degenerative neurological disease caused by degeneration of dopaminergic neurons in the substantia nigra; in the progression of the disease neuronal loss also occurs in the basal ganglia and the prefrontal cortex. Pharmacological treatment consists of substitution of dopamine by application of the precursor L-dopa. However, these medications lose their efficacy in the course of the disease progression and may even accelerate the disease's progress. Several behavioral strategies using a combination of learning based motor training approaches, including the application of portable electromyographic biofeedback neuroprostheses, were proven to considerably slow the disease process and improve quality of life and motor functioning in less-advanced Parkinson syndromes.[19] The treatment package for Parkinson disease included the use of a portable neuroprosthesis called 'physical-restraint therapy'.[20] First demonstrated in monkeys, Taub et al.[21] have shown in deafferented monkeys that despite intact motor innervations, movement of deafferented, painfully or otherwise affected limbs is avoided. Successful avoidance of the use of the pathological limb leads to overuse of the intact limbs and progressive non-use and atrophy of the deafferented or otherwise afflicted bodily function (Fig. 8.2). With physical restraint of the healthy body part patients are forced to use the deafferented or non-used limb. Increased use of the ignored or neglected body part positively reinforces its activation and restores the cortical and subcortical reorganization responsible for the maintenance of this behavior. Liepert et al.[20] have demonstrated that physical restraint therapy over several weeks with forced use of the pathologically affected limb leads to dramatic improvement of paralyzed body parts together with the recruitment of new cortical areas and remodeling of the overused brain systems.

Tinnitus

Tinnitus consists of a phantom-like noise in one or both ears occurring mostly after traumatic auditory experiences, such as long-term presence of extreme noise (such as disco music), infections or alterations of inner-ear blood flow. If acute medical treatment cannot eliminate the symptoms within weeks, permanent presence of the disturbing noise may be the consequence. The amount of suffering depends heavily on the psychological and social context of the patients (for a professional musician even a 30 db constant noise may end a career). Mühlnickel et al.[22] have shown that tinnitus is accompanied, comparable to phantom-limb pain, by a cortical reorganization of the tonotopic map in the primary and secondary auditory cortex. The disturbing tinnitus frequency is represented in an enlarged cortical area and a displacement of

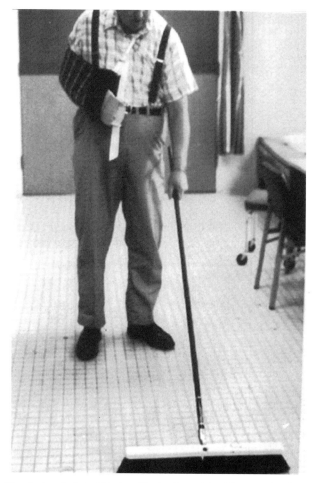

Figure 8.2   Physical restraint of the healthy body part, in this case the right arm. Patients are trained to use the non-used limb.

the cortical representation away from the tonotopic map. Consequently, a behavioral neuroprosthesis using long-term discrimination training of the tone frequencies adjacent at the tonotopic map may lead to an increase of the representation of the nearby tone frequencies and a restoration of the regularity of the tonotopic map. First systematic training devices based on cortical reorganization show promising results.[23]

Epilepsy

One percent of the population is affected by epileptic seizures. One-third of epileptic syndromes cannot be treated by drugs or surgical removal of the epileptic focus. Drug-resistant epilepsy consists mainly of temporal lobe epilepsy with secondary generalized seizures. These otherwise untreatable syndromes are the targets of recently developed behavioral neuroprostheses.[24–26] The neuroprosthesis consists of a training device for voluntary regulation of slow cortical potentials and, following training, helps patients to perceive seizures in an anticipatory fashion and in real-life situations. Physiological regulation of slow cortical potentials is directed toward the voluntary production of inhibitory potentials in and around the overactive brain areas. Electrically negative slow cortical potentials indicate an increase in cortical excitation; electrocortically positive slow cortical potentials do indicate an increase in inhibitory action of the relevant brain areas. Therefore, patients are trained to perceive seizure onset and block the accumulating hyperexcitation by voluntary regulation of positive cortical potentials. During behavioral training they observe their own slow cortical potentials on a screen and are reinforced for increase and decrease of the slow cortical potential amplitude. Usually 30–50 training sessions are necessary before patients develop perceptual sensitivity for their seizure dynamics. After the first training block subjects are trained in their social environment to reduce cortical negativity contingent upon seizure perception. Several controlled studies have proved the effectiveness of this approach: one-third of the patients became seizure-free, one-third showed considerable improvement, and one-third remained unchanged.[26]

Based on this neuroprosthesis for the treatment of epileptic syndrome a similar device was constructed to regain communication with patients suffering from locked-in syndrome: the intact brain is locked in a paralyzed body. The Thought Translation Device (TTD) controlled by slow cortical potentials of the brain is described in the remainder of the chapter.

THE TTD

Methodology

The TTD is a direct connection between the brain and a computer referred to as a brain–computer interface (BCI) (Fig. 8.3). A BCI uses the electrical, magnetic or metabolic activity of the brain to control an external application, which may be, e.g. a cursor to select letters, words or icons on a computer screen,[3,6] an orthosis to use a paralyzed limb[27] or a prosthesis to replace a paralyzed limb.[28,29] The 'EEG' (electroencephalogram), as it is commonly termed, refers to electrical activity arising from neurons in the cerebral cortex and is recorded non-invasively from the scalp. This includes spontaneous electrical activity of the cerebral neurons and the responses to external or internal events. In general, it is believed that spontaneous EEG activity results from the summation of excitatory and inhibitory postsynaptic potentials of underlying regions of the cerebral cortex with some contribution of granule and glia cell activity.[30]

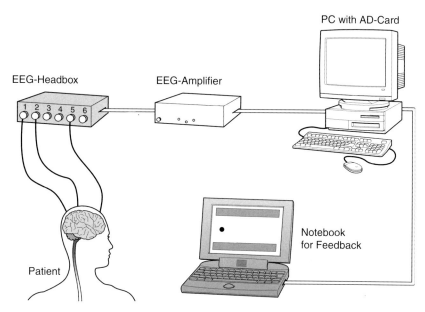

PC with AD-Card

EEG-Headbox   EEG-Amplifier

1 2 3 4 5 6

Notebook
for Feedback

Patient

Figure 8.3 Patients sit in front of a laptop, which provides them with online feedback of their SCP amplitude. The EEG is recorded from the scalp, amplified and transferred to a personal computer. On the PC the EEG is displayed online so that the trainer can check the quality of the EEG signal constantly. The PC converts the EEG into cursor movement on the laptop screen (from Archives of Physical Medicine and Rehabilitation,[7] with permission).

   The TTD is usually controlled by self-regulation of slow cortical potentials of the brain. Slow cortical potentials are shifts in the depolarization level of the apical dendrites of the cortex lasting from 300 ms up to 10 s. Negative slow cortical potentials are the sum of synchronized ultraslow excitatory post-synaptic potentials at the apical dendrites with the source in deeper cortical layers (III and IV) near or at the soma.[31] The depolarization of cortical cell assemblies reduces their excitation threshold. Firing of neurons in regions responsible for specified motor or cognitive tasks is facilitated. Whenever a task-relevant event is expected, cortical excitation thresholds are lowered in the corresponding cortical cell assemblies to facilitate neuronal firing resulting in negative slow cortical potential amplitudes. Negative slow cortical potential amplitude shifts can be recorded in the EEG using experimental paradigms that elicit cognitive or motor mobilization.[32,33] Negative amplitude shifts grow with increasing attentional or cognitive resource allocation. A strong relationship between self-induced cortical negativity and reaction time, signal detection, and short-term memory performance has been reported in several studies in humans and monkeys.[34–38] Tasks requiring attention are performed significantly better when presented after spontaneous or self-induced cortical negativity. For instance, Lutzenberger et al.[36] trained their subjects in slow cortical potential self-regulation by providing feedback and positive reinforcement of correct responses. Subjects were also presented with arithmetic tasks. In trials in which arithmetic tasks had to be solved no feedback (transfer trials) was provided, subjects were only asked to produce cortical negativity or positivity as in feedback trials. The arithmetic tasks were solved significantly faster after a preceding negative slow cortical potential shift. Self-induced cortical positivity usually reduces cognitive and motor performance. Cortical positivity can be caused by reduced afferent input to cortical layers I and II during periods in which no motor or cognitive operations are performed and, therefore, no neuronal resources are required.

To communicate with the TTD, patients must learn to self-regulate their slow cortical potential amplitude. The training procedure includes real-time visual feedback of slow cortical potentials, operant learning and shaping of behavior.[7] In patients who suffer from impaired vision, auditory feedback is provided additionally.[39] The EEG is usually recorded from the vertex (Cz: central, sagittal electrode position according to the international 10–20 system[40]) or frontal leads against both mastoids (electrode position behind the ears). The EEG is corrected online for artifacts caused by eye movement. The procedure of EEG recording, the algorithm which filters out the slow cortical potentials from the raw EEG and transfers this signal into cursor movement on a laptop screen and artifact correction is described in detail elsewhere.[7,41–43]

To enable patients to communicate by solely using their EEG, it is not only necessary to self-regulate the slow cortical potential amplitude, but to select simultaneously letters or words in a so-called language support program (LSP).[44] Moreover, when patients want to communicate individually (i.e. without preconceived expressions) they have to imagine what they want to communicate and how to write these words. Patients are trained to perform this rather difficult behavior by reinforcing successive approximations to that response, a procedure known as shaping. In order to achieve a behavioral response by shaping, it is necessary to know the topography of the required behavior the subject has to learn and then to train and reinforce every step in the correct direction.[45] Thus, communication by means of slow cortical potential controlled cursor movement on a computer screen is divided into several small steps of increasing difficulty: first, it is necessary to learn slow cortical potential self-control. Second, letters have to be selected and third, self-imagined words have to be communicated. These three components of the to-be-shaped behavior are, again, subdivided. We proceed from basic training to achieve slow cortical potential self-control to verbal communication in a series of small steps and with a slow increase of task complexity.[7]

Visual or auditory feedback, or both, is not provided continuously, but rather in separate trials. In each trial of basic training patients have to move the cursor toward a rectangle placed at the top or bottom of the screen,

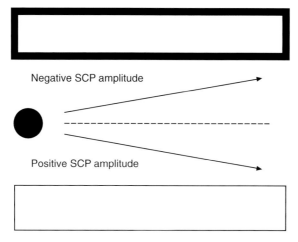

Negative SCP amplitude

Positive SCP amplitude

Figure 8.4   To learn self-control of slow cortical potentials patients are presented with two rectangles each at the top and bottom of the screen. At the beginning of the active phase the cursor starts moving from the left to the right margin of the screen. Vertical cursor movement occurs according to the slow cortical potential amplitude. Negative slow cortical potentials move the cursor upward, positive slow cortical potentials downward. The highlighted rectangle indicates the required direction of cursor movement (in this case the top rectangle).

respectively. The required direction is indicated by highlighting the corresponding rectangle (Fig. 8.4). Negative slow cortical potentials move the cursor upward, positive slow cortical potential shifts it downward. Whenever a slow cortical potential amplitude according to the task requirement is produced, a smiling face appears at the end of the trial to reinforce the correct response and to encourage patients to continue with the used mental strategy to control cursor movement. Patients are not provided with a specified mental strategy for cursor control, but are advised to watch the feedback attentively, to try all kinds of different thoughts and to find out the most suitable strategy. Patients and healthy volunteers report visual and verbal strategies. In order to produce cortical negativity one of our patients reported the image of carrying something heavy up a hill; another gave the command 'ball move up' (the cursor is a ball-like yellow-filled circle).

While healthy individuals learn to control their slow cortical potentials within 1–2 hours training,[46] patients diagnosed with neurological diseases usually require much longer,[3] probably because of brain damage. At the end of basic training to self-regulate the slow cortical potential amplitude, patients are able to produce two clearly distinguishable brain responses, i.e. a binary 'yes-no' signal (Fig. 8.5). With such a binary signal many, if not all, applications according to the individual patient's preferences may be controlled (e.g. switching television programs, ringing a bell to call attention, surfing on the Internet[47]). With 2-D cursor control two additional responses

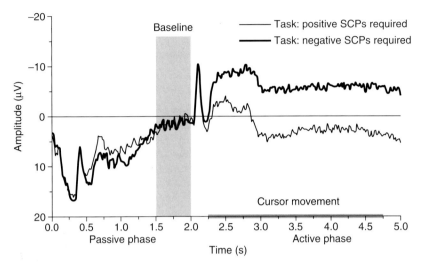

Figure 8.5 Course of slow cortical potentials averaged across 500 trials and separated according to the task requirement. The bold line shows slow cortical potentials (SCPs) when upward cursor movement is required, thin line when downward cursor movement is required. The two curves reveal a voltage difference of 10 μV during the active phase. The patient is therefore able to produce two clearly distinguishable brain responses according to the task requirement. The positive and negative slow cortical potential amplitudes are used as a binary (yes–no) signal to control external devices.

could be introduced (e.g. additional rectangles on the left and right margin of the screen). In several studies it was shown that healthy participants could learn to self-regulate slow cortical potential differences between the left and right hemisphere at electrode positions C3 and C4.[48–50] However, in healthy participants it proved to be rather difficult to achieve reliable control over interhemispheric slow cortical potential asymmetry within the timed trial structure of the TTD.[50] For this reason, until now, severely paralyzed patients have been trained to achieve 1-D cursor movement only, leading to a binary response.

After basic training, patients have to use the newly acquired skill to select letters or other options presented on the screen. As our main goal is to enable patients to communicate verbally, we provide patients with a LSP: the rectangles on the laptop screen are now used for letter or word presentation. Letters or words to be selected are presented in the bottom rectangle in a dichotomous manner.[44] To perform a selection, patients have to move the cursor downward by producing a positive slow cortical potential amplitude. The alphabet including umlauts (ä,ö,ü), space (-), and punctuation marks (, .) is split in two subsets, each containing 16 symbols. These two subsets are presented one after another until the patient selects one subset, which contains the target letter he has to select. After selection this subset is again split in two and this is continued until a single letter is presented for selection.

The LSP comprises two different versions: copy spelling and free spelling. In the copy spelling mode patients are required to copy letters or words presented in the top rectangle by the trainer. In the free spelling mode patients can write whatever they want to communicate. Using the ability to self-regulate slow cortical potentials to select items in an application controlled by a BCI is not trivial. In addition to producing negative or positive slow cortical potential amplitudes, respectively, patients have now at the same time to think about what they want to communicate, how to write the words and what to select on the screen in order to communicate their message. Thus, the usage of the TTD becomes more and more difficult from basic training, to self-regulate slow cortical potentials, to copy spelling, to free spelling.

   To facilitate the transfer from slow cortical potential self-regulation training to letter selection, patients are provided with a subset of letters only and they have to copy words preset by the trainer. At the end of training, patients are confronted with the entire alphabet. Patients have to practice each step in training until they reach a correct response rate of 75%. Then the next, more difficult step is introduced. The entire shaping procedure is described in detail elsewhere.[7,42]

OVERVIEW

BCIs depend on the interaction of three adaptive system elements: first, the electrophysiological activity of the user's brain that produces the input, second, the interface itself that translates the electrophysiological activity into the signals that control, third, an application, for example, a program to realize verbal communication. The user has to learn to use his or her EEG to control a device – an entirely new task for all users. The BCI has to be adapted to the patient's individual EEG pattern, physical abilities and individual circumstances (e.g. patients lying in bed or sitting in a wheelchair, BCI training at the patients' homes or in nursing homes, etc.). The application has to be adapted to the various needs, performance and learning progress of the individual user.[4]

   Over the past 15 years, productive BCI research programs have arisen.[51] This research has been encouraged by a better understanding of brain function, by more and more inexpensive computer hardware and software of high processing capacity, and by increasing insight into the needs of people with severe motor disabilities. The aim of BCI technology is to provide the user with new communication and control devices, which operate independently of any muscular activity. This fundamentally new communication technology is aimed mainly at people who suffer from severe motor impairment caused by neurological or muscular diseases, such as amyotrophic lateral sclerosis, infantile cerebral paresis, or stroke. Severe motor paralysis prevents such patients from using conventional augmentative communication methods, which depend on reliable voluntary muscular control. In the following paragraphs only those BCIs are reviewed which describe human use of the system in peer-reviewed articles, and which give the users control over a device and provide them with feedback. Studies from a vast group of researchers describing EEG phenomena that might be used as a control signal in a BCI are not considered.

According to Wolpaw et al.[51] current BCIs fall into two classes: dependent and independent. Dependent BCIs do not use the normal output pathways (speech, movement) of the brain to carry a message, but activities in these pathways are necessary to elicit the electrical brain activity that carries the message detected by the BCI. For example, the BCI developed by Sutter[52] used visually evoked potentials of the brain. Users are presented with a video screen displaying 64 symbols (e.g. letters) in an eight-by-eight grid. Subgroups of the grid undergo a fine red/green check pattern at 40–70 Hz. In order to select a symbol the user has to look at the symbol he or she wants to select. On-line comparison of the visual-evoked potential amplitude to a previously established template for the user enables the system to determine the symbol the user is looking at.[52,53] Another approach using visually evoked potentials presents the user with several items on the screen, which flash at different rates.[54] The users have to fixate their gaze on the item they want to select. The visually evoked potentials elicited by the flashing of items at a determined frequency can be recorded over the visual cortex as so-called steady-state visually evoked potentials. These steady-state visually evoked potentials have the same frequency as the item by which they are elicited. The BCI detects the frequency, compares it to the flashing frequency of the different items on the screen and decides from there on which item the user is looking at. Both systems depend on the user's ability to control gaze direction, which is a muscular activity, and belong, therefore, to the category of dependent BCIs.

Independent BCIs can be subdivided according to whether brain signals are recorded non-invasively from the scalp or invasively with subdural or intracortical electrodes. BCIs can also be categorized in terms of whether they use brain signals, which are present in the spontaneous EEG, or whether the brain signals are elicited by external stimuli.

The described TTD uses the slow cortical potentials of the brain, an electrical brain activity that can be recorded non-invasively from the scalp in the spontaneous EEG. BCIs, which use μ and β rhythms from the sensorimotor cortex, belong to the same category. The μ rhythm is defined as an arch-shaped 8–12 Hz activity over the sensorimotor cortex. In contrast to the α rhythm, it is not dependent on vision, but is blocked by motor activity, movement preparation, and motor imagery. The β band covers frequencies above 13 Hz mainly over frontal and central regions.[55] The BCI developed in the Wadsworth Center in Albany, USA[56–59] requires the users to learn to self-regulate the μ or β rhythm amplitude over sensorimotor cortex. Users are provided with feedback and mostly employ motor imagery to increase or decrease the μ or β rhythm amplitude thereby controlling a cursor on a computer screen. More than 80% of the subjects participating in training in the laboratory achieve significant control within 2–3 weeks of training (2–3 sessions per week).[51] The Graz-BCI, Austria, is also controlled by μ and β rhythms over sensorimotor cortex.[60–63] The research in this group has focused on distinguishing between the EEG associated with imagination of movement of tongue, arms, fingers or feet. In the standard training protocol, the users first participate in an initial session to select the most effective motor imagery. The EEG associated with movement is classified online thereby translating the user's motor imagery into continuous output, which is fed back to the user on a computer screen. Currently, the Graz-BCI is used by a tetraplegic patient after spinal-cord injury to control an orthotic device that opens and closes his paralyzed hand.[27] The Graz-BCI is the first to integrate a so-called telemonitoring system. Placement of electrodes and training situation can be observed via web cam and the BCI can be controlled online in the Graz laboratory.[64,65] Thus, the training itself can be conducted by a caregiver and supervised, and corrected online by the experts in Graz enabling them to train patients at a great distance. Currently, a severely paralyzed patient diagnosed with cerebral palsy in South Germany is trained by his attendant, supervised by the Graz laboratory and once a month visited by psychologists from the Tübingen group. For comparison: the TTD requires psychologists to travel to the patients' home two to three times a week. After patients have learned to control the TTD, we teach attendants to handle the system, but online supervision in the laboratory is not yet possible.

Farwell and Donchin[66] and, subsequently, Donchin et al.[67] introduced a BCI that uses the P300-evoked potential recorded non-invasively from the scalp over the parietal cortex.[68,69] The P300 is an evoked potential of positive polarity recorded 300 ms after infrequent or particularly significant auditory, visual or somatosensory stimuli interspersed with frequent or routine stimuli. In the P300 BCI the users are presented with a six-by-six symbol matrix, which contains the alphabet, numbers and a space symbol, resulting in a square containing 36 cells. Visual stimuli consist of flashing one row or one column of the matrix in random order. To select a letter, the users have to focus attention on the cell containing the target letter they want to select and count the number of times the row or column with that cell flashes. Each illumination of the target cell elicits a P300. All other flashes (rows and columns, which do not contain the target cell) do not elicit a P300. By detecting the P300 the system decides which letter the user wants to select.

Finally, an invasive BCI will be introduced. Kennedy and Bakay[70] use an intracortical electrode consisting of a hollow glass cone containing recording wires. Neurotrophic factors within the electrode stimulate adjacent neurons to grow into the tip of the glass electrode. The electrode then measures neuronal activity directly from the cortical tissue. The electrodes are implanted in motor cortices and have provided stable neuronal recordings for more than 1 year in monkeys and humans.[70–72] Because this method is invasive, the threshold for the clinical use is presumably higher than for methods based on scalp-recorded EEG activity.[51]

To communicate by using EEG signals, patients should be able to produce these signals rapidly and with high accuracy. These two criteria, accuracy and speed, are often used to evaluate the feasibility of a BCI. The reason for this seems to be obvious: the more rapid a BCI is controlled, the more communication is possible in a defined time interval. A high level of accuracy avoids false and unintended communication. One problem arising from speed as a criterion, is how it can be defined in a paralyzed person. When compared to speech, all other muscle-controlled devices are slow and most EEG-controlled responses are even slower. It must be considered, however, which output channels for communication are available in a particular situation. When speech is available, this is the most suitable way to communicate among individuals in daily life. When speech fails, e.g. due to paralysis of speech muscles, but fingers are available, a keyboard is probably the method of choice, although the communication rate is slow compared with speech. When control is reduced to few muscles only, for example, due to degenerative diseases, communication may only be mediated by a single switch. Compared with speech, the communication rate is very slow, but such a communication is still worthwhile even if it takes much longer to select an item. Neurological diseases can lead to total motor paralysis, which affects even eye movement. For such patients brain–computer communication is the method of choice, even though the communication rate is further decreased compared with single muscle switches. There are probably limits for the communication rate a BCI should not fall below. This limit is certainly dependent on the motivation and the patience of the individual patients and their social environments and cannot be defined as an absolute number.[4]

For the second criterion, accuracy, similar considerations have to be taken into account. A lack of accuracy is not a severe problem when error correction is possible. We define accuracy as rate of correct responses, i.e. correct selections per time interval; accuracy does not mean the correctness of the final communicative message. The accuracy of communication using speech or keyboards is far from 100%, but correct communication is possible because errors can be immediately eliminated. To avoid unintended brain–computer communication, the application must be equipped with options to correct wrong selections. It is obvious that less accurate control over the BCI results in larger numbers of errors, slower error correction and, consequently, slower brain–computer communication. When speed does not matter, 100% correctness of communication (e.g. no spelling mistakes when using an LSP) can be attained even if accuracy is below 70%. Although this is an open empirical question, one can assume that a BCI that enables the users to select only one correct option every few minutes may be not efficient enough to motivate the patient. Thus, the challenge is to find the optimal balance between accuracy and speed for the individual user.

FUTURE DIRECTIONS

Providing severely paralyzed patients with a BCI for communication is not simply a technological issue. The patient's individual life history and the current social and psychological situation have to be taken into account.[4] The conventional intervention in ALS focuses primarily on functional problems of the disease. Physicians and relatives concentrate first of all on the physical needs of the patients.[73] The necessity of psychological intervention, however, was indicated by McDonald et al. who showed that depressive mood shortens survival time in ALS patients.[74] In a sample of 76 patients with ALS, clinical relevant depressive symptoms have been found in more than 40% of the patients and more than 30% had mild depressive symptoms.[75] But compared to a sample of psychiatric patients diagnosed with major depression, ALS patients were significantly less depressed. Depression was assessed with Beck's depression inventory and a newly constructed questionnaire to assess depression in ALS patients.[75] In the same study, patients were asked to rate their quality of life using the Skalen zur Erfassung der Lebensqualität[76] and 80% rated their quality of life as 'good' or 'satisfying'.[77] As documented in the literature,[78] a highly negative correlation between the extent of depressive symptoms and quality of life was found in our patient sample. Many patients expressed the difficulties in communication as a major problem and a source of distress. Although correlation does not mean that depression and quality of life are causally related, one can assume that a reduction in depressive symptoms may improve quality of life and vice versa. As communication is important for a good quality of life in patients with severe motor impairment, it might be concluded that maintaining or re-establishing patients' communication abilities may maintain or improve patients' quality of life and – although this has yet to be proven – depressive symptoms may be prevented or reduced.

All currently available BCIs are not yet feasible for daily use at the patient's home. The equipment is – in most cases – bulky, and technically and psychologically skilled people are necessary to train the patients. Training may last for weeks or months.[1,65] The length of training depends first on the learning abilities of each individual patient. Some patients learn significant self-regulation of slow cortical potentials within few weeks of training only, others need more time or may not learn it at all. The reason for these individual differences is not yet known. The only predictor of successful learning in severely paralyzed patients, which was found until now, is whether or not patients achieve significant cursor control within the first 30 runs (about 6 training days in 2–3 weeks) of training.[79] If there is no learning within this early period of training, the probability that patients will ever learn self-regulation of slow cortical potential is low. Second, the length of training depends on how well the BCI can be adapted to the individual patient's EEG. It may be the case, for example, that the default EEG signal to control cursor movement is too low and that another EEG frequency, other electrode positions or other algorithms to filter out the EEG signal have to be used. Third, as the patient group is usually suffering from a severe disease, interruption of training, e.g. due to a stay in hospital, prolongs the training procedure. However, only the outcome of the early training phase is affected by interruptions. Patients who have learned successfully to self-regulate their slow cortical potentials are able to do so even after an interruption of 3–6 months.[7,80] Finally, an application that fits the individual patient's need has to be identified and controlled by the BCI.

Current BCI technology is limited to 25 bits of information (three characters) per minute,[29] which we consider sufficient for communication bearing the above-mentioned in mind. But with patients such a bit rate is often not achieved. In the TTD the number of characters selected per minute varies between 0.15 and 3 per minute,[4] and Obermaier et al.[64] report 0.95 letters per minute with their 'virtual keyboard'. Thus, the future value of BCI technology will depend substantially on how much the information transfer rate (bitrate) can be increased. Improving the bitrate depends on a number of crucial issues that include: BCI independence from normal neuromuscular communication channels and dependence on internal aspects of normal brain function; selection of signal acquisition methods, signal features, feature extraction methods, translation algorithms, output devices, and operational protocols; development of user training strategies (the first training schedule was described in this chapter);[7] attention to psychological and behavioral factors that affect user motivation and success;[4] and adoption of standards research methods and evaluation criteria.[51] Addressing these issues imposes interdisciplinary problems involving neurobiology, psychology, engineering, mathematics, and computer science. For a review of present-day BCIs and future directions and efforts that are currently undertaken see Kübler et al.[4] and Wolpaw et al.[51]

ACKNOWLEDGEMENT

Supported by the Deutsche Forschungsgemeinschaft (DFG) and the Bundesministerium für Forschung und Technologie (BMFT).

REFERENCES

1. Kübler A 2000 Brain–computer communication – development of a brain–computer interface for locked-in patients on the basis of the psychophysiological self-regulation training of slow cortical potentials (SCP). Schwäbische Verlagsgesellschaft, Tübingen
2. Bach JR 1993 Amyotrophic lateral sclerosis – communication status and survival with ventilatory support. American Journal of Physical Medicine and Rehabilitation 72(6): 343–349
3. Birbaumer N, Ghanayim N, Hinterberger T et al. 1999 A spelling device for the paralysed. Nature 398: 297–298

4. Kübler A, Kotchoubey B, Kaiser J et al. 2001 Brain–computer communication: unlocking the locked-in. Psychological Bulletin 127: 358–375
5. Neumann N, Kübler A, Kaiser J et al. 2003 Conscious perception of brain states: mental strategies for brain–computer communication. Neuropsychologia 41: 1028–1036
6. Kaiser J, Kübler A, Hinterberger T et al. A non-invasive communication device for the paralyzed. Minimally Invasive Neurosurgery 45: 19–23
7. Kübler A, Neumann N, Kaiser J et al. 2001 Brain–computer communication: self-regulation of slow cortical potentials for verbal communication. Archives of Physical Medicine and Rehabilitation 82(11): 1533–1539
8. Flor H, Birbaumer N, Fürst M 1994 Pavlovian conditioning in chronic pain. Psychophysiology 31–47
9. Flor H, Knost B, Birbaumer N 2002 The role of operant conditioning in chronic pain. Pain 95: 111–118
10. Flor H, Braun C, Elbert T et al. 1997 Extensive reorganisation of primary somatosensory cortex in chronic back pain patients. Neuroscience Letters 224: 5–8
11. Flor H, Turk DC, Birbaumer N 1985 Assessment of stress-related psychophysiological reactions in chronic back pain patients. Journal of Consulting and Clinical Psychology 53: 354–364
12. Fordyce WE 1976 Behavioral concepts in chronic pain and illness. In: Davidson PO ed. The behavioral treatment of anxiety, depression and pain. Brunner and Mazel, New York, 147–188
13. Flor H, Turk DC Psychopathology of pain. Plenum Press. In press
14. Birbaumer N, Flor H, Lutzenberger W et al. 1995 The corticalization of chronic pain. In: Bromm B, Desmedt JE eds. Pain and the brain. From notiception to cognition. Raven Press, New York, 331–343
15. Flor H, Elbert T, Knecht S et al. 1995 Phantom-limb pain as a perceptual correlate of cortical reorganization following arm amputation. Nature 375: 482–484
16. Birbaumer N, Lutzenberger W, Montoya P et al. 1997 Effects of regional anesthesia on phantom limb pain are mirrored in changes in cortical reorganization. Journal of Neuroscience 17(14): 5503–5508
17. Huse E, Preissl H, Larbig W et al. 2001 Phantom limb pain. The Lancet 358: 1015
18. Wiech K, Toepfner S, Kiefer R-T et al. Prevention of chronic phantom limb pain and pain-associated cortical plasticity by long-term regional anesthesia and memantine. Submitted
19. Mohr B, Müller V, Mattes R et al. 1996 Behavioral treatment of Parkinson's disease leads to improvement of motor skills and to tremor reduction. Behavior Therapy 27: 235–255
20. Liepert J, Bander H, Miltner WHR et al. 2000 Treatment induced cortical reorganization after stroke in humans. Stroke 31: 1210–1216
21. Taub E, Crago JE, Burgio LD et al. 1994 An operant approach to rehabilitation medicine: overcoming learned nonuse by shaping. Journal of the Experimental Analysis of Behaviour 61(2): 281–293
22. Mühlnickel W, Elbert T, Taub E et al. 1998 Reorganization of auditory cortex in tinnitus. Proceedings of the National Academy of Sciences 95: 10340–10343
23. Flor H, Schwartz MS. Nothing is as loud as a tone you try not to hear. In: Schwartz M, Andrasik F eds. Biofeedback. Guilford Press, New York. In press
24. Rockstroh B, Elbert T, Birbaumer N et al. 1993 Cortical self-regulation in patients with epilepsies. Epilepsy Research 14: 63–72
25. Birbaumer N, Rockstroh B, Elbert T et al. 1994 Biofeedback of slow cortical potentials in epilepsy. In: Carlson JG, Seifert AR, Birbaumer N eds. Clinical applied psychophysiology. Plenum Press, New York, 29–42
26. Kotchoubey B, Strehl U, Uhlmann C et al. 2001 Modification of slow cortical potentials in patients with refractory epilepsy: a controlled outcome study. Epilepsia 42: 406–416
27. Pfurtscheller G, Guger C, Müller G et al. 2000 Brain oscillations control hand orthosis in a tetraplegic. Neuroscience Letters 292: 211–214
28. Nicolelis MA 2001 Actions from thoughts. Nature 409 (suppl): 403–407
29. Craelius W 2002 The bionic man: restoring mobility. Science 295: 1018–1021
30. Speckmann EJ, Walden J 1991 Mechanisms underlying the generation of cortical field potentials. Acta Otolaryngologica 491(suppl): 17–24
31. Speckmann EJ, Caspers H, Elger CW 1984 Neuronal mechanisms underlying the generation of field potentials. Springer; Berlin

32. Birbaumer N, Elbert T, Canavan AGM et al. 1990 Slow potentials of the cerebral cortex and behavior. Physiological Reviews 70(1): 1–41
33. Rockstroh B, Elbert T, Canavan A et al. 1989 Slow cortical potentials and behavior. Urban & Schwarzenberg, Baltimore
34. Birbaumer N, Elbert T, Lutzenberger W et al. 1981 EEG and slow cortical potentials in anticipation of mental tasks with different hemispheric involvement. Biological Psychology 13: 251–260
35. Lutzenberger W, Elbert T, Rockstroh B et al. 1979 The effects of self-regulation of slow cortical potentials on performance in a signal detection task. International Journal of Neuroscience 9: 175–183
36. Lutzenberger W, Elbert T, Rockstroh B et al. 1982 Biofeedback produced slow brain potentials and task performance. Biological Psychology 14: 99–111
37. Lutzenberger W, Roberts LE, Birbaumer N 1993 Memory performance and area-specific self-regulation of slow cortical potentials: dual-task interference. International Journal of Psychophysiology 15: 217–226
38. Rockstroh B, Elbert T, Lutzenberger W et al. 1982 The effects of slow cortical potentials on response speed. Psychophysiology 19(2): 211–217
39. Hinterberger T, Neumann N, Pham M et al. A multimodal brain-based feedback and communication system. Submitted
40. Jasper HH 1958 Report of the Committee on Methods of Clinical Investigation of EEG. Appendix: the ten twenty electrode system of the international federation. Electroencephalography and Clinical Neurophysiology 10: 371–375
41. Gratton G 1998 Dealing with artifacts: the EOG contamination of the event-related brain potential. Behavior Research Methods, Instruments & Computers 30(1): 44–53
42. Kübler A, Winter S, Birbaumer N The Thought Translation Device: slow cortical potential biofeedback for verbal communication in paralysed patients. In: Schwartz M, Andrasik F eds. Biofeedback. 3rd edn. Guilford Press, New York. In press
43. Hinterberger T, Kübler A, Kaiser J et al. 2003 A brain–computer interface (BCI) for the locked-in: comparison of different EEG classifications for the Thought Translation Device (TTD). Clinical Neurophysiology 114: 416-425
44. Perelmouter J, Kotchoubey B, Kübler A et al. 1999 Language support program for thought-translation-devices. Automedica 18: 67–84
45. Leslie JC 1996 Principles of behavioral analysis. 1st edn. Harwood Academic Publishers, Amsterdam
46. Kotchoubey B, Schleichert H, Lutzenberger W et al. 1997 A new method for self-regulation of slow cortical potentials in a timed paradigm. Applied Psychophysiology and Biofeedback 22(2): 77–93
47. Hinterberger T, Kaiser J, Kübler A et al. 2001 The Thought Translation Device and its applications to the completely paralysed. In: Diebner HH, Druckrey T, Weibel P eds. Sciences of the interface. Genista, Tübingen, 232–240
48. Birbaumer N, Lang PJ, Cook III E et al. 1988 Slow brain potentials, imagery and hemispheric differences. International Journal of Neuroscience 39: 101–116
49. Rockstroh B, Elbert T, Birbaumer N et al. 1990 Biofeedback-produced hemispheric asymmetry of slow cortical potentials and its behavioral effects. International Journal of Psychophysiology 9(2): 151–165
50. Kotchoubey B, Schleichert H, Lutzenberger W et al. 1996 Self-regulation of interhemispheric asymmetry in humans. Neuroscience Letters 214: 91–94
51. Wolpaw JR, Birbaumer N, McFarland DJ et al. 2002 Brain–computer interfaces for communication and control. Clinical Neurophysiology 113: 767–791
52. Sutter EE 1984 The visual evoked response as a communication channel. Proceedings of the IEEE Symposium on Biosensors 1984, 95–100
53. Sutter EE 1992 The brain response interface: communication through visually-induced electrical brain responses. Journal of Microcomputer Applications 15: 31–45
54. Middendorf M, McMillan G, Calhoun G et al. 2000 Brain–computer interfaces based on the steady-state visual-evoked response. IEEE Transactions on Rehabilitation Engineering 8(2): 211–214
55. Niedermeyer E, Silva FLD 1993 Electroencephalography: basic principles, clinical applications and related fields. Williams & Willkins, Baltimore

56. McFarland DJ, Neat GW, Read RF et al. 1993 An EEG-based method for graded cursor control. Psychobiology 21(1): 77–81
57. McFarland DJ, Lefkowicz AT, Wolpaw JR 1997 Design and operation of an EEG-based brain–computer interface (BCI) with digital signal processing technology. Behavioral Research Methods, Instruments, & Computers 29(3): 337–345
58. Wolpaw JR, McFarland DJ, Neat GW et al. 1991 An EEG-based brain–computer interface for cursor control. Electroencephalography and Clinical Neurophysiology 78(3): 252–259
59. Wolpaw JR, McFarland DJ, Vaughan TM 2000 Brain–computer interface research at the Wadsworth Center. IEEE Transactions on Rehabilitation Engineering 8(2): 222–226
60. Pfurtscheller G, Flotzinger D, Neuper C 1994 Differentiation between finger, toe and tongue movement in man based on 40 Hz EEG. Electroencephalography and Clinical Neurophysiology 90: 456–460
61. Pfurtscheller G, Flotzinger D, Pregenzer M et al. 1996 EEG-based brain–computer interface. Medical Progress through Technology 21: 111–121
62. Pfurtscheller G, Neuper C, Guger C et al. 2000 Current trends in Graz brain–computer interface (BCI) research. IEEE Transactions on Rehabilitation Engineering 8(2): 216–219
63. Neuper C, Pfurtscheller G 1992 Event-related negativity and event-related desynchronization during preparation for motor acts. Zeitschrift für EEG-EMG 23: 55–61
64. Obermaier B, Müller G, Pfurtscheller G 2001 'Virtual keyboard' controlled by spontaneous EEG activity. In: Dorffner G, Bischof H, Hornik K eds. ICANN 2001, LNCS 2130. Springer, Heidelberg, 636–641
65. Neuper C, Müller GR, Kübler A et al. 2003 Clinical application of an EEG-based brain–computer interface: a case study in a patient with severe motor impairment. Clinical Neurophysiology 114: 399–409
66. Farwell LA, Donchin E 1988 Talking off the top of your head: toward a mental prosthesis utilizing event-related brain potentials. Electroencephalography and Clinical Neurophysiology 70: 512–523
67. Donchin E, Spencer KM, Wijesinghe R 2000 The mental prosthesis: assessing the speed of a P300-based brain–computer interface. IEEE Transactions on Rehabilitation Engineering 8(2): 174–179
68. Donchin E 1981 Surprise! … Surprise? Psychophysiology 18: 493–513
69. Donchin E, Coles MGH 1988 Is the P300 component a manifestation of context updating? Behavioral and Brain Sciences 11: 357–374
70. Kennedy PR, Bakay RAE 1997 Activity of single action potentials in monkey motor cortex during long-term task learning. Brain Research 760: 251–254
71. Kennedy PR, Bakay RAE 1998 Restoration of neural output from a paralyzed patient by a direct brain connection. Neuroreport 9: 1707–1711
72. Kennedy P, Bakay RAE, Moore MM et al. 2000 Direct control of a computer from the human central nervous system. IEEE Transactions on Rehabilitation Engineering 8(2): 198–202
73. Lange DJ, Murphy PL, Roger MS et al. 1994 Management of patients with amyotrophic lateral sclerosis. Journal of Neurologic Rehabilitation 8(2): 75–82
74. McDonald ER, Wiedenfeld S, Hillel A et al. 1994 Survival in amyotrophic lateral sclerosis. The role of psychological factors. Archives of Neurology 51: 17–23
75. Kübler A, Winter S, Kaiser J et al. ADF-12: Item Fragebogen zur Messung von Depression bei degenerative neurologischen Erkrankungen (amyotrophe lateralsklerose). Zeitschrift für Klinische Psychologie. Submitted
76. Averbeck M, Leiberich P, Grote-Kusch MT et al. 1997 Skalen zur Erfassung der Lebensqualität (SEL) – Manual. Swets & Zeitlinger BV, Swets Test Services, Frankfurt
77. Kübler A, Winter S. Depression and quality of life in patients with amyotrophic lateral sclerosis. In preparation
78. Badger TA 2001 Depression, psychological resources, and health-related quality of life. Journal of Clinical Gerontopsychology 7: 189–200
79. Neumann N 2001 Gehirn–Computer Kommunikation: Einflussfaktoren auf die Selbstregulation langsamer kortikaler Hirnotenziale. Schwäbische Verlagsgesellschaft, Tübingen
80. Kotchoubey B, Blankenhorn V, Fröscher W et al. 1997 Stability of cortical self-regulation in epilepsy patients. Neuroreport 8: 1867–1870

WEBSITES OF INTEREST

Help and information: http://www.muscular-dystrophy.org/

Information on amyotrophic lateral sclerosis: http://omni.ac.uk/browse/mesh/detail/C0002736L0002736.html

Information on chronic pain:
http://www.ninds.nih.gov/health_and_medical/disorders/chronic_pain.htm
http://www.efic.efic.org/eap.htm

Institute for Medical Psychology and Behavioral Neurobiology, University of Tuebingen. Development of Brain–Computer Interfaces: http://www.uni-tuebingen.de/medizinischepsychologie/

PART 3

Technology of replacement

9

Reaching with electricity: externally powered prosthetics and embodiment

David Gow   Malcolm MacLachlan
Campbell Aird

SUMMARY

Recent years have witnessed dramatic improvements in prosthetic technology. We trace the history of the development of the Edinburgh Arm and contrast one person's experience of using a traditional muscle-powered arm prosthesis with that of using the Edinburgh Arm; one of the most advanced externally powered prosthetic arms in the world. While the public's imagination has been fired by media reports of the 'bionic arm' we describe the innovative, but less dramatic mechanism responsible for its functioning. As well as elucidating the biomechanics of the Edinburgh Arm, we also explore the psychological significance of the two types of prostheses described. In particular, we consider the relationship between prosthetic functioning and the extent and nature of embodiment that may occur with a prosthesis. Development in prosthetic technology and the understanding of its psychological ramifications may not only improve psychological well-being and physical functioning, but also provide insight into mind–body relationships.

CASE STUDY

The case study reported here describes the experiences of our co-author, Campbell Aird. On the 18th of December 1982, Campbell had his left arm amputated at the shoulder. Only a few days previously, following the results of a biopsy, he had learnt that he had a rare form of cancer. On the 24th of December 1982 Campbell checked himself out of hospital, in order to be home for Christmas. At home he 'lived on morphine' for about 2 weeks and returned to work (in the hotel industry) within 3 weeks of the amputation. He says: 'The company appreciated it, but I think there was more to it: I wanted life to be as normal as possible, because then I had two children that were quite young and I didn't want them to see things in the family changing'.

Campbell talked 'an awful lot' with his very understanding GP and says: 'We had a theory that I should take vitamin C in massive doses, 14 mg a day. We [also] had a theory that the chemical make-up of the body changes every 7 years, aged 1–7, 7–14 (puberty), 21 (the key to the front door), so on and so forth, right up to 42. I was 32 at the time … and so if I could get through the next 3 years without getting secondary cancer, hopefully after that 7-year stint, the chemicals would either remix within your body or you've got what you need to combat cancer'.

Within 6 weeks of the amputation '… I had an arm fitted, in fact, this is the arm here (the one he is wearing), I rather like it, so much it's a part of me now: if you touched it and I wasn't looking at it, I'd know you touched it. So I started wearing it and it had its functions; it helps me tie my tie in the morning, it helps me tie my shoelaces, whatever, and I've mastered it over the period, I never take it off. … This is twenty years old, it's the myo-hand which is externally powered with a body powered, cable-operated elbow. Anyway, I've disciplined myself to wear the arm because I want to look natural'.

Campbell described how the challenge of just being able to wear the arm passed long ago and how the challenge became '… to prove to yourself and other people that you're not as disabled as you and they think you are. I don't know which one comes first, to prove it to yourself or to prove it to other people, but anyway, you get on with life'. Subsequently, Campbell windsurfed the English Channel in 2 hours and 20 minutes, in 1986. Later, he windsurfed the Firth of Forth (an even greater distance), laid a patio and walkway, and built a garden wall, all on his own. He learnt to fly an airplane and took up clay pigeon shooting – at which he won fourteen trophies. In terms of work, Campbell says his aim was to '… try and convince your directors that you're as good with one arm as you are with two, because they're paying you for your mind, not your arm'. Unsurprisingly, Campbell was highly successful in his chosen career and now owns his own hotel in the Scottish Borders. Campbell contends that he would not have got on so well in life, if he had not lost his arm: 'I had ambition, but the ambition got worse when the arm was lost'.

Campbell has had phantom sensations of his missing limb since the amputation. His phantom arm has now telescoped into his shoulder so that his phantom hand is felt to stick out from his shoulder and he can feel finger movements. He is aware of the presence of the phantom through a sort of tightness around the shoulder – the sort of feeling one gets when having blood pressure recorded by a sphygmomanometer. He can, when he wishes, control the sensation of finger movements, and make various gestures with his fingers! Although initially frequently very painful, Campbell's phantom-limb pain is now rare and experienced '… as if someone comes up to the back of me and takes a knife and sticks it in the shoulder, and I jump!'

Although Campbell's original prosthetic arm helped him in many ways and he felt a certain emotional attachment to it, in other respects he was frustrated by its limitations. As a result, over the past 10 years he has been a participant in the development of the world's first *externally powered prosthetic arm*. The current model in this project not only allows for electronic-mediated movement of the whole arm, it has a rotating wrist and elbow and allows the wearer to reach upward, it also allows for individual finger digit movements (see Gow et al.[1] and below). The mechanical part of the arm is covered with a silicone cosmesis and so the arm looks very realistic.

Interestingly, although the externally powered prosthetic arm looks and can behave in a more authentic fashion, Campbell says it does not yet feel a part of him in the same way as his original prosthesis does. There are probably several reasons for this greater identification with the lower-tech prosthesis, including greater familiarity, sense of 'safety' having mastered it, and, quite simply, because it does less there is less to go wrong with it and it is, therefore, more reliable. Thus, at this stage of development of the externally powered prosthetic arm, the original can be relied upon to a greater extent. Furthermore, Campbell explained that '… the thinking required to make it [the externally powered prosthetic arm] work is very different, you have to flick a lot of different areas of your shoulder to make it work, so you're conscious of making it work all the time'. Campbell suspects that if he had had the opportunity to wear the externally powered prosthetic arm from the start (that is, soon after the amputation), it would now feel as much 'a part of him' as his original prosthetic arm does. According to himself, he rarely takes the myo-hand off, only having the inclination or opportunity to wear the externally powered prosthesis sporadically.

When asked 'What would it take to make the externally powered prosthetic arm really feel as if it were a part of you?', Campbell replied: 'Notice what you're doing, you're talking to me but using your hands to express yourself, you're probably not even aware you're doing it … until you are not aware you're doing it [gesticulating with a prosthesis], then you'll never achieve what was lost'. Summarizing the technological advances in terms of its impact on him personally, Campbell says: 'We have something that's going in the right direction, … we've gone up in the air 150 feet – think how people felt before we mastered flight, it's tremendous – we haven't been to space yet with prosthetics, but we've got off the ground'.

As a final aspect of this case study, it is important to mention that Campbell has been closely involved with the engineer who has developed the externally powered prosthetic arm, David Gow, in marketing and attracting research funding, in order to further develop the technology. It has been most advantageous to have such a close alliance between the engineer and the end user.

INTRODUCTION

This case study hopefully illustrates not just the nature of the technology that has been developed, but also the importance of considering the nature of the user of that technology,[2] and possibly also of carefully selecting the 'right type' of person to become involved in trialing such pioneering techno-logy. For instance, Campbell's reaction to his limb loss is clearly not typical and he has also, quite obviously, been driven by the desire to compensate – not just physically but also psychologically – by showing what he is cap-able of doing. Ironically, while he may have had the capability – and was undoubtedly *more physically able* – to do these things before having had an amputation, he may never have exploited this capability had he not had that misfortune. Thus, technology's ability to help people combat impair-ments may exceed simple compensation and actually help them to *reach beyond themselves*. However, while this is an idealistic goal we are conscious that many people, especially the elderly, simply want to regain some of the functional ability that they lost as a result of having an amputation. At the same time it is important to recognize the value of having an end user involved in the early trialing of a prosthesis who is tenacious and motivated enough to work through some of the inevitable early hitches.

Our discussion is partitioned below into two sub-sections, the historical development and contemporary biomechanics of the externally powered prosthesis is outlined first, and then we consider the broader psychological implications of such prosthetic devices, especially as regards how they may influence a sense of embodiment. We are, however, keen to emphasize the importance of these two dimensions informing each other, and in turn being informed by the experience of the technology's users.

THE BIOMECHANICS OF PROSTHETICS AND THE EDINBURGH ARM

Prosthetic devices come in three types, passive or cosmetic limbs without function, which are used for esthetic purposes; and body-powered limbs, which are motivated by the muscular strength of the body via cables and pulleys attached to a harness. These devices, such as hooks or hands and elbows, require no external power and are simple and reasonably rugged. Finally, there are externally powered limbs, driven by battery power or other stored energy, such as carbon dioxide gas. These allow greater functionality, but they are heavier, more expensive, more complex and so are more prone to breakdowns. There can, of course, be combinations of the above; for example, Campbell's 20 year old prosthesis is an externally powered hand, with a body-powered elbow. Such a device is known as a 'hybrid prosthesis'.

Prosthetic developments of the types of prostheses mentioned above are at once incremental, chaotic and diverse. They are often produced in different countries at different times by various companies, laboratories or university departments. Catalysts for development are often warfare and conflict resulting in the need to invest in the rehabilitation of the war heroes. In Edinburgh's case, the advent and social impact of Thalidomide was the prime mover for its pioneering work into powered prostheses.[3] This drug, taken to alleviate the symptoms of morning sickness in pregnancy, had a profound effect in Britain when its results became obvious. Major centers in London, Oxford and Edinburgh contributed to prosthetic research and development, and this was driven by the political will to see progress in real time. The developments also had to match the pace of the children's own growth.

Edinburgh then became a center of excellence for the surgical and prosthetic work related to Scottish and Northern Irish children affected by Thalidomide. The work concentrated on developing prostheses for children with bilateral absence. At that time, carbon dioxide as a power medium was considered state-of-the-art technologically. This lightweight gas allowed the team to develop light and functional actuators to power the hand, wrist, elbow and shoulder of the children's prosthesis. As the program developed, a second series of prostheses was developed for adolescent patients. This then established the background to Edinburgh's prosthetics program from 1963 to the late 1970s. However, over the same period, the rest of the prosthetics world had concentrated on electrical prosthetic developments with hand prostheses, followed by wrist-rotation devices and elbows.[4] In the early 1980s Edinburgh moved into the mainstream and attempted to transfer its experience with gas-powered limbs to electrically powered devices. This took a major step forward in 1990, when work was funded to develop an electrical version of the gas-powered limbs of the 1970s. This eventually led to a unilateral version of the arm with electrical motors and gearboxes instead of pistons and cylinders being built in 1993, and requiring a willing 'test pilot'.

Campbell practically selected himself for the trial of the Edinburgh arm. He was already known within the prosthetic community as a willing participant in the uncertain world of research and development. In Campbell's case he represented a major challenge for the Edinburgh team. Their previous experience of highly functional arm prostheses had been in developing gas-powered limbs for children/young adults with bilateral absence. This was a markedly different challenge for the following reason: these children had been born without upper limbs and had no experience of upper-limb function. The prostheses were designed to give one functional limb and one counter-balancing passive arm, which would also contain the gas power supply. To wear these arms the children needed to be fitted with a steel frame to support the prostheses. Thus, giving these children some upper-limb function was above all other considerations. This is clearly inappropriate and undesirable in an unilateral arm absence such as Campbell's. Firstly, he has a perfectly good remaining arm, which, since it is infinitely 'smarter' than any prosthetic device, can do about 90% of tasks achievable with two arms. The functional role of the device is, therefore, as a *support to the natural arm* and not a replacement. Secondly, the natural arm should not be constrained by the prosthesis, which would be the case if we tried to use its shoulder movements as control sites.

Historically, researchers in Edinburgh and beyond have tried a number of control methods to operate the Thalidomide prosthetic limb in space. They had discovered that unless they could reduce the mental load on the user, the task of simultaneous real-time control of multiple joints was beyond the user's capabilities. Fortunately, they developed a simple control strategy that worked well enough to allow meaningful use of the devices. They had found that by linking the individual residual movements of the children's shoulders to individual joint movements in the prosthesis, there was sufficiently good correspondence in the children's minds to permit good proportional control of the joints. The movement of the shoulder vertically upwards (as in the action of shrugging), for example, was repeatable and independent from other shoulder movements. A second shoulder movement at 90° to the first, that is, in the horizontal direction, was also found to be useful. Both shoulders were thus harnessed to the task of controlling the single functional limb (each shoulder provided two movements to give a total of four independent spatial control inputs). These controlled the wrist rotation, elbow flexion and shoulder elevation, and cross-body rotational movements of the prosthesis.

Initially, these separate shoulder movements were not successful in simultaneously controlling the complex movements of the gas-powered arm. However, gas control switches (one per joint) had been fitted around the shoulder girdle, attached to the steel frame. Apart from the single degree of freedom control, this configuration had been found not to work well because the children could not cope with the 'data processing' of simultaneous control tasks. The Edinburgh team succeeded where others had failed by realizing that subtle changes were necessary in this arrangement. By effectively removing the gas switches from around the shoulder girdle, placing them on the arm itself (one at each joint), and linking them by simple cable to straps that were connected to the shoulder movements, they could create what engineers grandly term servomechanisms. In short, each movement of the prosthesis is a powered slave to the anatomical movement controlling it. Not only did this give a logical, repeatable and proportional linear relationship, but it also produced an effect called extended physiological proprioception (EPP).

EPP can be thought of as the tennis racket or golf club effect: in using these devices we can extend the human body's area of influence outside its natural physical limits. The fact that we can hit a moving or static ball with extensions of our arms is largely because we are extending the innate sense of proprioception present around joints such as the shoulder and elbow, down into the racket or club. Importantly for the Edinburgh prosthetic wearers, their proprioceptors were intact and, thus, their improved control was attributable to having this spatial feedback mechanism. Thus, they knew if they moved their natural shoulder halfway the prosthetic joint linked to that movement was also moved to halfway in its travel. Crucially, this enhanced feedback cut down on the amount of visual monitoring required by the user and produced startling improvements in control. Training of the children to use more than one movement simultaneously became easier and some could demonstrate simultaneous control of all four degrees of freedom at once. Interestingly, the children when tested in spatial positioning tasks, such as drawing a line on a blackboard, could reproduce the lines to an acceptable degree, even when blindfolded. The control had practically, at least in some cases, become subliminal. It is important to note that this was all due to the simple cable linkages.

When people see Campbell controlling the Edinburgh arm, they believe it is bionic technology that makes it possible. The secret, then as it is now, is down to the body's own natural feedback mechanisms and a simple linkage to the body. The Edinburgh philosophy, so carefully developed over the years, to use residual body movements because of the inherent feedback and improved control, is at odds with practice in other places. In American prosthetics, myoelectric control by the use of electrodes placed over the skin to sense the underlying muscular electrical activity (the myoelectricity) would be the norm. This method is more sophisticated and requires no movement or force sensors, but it lacks the type of feedback mentioned above. The body simply has no awareness of this electrical phenomenon. For this reason, despite many gallant and elegant control schemes, simultaneous control of multi-degree-of-freedom prostheses using myoelectricity is still largely unrealized.

The challenge with Campbell was, therefore, to find enough independent control sites from, effectively, one side of his body and thereby not restrict the natural arm. Campbell from the outset, however, surprised the research team with his control capabilities. He retained a small amount of movement of the musculature around the residual bones in his shoulder. With this he could operate micro switches or pressure pads to control the power of the electrical shoulder going up and down. We also tried to mimic his prosthetic experience with his body-powered limb and used scapular movement to control the elbow function. He achieved a complex combined movement of the shoulder and elbow within minutes of his first laboratory fitting. Eventually, we added another switch control for the wrist and hand. Campbell proved he could harness the four movements of the arm efficiently in front of the world's press in August 1998 when he became the living embodiment of 'bionic man' and demonstrated the world's first all electrically powered artificial arm complete with powered shoulder (see Gow et al.[1] for a fuller account, and Fig. 9.1). Clearly the ability to have a controllable locus of movements above the head is very important in increasing the functionality of an arm prosthesis. One of the things, which attracted Campbell to the development, by his own account, was this enhanced functionality offered by the externally powered prosthesis, both relative to his own original

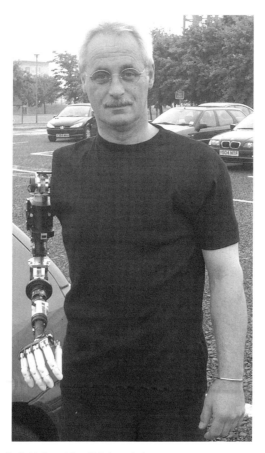

Figure 9.1 Campbell Aird and the Edinburgh Arm.

and body powered elbow myohand and to the gas-powered prostheses that existed at the time.

Campbell has given a myriad of interviews on the subject of controlling his 'bionic' limb. His explanation about how he thinks about controlling the arm, his 'phantom image' and the electrical activity that initiates movement has been widely, and wrongly, interpreted by a number of journalists and media. The general media ignorance about technology ascribes much to the operation of the arm that is akin to magic. In short, many reports misinterpreted Campbell's explanation as some clever invention or microchip, which translated his thoughts into bionic signals. Many academics, journalists and film crews have made the pilgrimage to Edinburgh to see the magic thought-control invention for themselves. The truth is out there and it is much more banal!

Since 1998 the arm has progressed to smarter control and refined movements with other functions added, such as wrist flexion and smoother control. A microprocessor-based control system is now available to build in intelligence to the arm and to help those not as coordinated as Campbell to gain good control. Campbell has also helped form a charity and is fundraising to help drive forward the development of the work. This has successfully led to a full-time development program that began in summer 2003 and the formation of a commercial company to build and market the arm in years to come.

Currently, the arm program has three test pilots with another adult and a young boy assisting the team in moving the work forward and producing a realistic and rugged set of devices. Campbell and his co-workers, can not only evaluate the technology and the functionality within the Edinburgh arm, but also can influence its future and change its development. More power to their elbows!

PSYCHOLOGICAL CONSIDERATIONS

There are different ways in which psychology can make a contribution to the rehabilitation of people with prostheses. This may range from assessment of how quality of life is affected,[5] to exploring which coping strategies may be most effectively employed,[6,7] to being involved with direct therapeutic interventions for an array of possible psychological sequelae (e.g. pain, depression, anxiety, post-traumatic stress disorder, sexual difficulties and drug abuse[8]), as well as less direct adjunctive interventions.[9] While these aspects are important and have been a particular concern of the *Trinity Psychoprosthetics Group*,[10,11] they are beyond the scope of what we wish to discuss here.

We are interested instead in exploring how the aforementioned exciting developments in prosthetic technology might influence the 'sense of self' that someone with an amputation has to renegotiate. This 'renegotiation' is not a straightforward activity, for it is not simply an objective loss of the physical limb that the person has to accommodate to, but also, commonly, the phenomenological experience of that limb – the phantom limb – continuing to exist. Furthermore, to literally add insult to injury, the absent – phantom – limb may be experienced along with great pain, pain that lasts many years, or even decades.[12–14] While a detailed discussion of phantom limb and phantom-limb pain is beyond the scope of this chapter, there are nonetheless some interesting phenomena relating prosthetics and phantoms. For instance, it is commonly reported by people who have had a leg amputated, and who subsequently experienced their phantom limb telescope (retract) into the limb stump, that they feel their phantom reoccupy the space of their leg whenever they put on their prosthetic leg. The phantom limb can be such a compelling experience that a participant in one of our research studies[15] reported being able to get relief from an itch on his phantom ankle, by bending down to scratch his prosthetic leg, in the same place!

This compels us to consider, as he must, 'what is me' and 'what is not me'. Where do 'I' stop and where does the prosthesis begin. Ramachandran and Blakeslee[16] suggest that one could even think of the whole body as a phantom itself, but equally, the body may be construed as a prosthesis. Another participant in one of our studies, a young woman who had to have both her legs amputated after she was caught in a fire, described her anguish at having to replace her prosthetic legs, as being *more* disturbing than the loss of her 'own' legs, because at least she did not know in advance she was going to lose them. Just as Campbell described above, for some people, and no doubt to varying extents, a prosthesis can become a 'part of you'. This can be described as *prosthetic embodiment*.[14,17] Here embodiment refers to the idea of identifying some aspect of the self with an object. On the one hand this could be an emotional identification with, for instance, a wedding ring, or on the other hand, a functional identification with, for instance, knowing that you will need a wheel chair to go shopping. The instances of prosthetic embodiment, described above, in some ways incorporate both of these elements: there is a functional as well as an emotional 'attachment', and the boundaries of 'the self' are somewhat ambiguous.

Groz[18] notes that 'inanimate objects when touched or on the body for long enough become extensions of the body image sensation'. Amputation requires a renegotiation of the body image. We use the term negotiation because the boundaries are not necessarily discrete and the person with an amputation must find a resolution to competing experiences that allows them to re-establish a coherent sense of self. This will require incorporation of the loss of the amputated limb, the phantom limb image they will probably experience, the prosthesis they wear, and possibly also the use of canes and crutches, at least for a time.[19] The way in which a person with an amputation experiences him or herself and how they construct meaning out of their experience will, of course, influence their attitude towards prosthetic use. A given prosthesis may embody *ability* for one person because of what it enables them to do, while for another person, or the same person at another time, the same prosthesis may embody *disability* because it represents what they are unable to do.

In terms of the externally powered prosthetic arm described above, and used by Campbell, what are the psychological implications for this technology in terms of body image and body function? The externally powered prosthetic arm has the obvious 'advantage' over the traditional myo (hybrid) prosthesis of being primarily electrically powered. However, it is still directed by muscle movement. Minute muscle contractions are used to indicate which aspect of the prosthesis Campbell wants to raise, lower, extend, or whatever (as described above). While this control over the prosthesis is obviously also modulated through the nervous system – in that this is necessary to make the appropriate discriminations in muscle tension – it is neither direct nor subconscious neural control. If we think about moving an arm we can do it, but if we think about picking up a pen, we can still move the arm but without being conscious of the neuronal and muscle activity required to control it. Being able to talk and gesticulate with hands is perhaps an example of ultimate embodiment, where a prosthesis can be used functionally and expressively (emotionally), and the user need not be consciously directing its movement.

While the externally powered prosthetic arm is a significant advance in terms of body function, the challenge of people being able to fully integrate it into a coherent body image remains. There are at least two aspects to this. Firstly, it may be that in time it is possible to develop a prosthesis that responds so 'intuitively' to the thoughts and intentions of its wearer, that the sense of it being 'other' is negligible. Secondly, we should not assume that because people have an arm that is obviously not their biological arm, that they cannot still have a very positive body image and, indeed, have this strengthened by the sense of being able to master a prosthesis that is very clearly not a part of their self. Creating a sense of *prosthetic embodiment* will not necessarily result in a more positive body image or a better quality of life in itself. Wearing a prosthesis is only one aspect of how a person with an amputation responds to their situation (see Chapter 15).

DISCUSSION

Routhier et al.'s[20] recent review of the literature pertaining to use and abandonment of pediatric myoelectric fittings identified a range of personal, environmental and technical factors. Three personal factors (including 'needs and expectations') were identified, along with six environmental (including social acceptance, family attitude and the cultural environment) and 12 technical (including appearance) factors. Routhier et al. state: 'More often than not, expectations regarding needs or technical possibilities are not realistic'.[20] It is, of course, difficult, even for a well-resourced multidisciplinary team, to work on all aspects of the 'matching the person to technology model'.[2,21] It can be frustrating and, indeed, disempowering for clinicians to be presented with clients seeking a level of technology that their services do not have the resources to provide. But in a sense, such 'unrealistic' expectations provide at least part of the impetus for continued research and development in the field of prosthetics. While we may never be able to replace the limb that was lost (but see Chapter 10 for a discussion of limb transplantation), we should aspire to being able to replace it with something as close to it as possible.

It is, however, important not to fall into the self-congratulatory rhetoric of 'technoculture' that so many of us are familiar with. Technologies also bear negative meanings and implications for the disabled.[22] In essence, technologies that represent a normalization or correction of impairment, and in doing so allow people to 'overcome' their disability, effectively 'buy into' a *deficit model* of physical impairment. As such, enabling technologies can be somewhat 'double-edged'.[23] On the one hand they offer disabled people the opportunity to diminish the functional significance of their impairment, while on the other hand technologies, by their very presence, emphasize the existence of that impairment, which may be in turn attributed to the 'owner' of the impaired body. As Lupton and Seymour[22] put it: 'Technologies have the potential both to exacerbate disability and to enhance selfhood and embodied capacities'. Later on Lupton and Seymour state that: 'Some people reject these technologies outright, seeing them as barriers to presenting their preferred self even though they may have enhanced bodily capacities'.

At a recent international prosthetics conference in Glasgow some of the demonstrations emphasized the importance of 'letting your prosthesis show', while others emphasized the importance of providing realistic cosmetic coverings for prosthetics limbs. There is currently a movement within the USA that feels the desire to wear a cosmetic covering over a prosthesis is driven largely by the felt need to conform to the 'non-disabled' expectations of society and that society should instead learn to recognize the value of disabled people, and, thus, that showing the 'hardware' of one's prosthesis is taking an affirmative stance. As with so much else, the personal and cultural meaning of technology is not specific or constant, rather it is negotiable and dynamic.[17]

FUTURE PROSPECTS

The next stage of development of the externally powered prosthetic arm may be to incorporate these into the nervous system. So instead of micro switches, or pressure pads, being operated through fine movement of the remaining musculature, control could be achieved through directly wiring the prosthesis into the nervous system (see Chapter 12).

If myoelectric and externally powered prostheses were a leap forward in prosthetics, then the linking-up of this technology with the nervous system surely offers another. If an arm can be moved not only 'at will', but also without awareness and expressively, and one adds to this the possibility of incorporating touch-sense detection in the fingers, then at what point might that arm become a 'part of the user' rather than an external appliance? We are now on the cusp of just such advances in biomedical engineering.

Another area in which technology can be brought to the fore in the rehabilitation of people who have had amputations is in the treatment of phantom-limb pain. Ramachandran ingeniously used a simple 'mirror box' to treat phantom-limb pain: the mirror image of the remaining arm of someone with an upper-arm amputation can be used to create the visual illusion of the amputated arm still being present. For some, but not all, people with amputations, carrying out certain procedures in the 'mirror box' has been found to reduce their phantom pain experiences. MacLachlan et al.,[24] have shown that various psychological factors, such as ratings of 'body plasticity' (how rigidly or fluidly one views the boundaries of one's body), degree of somatic preoccupation and creative imagination are associated with the occurrence of such illusory body experiences. Based on Ramachandran's original work, virtual- and augmented-reality systems that will allow people to view their 'phantom limbs' in real-time are now being developed. It is hoped that these will provide a more authentic intervention based on the 'mirror box' rationale.[25] In the case of non-traumatic amputations, when a patient's amputation can be planned for and they can be prepared for it, we also intend to use this same technology to allow people needing prosthetics to experience how their body will look after an amputation and to subsequently try out different types of 'virtual prostheses'.

In Campbell Aird's case, the use of an externally powered whole-arm prosthesis has allowed him to *reach with electricity*. However, it is noteworthy that his older and more trusted myoprosthesis has allowed him to, or perhaps propelled him to, *reach beyond himself*, in the sense that he rose to the challenge of an amputation by exceeding what he might have achieved without this 'challenge'. While the technological achievements of the externally powered prosthesis are impressive, perhaps even more impressive is the way in which the human spirit can become embodied in rising to both physical and mental challenges brought about by physical impairment. Technology that facilitates such a response could be truly augmentative rather than simply restorative or facilitative. Furthermore, such advances offer not only the possibility of greatly improved rehabilitation, but also of illuminating in new and dramatic ways some of the most ancient, perennial and intractable debates about mind–body relationships and the essence of personal identity.

REFERENCES

1. Gow DJ, Douglas W, Geggie C et al. 2001 The development of the Edinburgh modular arm system. Proceedings of the Institute of Mechanical Engineers 215(H): 291–298
2. Scherer MJ 2000 Living in the state of stuck: how assistive technology impacts the lives of people with disabilities. 3rd edn. Brookline Books, Cambridge, MA

3. Simpson DC 1968 An externally powered prosthesis for the complete arm. Proceedings of the Institute of Mechanical Engineers 183(J): 11–17
4. Childress DS 1985 Historical aspects of powered limb prostheses. Clinical Prosthetics and Orthotics 9: 2–13
5. Gallagher P, MacLachlan M 2000 The development and psychometric evaluation of the Trinity Amputation and Prosthesis Experience Scales (TAPES). Rehabilitation Psychology 45(2): 130–154
6. Gallagher P, MacLachlan M 1999 Psychological adjustment and coping in adults with prosthetic limbs. Behavioral Medicine 25: 117–124
7. Pucher I, Kickinger W, Frischenschlager O 1999 Coping with amputation and phantom limb pain. Journal of Psychosomatic Research 46: 379–383
8. Fitzpatrick MC 1999 The psychologic assessment and psychosocial recovery of the patient with an amputation. Clinical Orthopaedics and Related Research 361: 98–107
9. Gallagher P, MacLachlan M 2002 Evaluating a written emotional disclosure homework intervention for lower limb amputees. Archives of Physical Medicine and Rehabilitation 83: 1464–1466
10. Desmond D, MacLachlan M 2002 Psychosocial issues in the field of prosthetics and orthotics. Journal of Prosthetics and Orthotics 12(2): 12–24
11. Desmond D, MacLachlan M 2002 Psychological issues in prosthetic and orthotic practice: a 25 year review of psychology in 'Prosthetics and Orthotics International'. Prosthetics & Orthotics International 26: 182–188
12. Gallagher P, Allen D, MacLachlan M 2001 Phantom limb pain and stump pain: a comparative analysis. Disability and Rehabilitation 23: 522–530.
13. Desmond D, MacLachlan M. A study of 1,250 British war veterans who suffered limb loss. In preparation
14. Sherman RA 1997 Phantom pain. Plenum, New York
15. Horgan O, Coakley D, MacLachlan M. A longitudinal study of psychosocial rehabilitation of people with amputations. Submitted
16. Ramachandran VS, Blakeslee S 1998 Phantom in the brain. Fourth Estate, London
17. MacLachlan M 2004 Embodiment: clinical, critical and cultural perspectives. Milton Keynes, Open University Press
18. Groz E 1994 Volatile bodies: towards a corporeal feminism. Allen and Unwin, Sydney
19. Novotny M 1991 Psychosocial issues affecting rehabilitation. Physical Medicine and Rehabilitation Clinics of North America 2(2): 373–393
20. Routhier F, Vincent C, Morissette MJ et al. 2001 Clinical results of an investigation of paediatric upper limb myoelectric prosthesis fitting at the Quebec Rehabilitation Institute. Prosthetics and Orthotics International 25: 119–131
21. Scherer MJ 2002 The change in emphasis from people to person: introduction to the special issue on Assistive Technology. Disability and Rehabilitation 24(1–3): 1–4
22. Lupton D, Seymour W 2000 Technology, selfhood and physical disability. Social Science and Medicine 50: 1851–1862
23. Oliver M 1990 The politics of disablement. MacMillan, London
24. MacLachlan M, Desmond D, Horgan O 2003 Psychological correlates of illusory body experiences. Journal of Rehabilitation Research and Development 40(1): 59–66
25. MacLachlan M, de Paor H, McDarby G et al. 2002 Development and evaluation of augmented reality technology for the treatment of phantom limb pain and to facilitate adaptation to use of a prosthesis. Trinity Psychoprosthetics Group, Trinity College Dublin

WEBSITES OF INTEREST

International Society for Prosthetics and Orthotics: http://www.ispo.ws/

Rehabilitation Engineering Services: http://www.rehabtech.org.uk/

The Trinity Psychoprosthetics Group: http://www.tcd.ie/psychoprosthetics

10

Psychology and hand transplantation: clinical experiences

Gabriel Burloux   Danièle Bachmann

SUMMARY

Hand grafts pose different problems to other grafts, due to the visibility factor and because of the lack of immediate functionality that results in a long period of rehabilitation. This chapter will present the different criteria that we take into consideration when future candidates for this type of graft are being evaluated. This evaluation consists of psychometric testing and a clinical evaluation undertaken by two different analysts, who can subsequently compare their points of view. This process permits a better expression of the *Splitting*, which for this type of visible graft is a central and, at first, necessary mechanism that involves denial and acceptance.

The candidate's evaluation, however, cannot be separated from a simultaneous psychological preparation for the graft. This preparation makes it possible, inter alia, to elaborate upon the original trauma that was experienced at the time of hand loss. This is important given the potential for the re-emergence of this trauma after the graft. The follow-up continues during the post-graft phase in the form of repeated interviews where the goal is to allow the patient to integrate the grafted hands, in line with the progressive recovery of functionality. This chapter discusses the possible psychological disorders that may occur postoperatively and, in particular, the process of denial. Our clinical experiences demonstrate that the follow-up slowly reduces the necessity of splitting and the original denial of the foreign aspect of the hands. The family is also considered important in the patient's recovery and adjustment to the graft.

CASE STUDY

Having received a double hand graft, the period immediately following the graft was difficult for Mr GH. Just after the operation, he displayed a confused state where he saw scary scenes in which there were hands flying above his head, and he thought he was having perfusions of toxic products (he was actually having blood transfusions). As he did not know where he was, it was necessary to use sedatives (high doses of benzodiazepine, a tranquillizer) in order to reduce the major anxiety expressed in this hallucinatory mode. The reasons for this hallucinatory period were discussed by the surgeon, the intensive care unit doctor and the psychiatrists. It seemed to have a multi-factor origin: operating shock, multiple drugs, mental reactivation of the initial trauma, a short-lived grafted-hand reaction against the host, and, probably, a serum reaction causing a high temperature and his whole body to itch.

These symptoms disappeared in less than a week. The patient was then hospitalized in a less intensive care unit, where he was well supported by the nursing staff who fulfilled all his needs. Indeed, he was incapable of any gesture; for instance, he could not even scratch himself on his own. He seemed to be quite calm despite this state of extreme dependence that was akin to that of a newborn baby, and was similar to the period that followed the original trauma where an explosion resulted in the loss of both hands. This period, where he was in the same situation of total dependence, lasted for several months.

Just after the graft, he could see the ends of the fingers of the grafted hands appearing at the edge of the dressing and he thought that the professor had put his hands back on. In response to our amazement and when we mentioned the fact that they were donor's hands, he strongly asserted that they were his own hands, and that he knew since the accident that one day he would have them back. In spite of this delirious-like assertion, we noted that his behavior was otherwise perfectly adjusted, notably with the members of the nursing staff. On the other hand, the first dressing caused major anxiety, all the more since he could then see the demarcation between his forearms and the donor's hands. The grafted hands were lifeless and the donor's skin color was slightly different from the receiver's. Furthermore, although grafted hands are warm, the evidence of their cadaveric aspect reaches its climax because the limit between the two bodies is obvious as a result of the stitches, swells, and seams. At this stage the patient's anxiety was never verbally expressed. It showed through abundant sweats, some agitation, somatic complaints about difficulties swallowing, and the obvious refusal to verbally express what he felt. With our cautious encouragement, he was able to mention it a few days later, saying that the most striking element was the stitches and the apparent seams, which he feared might come unstitched. As a result of this fear of losing the newly grafted hands, and the return of traumatic dreams about the explosion that caused the loss of his hands originally, the initial trauma felt at the time of the hand loss reoccurred and was acutely felt.

Six weeks after the graft, the patient entered the rehabilitation center. The aim was now to actively recover motility functions. We were surprised with the natural way in which the patient scratched his head and caressed his face, despite the fact that the mobility and sensitivity of the fingers had not yet appeared. An episode of great importance for the psychological integration of the hands happened during the patient's first return home, about 3 months after the graft. One of his sons, aged 2 years, immediately noticed the difference between the grafted hands and the prostheses, and he caressed his father's hands saying 'hands, daddy', and kissed them, amazed and delighted. Back at the rehabilitation center, the patient talked emotionally about this moment, which greatly reassured him about his relatives' acceptance of the grafted hands, although, he still insisted that these hands were his own. However, one day he said, 'I am not sure Professor Dubernard grafted my own hands on me', which paradoxically attested the reality of the denial and a mental doubt about it. It is also important to remember that both journalists and some members of his family circle highlighted that they were, in fact, grafted dead man's hands. These remarks, which demonstrated an external return of the foreign nature of the hands, caused major anxiety every time. These anxieties showed through physical feelings of illness that went as far as vomiting. However, the patient preferred not to talk about it, as verbally discussing those difficult moments would reactivate the anxiety. At this point we respected his denial and tried to reassure him by emphasizing how unique and shocking such an experience was for any human being.

Between the 3rd and 9th month after the graft, the patient recovered voluntary movement activity little by little thanks to the rehabilitation. An element important in the integration of the grafted hands was the MRI. An MRI shows the moving of the cortical motility areas as the patient recovers this motility. These MRI show the cerebral flexibility on a scientific level, but they also have a major psychological part to play: the patient uses the imagery as a sign that the hands are becoming his own since his brain activates them. From this moment on, the necessity of denial becomes less fundamental. The simple fact of saying that the hands become his own through the cerebral activity visualized by the MRI suggests that the patient has a more realistic conscience of the foreign origin of the grafted hands.

About 10 months after the graft, the patient could spontaneously talk about the donor and publicly thank the latter's family in a very moving way, he brought a flower to a place of pilgrimage, in memory of the unknown donor. Denial was no longer necessary and the psychological integration of the hands was progressing, along with a more obvious sensitivity and motile activity.

INTRODUCTION

Hand grafts pose problems not only on a somatic level (composite tissue), but also on a psychological level. Heart or liver transplants are vital, and kidney or pancreas transplants can be replaced by substitutive techniques or treatments (e.g. dialysis, insulin). Hand or hands grafts are, however, a special case because of their symbolic nature that gives the human being its uniqueness; because of the visibility of the graft and of the very long delay before it becomes functional. For these reasons, the fantasies that haunt the grafted patients' imagery and psyche are much more intense and felt much deeper in cases of hand graft. Hence the first hand graft attempt in Lyon in September 1998 by Professor Dubernard (Lyon, France) and an international team, including Professor Hakim (England), Professor Lanzetta (Italy) and Professor Owen (Australia), produced massive media and popular attention, and was almost as important as when the first heart transplant was performed in South Africa in 1967. Indeed, it was only after considerable ethical reflection and the legal definition of the cerebral death, that Professor C. Barnard was permitted to perform this first heart transplant.[1] Similar issues also emerged before the first hand graft was undertaken in Lyon.

If the story of humanity starts with the practice of burying the dead, the graft of an organ taken from a corpse is somehow a transgression. In primitive societies, the dead were guided to their supposed new life: symbolic or non-symbolic objects and food were put in their grave in order to help their journey in the afterlife. Beliefs, funeral rites and religious ceremonies also show the fear of seeing the dead come back.[2] Whoever desecrates a tomb can expect a malediction, a vengeance from the corpse. Do we have the right to take his or her hands? This ethical aspect is important. The Etablissement Français des Greffes (French Grafts Establishment) was consulted and gave its agreement for a restricted number of hand grafts. Outside France, the law allows grafts almost everywhere around the world, under specific conditions. Strangely, it seems that in France the changes that were made to the legislation in order to favor the possibility of organ acquisition, actually have had the opposite effect. This shows the resistance to the idea of organ procurement after the death of another. Hence, the surgeons who offered to perform the first graft also asked for the religious authorities' agreement, which they obtained.[3,4]

The corpse seems to be more taboo than the fetus, although each is on the extreme end of life. The legislation may be out of date on this subject, probably because the 'chimera' of the living-dead is currently more likely to be achieved, but problems posed by the fetus are yet to come. But they will. For example, how legal is it to experiment on a human fetus or embryo or to collect stem cells from them for therapeutic purposes? Are the rights of the fetus or embryo accurately defined by law? Science advances quickly. Ethics and law need to catch up.

These brief considerations show us how sensitive the human psyche is to this question, and, furthermore, the psyche of the candidate for the hands graft. In the latter case this is particularly pertinent because the foreign organ will remain forever visible; therefore, the feeling of having something alien to oneself will not be forgotten very easily. Hence it is necessary to psychologically evaluate candidates for hand grafts with the greatest rigor possible.

EVALUATION
The necessity of the graft in terms of life quality

It is necessary to evaluate what quality of life was like before the graft, and what it could be like afterwards. This becomes a pertinent issue in the case where both hands have been lost. Indeed, the loss of a single hand is infinitely less harmful than the loss of both hands. In our opinion the only graft that should be performed is the one where there has been the loss of both hands, and in France, the 'Etablissement Français des Greffes' (French Establishment of Grafts) has expressed the same idea. Quality of life with the graft needs to be evaluated against the alternative benefits brought by the use of prostheses, knowing that the graft will only reach the same level of life quality after approximately 1 year, but that afterwards it can be incomparably more efficient. Another point to be taken account of, in our experience, is the sensitivity of the stumps. Some candidates for graft have acquired a degree of functional autonomy by alternating the use of prostheses, and the use of both stumps; used alternately as pliers or as sensitive organs to touch, feel, etc., which prostheses cannot do. The graft candidate must know and understand what they will lose because of the graft, what they will gain thanks to it, but at what price, at what level, and after how much time.

Some candidates ask for a graft to recover the sensitivity that prostheses do not allow, while for others the motility is more important. Should a blind man be grafted whose stumps' sensitivity is essential to find his bearings in life, when it is not sure that he will recover the same sensitivity after grafting? Of course, the decision belongs to the patients, but it is essential that they have the most accurate picture of what to expect. The active and passive dimensions are found in these two poles: voluntary motility and sensitivity. The value patients give to the sensitivity differences between prostheses, stumps and graft belongs to them only. However, these nuances are not clear in their mind and it is essential to know how to update them and provide them with useful information.

Motivation: of two types, narcissistic and functional

Narcissistic motivation refers to the difficulty in accepting the loss and, having sufficiently mourned the loss, being able to bear the glances of others, not feeling too demeaned, not overly investing the situation due to the amputation in a masochistic or narcissistic way. Although masochistic and narcissistic aspects are linked, they also need to be appreciated separately. Body image and the feeling of identity are deeply revised after the amputation. The mourning this involves makes psychological work necessary that might never be finished. The desire to have new hands, however legitimate, can be the sign of impossible mourning. It is, therefore, essential to evaluate the status of the lost hands in one's psyche, resulting from the mourning, as well as the quality of this mourning. There can be narcissistic mourning: 'I am the miserable hero! Pity me!' In other cases the mourning has a masochistic dimension where the patient invests too much in pain, giving him a new, demeaned image that is used in a melancholic way.

In a sense, mourning is never complete, probably because it is endlessly recalled by the visible absence of hands and by the constant functional limitations in everyday life with regard to even the most banal gestures. However, if mourning is incomplete, denied or intellectualized, it can be revived in the immediate postoperative phase following the graft, coupled with the return and resumption of the trauma associated with the initial cause of the amputation.

Functional motivation refers to the legitimate desire to recover satisfying motility and sensitivity thanks to new hands. Except with the most advanced myoelectric prostheses (Chapter 9), the recovery of movement is impossible because most prostheses only allow thumb-palm pliers. Moreover, they are very heavy, whereas grafted hands provide much better comfort. Prostheses can also cause rubbing and pain in the junction between the prostheses and the stump and, if they are myoelectric, proximity and contact with any electronic equipment is restricted in everyday life (e.g. one patient made an alarm go off in an airport).

Furthermore, on a strictly functional level, the recovery of sensitivity provides a better adaptation of the voluntary motility movements thanks to the recovery of different modes of this sensitivity (protective, tactile, pain, epicritic [discriminating], proprioceptive).

Both narcissistic and functional values always co-exist. We did think that it was important that the functional value predominated the narcissistic value.

However, this is not always the case, for example, with gastric surgery per-formed to treat obesity, the narcissistic dimension is the driving force.[5] In the case of hands, it is possible that, paradoxically, the intense desire to have new hands, coupled with the obstinate refusal to mourn them, is a favorable element giving the patient an unshakeable will stimulating them to build defences, but with the danger of depressive or psychotic breakdown if they collapse. That is to say, that choosing a candidate is not always easy, and we must know that a patient can, and has the right to change their mind. As for the psychiatrist or psychologist, the question is asked: do they have the right to be mistaken?

Patient understanding

The understanding the patient has (or has not) of constraints, difficulties and possible pain linked to the graft is important; particularly the necessity, dan-gers and secondary effects of the anti-rejection treatments, the long waiting for a functional result and the tedious rehabilitation. Even if the patient has a proper rational knowledge of all these aspects, their imagination will tend to skip over the long period of time existing between the graft and the moment when the first signs of functionality and life appear. Not anticipating the graft's traumatic aspect on a psychological level can reactivate the initial trauma that led to the loss of the hands. The request for the graft can be made to deny and cancel the accident, as if it could be erased, giving the surgical gesture an extraordinary and omnipotent aspect.

The degree of idealization

Idealization linked with the desire to have hands again, and too much enthu-siasm can lead to disappointment. What is asked of a heart or a liver is to work, which happens immediately after the graft. However, for a hand graft, there is a risk that the patient might desire to recover the precision of a professional gesture, or the mastery of playing a musical instrument, while the doctors will only aim for the recovery of the elementary possibilities of life with the hand. Hence, there may be disappointment leading to a re-evaluation of the necessity of the treatment and the need for rehabilitation; thus, the formation of a vicious circle leading to a worsening condition. If too strong, this disappoint-ment can be the cause of true depressive states, with a self-destructive dimen-sion involving the patient's earlier personality. This may possibly result in the patient giving up the rehabilitation or the anti-rejection treatment.

The candidate's general personality

Personality, that is to say the characteristics of their mental processes must be considered. It is first necessary to evaluate their possible traumatophilia, that is their 'proneness' to be in difficult, repetitive, similar circumstances, for example, to have further accidents (accident-prone patients). In psychiatry, this is called 'fate neurosis' or traumatic neurosis. This type of patient is pushed to repeat unconsciously acts or situations, like accidents that they attribute to coincidence or fate. According to our experience, this seems quite frequent with hand amputees. This is a delicate point. It is essential to spot both physical and psychological traumatic events that the patient has suffered in their history, the links they were able to establish between them, and the meaning it had for them. However, such an approach must not create too much guilt or other emotional reactions. It is also important to remember that the preliminary evaluation work also has a therapeutic function: psychologically preparing the patient for the graft.

Indeed, such a process leads the candidate to talk about the initial trauma again and, therefore, to relive the accident scene. This remembrance can help candidates integrate the trauma psychologically. Do they consider it as a peculiarity or have they made it another link in the chain of their traumas, which might demonstrate some reflective recovery? Some patients are very keen to describe the accident scene while others refuse to talk about it. Their story can be stereotyped or, on the contrary, include many variations. It is essential to see what those variations signify: a psychological necessity to protect oneself from the trauma, or the ability to work on it in order to exorcise it. The remembered details sometimes have a hallucinatory dimension showing the persistence of the impact of the trauma or traumas. We can be of some help to the patients in their 'working through' the trauma, that is, according to psychoanalysts, to help them integrate it in their mind and to prevent it from repeating (i.e. repetition compulsion).[6]

Other aspects of the personality are also important to evaluate: first the personality's solidity or fragility, the specificities of the defense modes, the types of anxiety the defences have been built against, the quality and diversity of the cathexis, and the possibilities of adaptation, etc. These aspects are important because the experience of a hand graft is also a trauma, and the patient will use the modes of defence they usually have.

In summary, the general psychological examination must consider that the mourning and trauma of hands loss have modified the psyche. Yet it must estimate how this psyche will face the difficulties of the graft. In order to achieve this, our method includes using both tests and interviews.

METHOD

Tests

The tests that one can use are either personality tests (e.g. Rorschach,[7] Minimult,[8] and Somatic Inkblot Series[9]) or Intellectual Quotient (IQ) tests (e.g. Raven's progressive matrices[10]).

The Rorschach test is a projective test. It is well established and provides information on the patient's resources and vision of the world, on the capacity to organize information efficiently, resistance to stress, adaptation strategies, affectivity, self-esteem, appreciation of own body image and of other people's, the ability to invest the other, identification possibilities, management of interpersonal relationships, and psychological maturity.

The Minimult[8] is a personality test. It is processed by computer and is very easy to take. It allows testing of the patient in a repeated way, which allows any changes to be tracked.

The Somatic Inkblot Test[9] is very important because it is centered on the body and its relationship with the mind, and also centered on the possible linked anxieties (e.g. fear of mutilation, of being devoured).

We have not used Raven's progressive matrices[10] yet, nor performed any intelligence test, as this seemed discriminatory and unfair to us. However, the question of the candidate's intelligence can be posed, and it is not only the psychiatrist's or psychologist's responsibility to answer this, as it is an ethical matter.

Clinical interviews

Clinical interviews can identify more nuances and be more precise than psychometric tests, as they have not only a diagnostic value, as we have seen earlier, but also a therapeutic and evolutional value. They permit the patient to integrate the trauma of the amputation better, and provide a protective and reassuring shield. Indeed, they allow for the provision and specification of information, which enables the patient to acquire a greater knowledge and to be better psychologically prepared. Of course these interviews must happen before the graft, but they must also continue afterwards as a therapeutic framing for the patient. Furthermore, it is more beneficial if the interviews are performed by two specialists, who can then compare their impressions and opinions.

The technique used for these interviews varies. First it is non-directive and the patient is allowed to express himself freely, in an associative way. However, experience has shown that it is important to probe the patient at times, and to ask him questions, not only on an information level, but also in order to explore a badly elaborated, vague, or under-evaluated aspect. Some interviews are performed by both psychiatrists at the same time, which is important to provide a coherent vision of the psychological treatment. Other interviews are performed by one psychiatrist, in order to differentiate between practitioners. Of course it is necessary that the psychiatrists exchange their impressions and opinions.

Besides the benefit of having two different points of view, there is yet another advantage. As we shall see later, hand-graft patients show important psychological splitting mechanisms. It may be interesting for the patient to use each psychiatrist differently, for example, by not talking about the same things, which can be very meaningful. Indeed, splitting is accompanied with projections of parts of oneself on different poles of the environment. A similar phenomenon happens to different members of staff, who receive different messages, hence the importance of good communication between clinical staff. This may allow for the expression of a certain inner conflict as well as expressing the splitting. For instance, the patient may explain to one psychiatrist that they feel pretty well, but to the other they may express the reasons for their anxiety. Thus, one side of the splitting may be expressed to one psychiatrist and the second side to the other. This can then provide a more global and therapeutic understanding of the patient.

THE FAMILY CIRCLE

Our experiences have shown how important the feelings and reactions of the family circle are. What is true for the patient is also true for the family (for instance, the hand deemed as that of a corpse, non-functionality, etc.). Moreover, if the family does not live in the location where the graft is performed, the patient cannot share with them all the difficulties and pain they may go through, and this results in them living in two different worlds.

It should be remembered that the hand has a symbolic and social aspect to it and is a tool for contact and relationships, mainly with the family. It is a factor of autonomy for the person and it allows exchanges with others, including sexual relations. Even though everybody in the family circle wants the patient to recover sufficient autonomy and escape the dependency suffered before the graft, how do they accept this new hand, which is dead, strange and alien, slowly coming back to life in such an odd way?

In terms of relationships in day-to-day life and also in intimate, particularly sexual life, the problem of touch is very delicate, whether it is considered from the grafted patient's side (fear of provoking reactions of repulsion) or from the touched person's side (apprehension and disgust). We will return to this aspect again later on in the chapter.

Proper acceptance of the graft by the people around the patient is very helpful in the process of 'taming' the transplanted hands. Their reaction can facilitate the inevitable and psychological aspects of denial; denial of the origin and of the unpleasant appearance of the hand. Consequently, the patient and the family are able to gradually integrate together in their minds all the aspects of the new hands, and questions like 'did the donor die?' that halt the process of denial are prevented.

FOLLOW-UP

The framework for follow-up involves seeing patients every day, sometimes more if something happens (delusion, anxiety, crisis) at the beginning and then less and less often, depending on how the case evolves. As far as possible, we get in touch with the patient's family and the social environment of the patient. Furthermore, the whole medical team meets together once a week to provide doctors with the opportunity to exchange their points of view.

POSTOPERATIVE DAYS AND POSSIBLE PSYCHOLOGICAL DISORDERS

Anxiety

As this type of graft can be described as 'visible', anxiety in this case takes the form of de-personalization. It is linked to the alien nature of the grafted hand, its cadaveric aspect, but also to the apparent boundary between the receiver's arm and the donor's hand, symbolic of the troublesome coexistence of the dead and the living, between the familiar and the unfamiliar.

This type of anxiety usually occurs right after the operation, and more so with the first dressing change, but fails to be expressed as such: it can take the form of vagal disorders or of any kind of physical symptom, or even a recurrence of acute pain. It can continue erratically until the psychological process of appropriation of the grafted hands is completed.

The anxiety is, in fact, pre-existent to the graft and linked with the horror induced by the idea of mix or coexistence, or even of confusion between the living and the dead. With the first dressing change, it is crystallized as a fear when the patient is faced with the vision of a dead hand hanging from their healthy elbow. This vision may bring to the fore their state of mortal being.

Regression

This is a necessary and desirable step, at least to a certain extent, especially in the immediate aftermath of the transplantation when the patient is extremely dependent and back in a state in which they have few of the functional abilities they had gained before the graft using their stumps or prostheses. This regression is temporary and its duration should not be long enough to prevent active physiotherapy. This state disappears when the body becomes a vehicle for the patient's anxiety and when thought becomes animistic, with fantasies of the hand taking on a life of its own and doing things beyond the patient's control. This point will be developed later on.

Depression

As with idealization, the risk of depression is dependent on the fragility of the personality of the patient, but also on the possible discrepancy between how the patient imagined their life after the graft and what they are capable of in reality. As we have indicated, the greater the difference between the two, the greater the risk of depression.

Multi-factor delirium

Postoperative shock, steroid therapy, serum reactions or a reaction of the grafted hand against the native body are elements that can induce a confusional type of delirium. The risk is even more acute in the first postoperative days, and compounded by a certain number of factors linked with the personality of the patient and by the reactivation of the initial trauma, which is common.

Reactivation of the initial trauma

The postoperative conditions can remind the patient of the trauma and the circumstances that occurred after the original accident that resulted in the loss of the hands. These conditions include the bandages on the forearms (even though the tips of the fingers are visible after the transplant, which of course is not the case after the amputation). They also include the regression associated with the state of total dependency for all the ordinary gestures of everyday life. Immediately after the transplant, the patient is totally unable to make use of the new hands attached to their forearms, and find themself in a state of even greater dependency than just before the transplant, particularly if the patient had learnt to master the use of their artificial limbs.

It is at this time that certain psychological phenomena may reappear, that is if they had disappeared in the first place. They are reactivated acutely, under the form of visual 'flashes' of the initial accident, anxiety, nightmares reliving the accident, etc.[11] This occurred with one of our candidates even before the graft. After our first interview, he relived all the symptoms he had experienced after his accident and the surgery that followed. He actually *saw* the circumstances of his accident, felt the same anxieties, and remembered the hallucinations he had had in the hospital as if they were happening again.

However, in contrast, the enduring dependency throughout the period between the initial accident and the possible use of prostheses and the associated state of regression can make the adaptation period after the transplant somewhat easier.

WHAT THE THERAPIST MUST FACE

The fantasies and psychological reactions to the hand grafts are linked to its visible aspect and also to the very long non-functionality of the grafted hands. The intensity of the regression experienced can also be explained by the necessary constraints of the life-long anti-rejection treatment and rehabilitation, and also by the patient's renewed passivity that results in them reliving their post-amputation experience. Moreover, this regression can be useful in allowing the patient to receive treatments passively from the active therapist. However, this regression must not be too long or too deep, otherwise there is the risk of depression. It is, therefore, essential that the patients are followed by the psychiatrist, all the more since the normal anxiety they experience must be taken into account. However, the most important fantasies, although they are not always directly expressed, are those that arise from having a corpse's hands at the end of one's arms (and to see it). It is important for the psychiatrist to be aware of this, as everything that surrounds this fantasy necessitates a specific type of defence system for the patient: denial, before and mainly after the graft, when it is then harder to maintain.

DENIAL

Denial consists of a patient saying simultaneously: 'I know that the grafted hand is a corpse's hand' and 'I don't want to know it'. So there is a splitting of the psyche into two parts, as this is the only way to avoid contradiction. Yet this contradiction exists, and reality will incessantly attack this psychological position. For example, the medical team will talk of 'the' hand while the patient will say 'my' hand. However, the fantasy of the corpse and, therefore, of the donor, is complex. Even if it is artificial and simplistic to differentiate some of these aspects, it is necessary to do so in order to understand them. This is because they are fantasy aspects that have always been repressed in the depths of humanity.

The 'Frankenstein' aspect

The path of the stitches, the threads, the swelling and the additions, the different color of skin, etc. remind one of Mary Shelley's[12] hero, and thrust the patient into the midst of his denial. The fantasy procession evokes the horror of the tomb, the world of shadows, the unnamable. This traumatic perception revives the idea of the lifeless coming back to life and becoming autonomous again, which poses the worrying question of the grafted hand taking control. What is the hand going to do? Will it do something unmentionable that may be a secret desire? Will one inherit its qualities or its defects? This reminds one of Maupassant's novels,[13] the story of Goetz von Berlinchingen's hand,[14] or of the American television series the Adam's family. Sometimes literature is prophetic. In a television program, a young patient about to receive a graft (a bone-marrow graft I believe) asked about the donor: 'If it's a girl then will I be a girl? If he doesn't like school, then won't I like it? But he's American, so I'll speak American!'

The fantasy of the donor taking control of the receiver's personality is frequent in all types of graft, but it is more conscious in the case of a hand graft. This fantasy attacks the continuous, reassuring sensation that we have of our own body, and also the continuous defence we exert against what is strange, alien, and non-familiar, which can both threaten and attract us. Like children who are afraid of wolves but who are fond of wolf stories and see wolves everywhere. It is the reason why phantom stories are so popular. The ambivalence expresses an inner conflict between the projection of repressed desires and being guilty about it. We must incessantly defend our identity, which is why denial is essential.

This denial necessitates that a certain psychological energy be maintained. It can give way under the pressure of anxiety or under the pressure of unconscious desires. For example, a patient may wonder what his wife's reaction will be when 'the other person's' hand touches her, if the grafted hands are a woman's hands, or if the hands are his own given back to him, even though he knows perfectly well that this cannot be the case.

Denial can also be attacked from the outside, for example, by the family or social circle. A patient who was holding out his hand to someone was told: 'I am not touching a corpse's hand!' It is particularly shocking in sexual or friendly circumstances, and even more when the medical team is involved. We remember the horrified reaction of a team member when a grafted patient started biting his nails!

Appropriating the hand

The process is not completed when the physical graft is achieved, as then the psychological graft begins. The patient needs to tame the hand in the same way as teenagers must tame and discover their new body. This is difficult while there is no sign of sensitivity or motor-function, and when there is no functionality. At this stage the social environment and the psychological framing must be careful and anticipative. Indeed, it is essential to remember that all the psychological impressions and fantasies that we have described are beneath the surface, hardly conscious. They rarely show themselves explicitly, but rather in an allusive or confused way. Much more often they are expressed through symptoms: Freudian slips, negations, doubts, anxiety, depression, even hallucinations and delirious ideas. These must be detected and understood, not to bring them into the open, which would be like materializing them, but rather to appease and to treat them. In fact, it is necessary to appreciate the situation and to evaluate if talking about the fantasies can dissolve them or, on the contrary, worsen the anxiety. Eventually, the moment comes when the alien hands are sufficiently tamed. A patient told us one day: 'I touch my hand, and it is like an old friend'.

So when the patient can retake, or rather take control of the grafted hand and start using it, the necessity of denial is lessened and the thought of the donor's existence, being less dangerous, can then become conscious.

The relationship with the donor

The relationship with the donor is greatly ambivalent. On the one hand, the patient experiences gratitude and feels in a position of debt towards the donor.

They experience the wish to meet the donor's family, which is forbidden by French law. This is not the case in Italy, for example, where such meetings are possible and seem to go well. However, alternatively, they also experience a deep guilt at the idea that a human being died for the hand graft to be possible and, although it is not the case, they may see themselves as a murderer. Then the natural balancing aspect to guilt appears, that is aggressiveness, with the necessity to repress it because it is even less confessable. The patient must be encouraged to talk about their gratitude and to express themself, in order to elaborate and metabolize their aggressive instincts by somehow dissolving them in the totality of their psyche (psychological elaboration).

Generally, in cases of non-vital organ grafts, the impact of the fantasy to having killed the donor in order to take his organ is not as important, because the question of life or death is not central. In hand grafts, this impact remains strong because the grafted organ is continuously visible, so they may wish or even have a definite need to erase the donor's characteristics because they have become traumatic (skin or hair color, nails, etc.). This can lead to a psychological rejection of the grafts that have become incompatible.

THE DONOR'S FAMILY

We have seen the loneliness of the donors' families. They find themselves isolated, and without any official psychological support, as if they were being intentionally ignored. Much is known about the bond existing between the donor and the receiver in other graft cases where anonymity is neither required nor possible, like kidney or bone-marrow donorship between parents and children for example. The desire to meet the receiver must exist in many cases. Since this desire is impossible to satisfy in our country, it should be possible to at least offer the donor's close relatives official psychological support, performed by different psychiatrists from the ones treating the grafted patient. Indeed, it must not be forgotten that they are in the process of mourning, which is certainly made more difficult or more unique because of the circumstances. Some donors' parents have the fantasy that a part of the deceased person still lives somehow, and that the receiver's behavior must not become estranged from the dead person's, which perpetuates this survival fantasy. They want to keep control all the more since the grafts produce a large media attention.

Likewise, let us repeat that psychological support should be provided for the grafted patients' families, as they may not be in harmony with the patient's deeply modified inner world, especially if they are living very far from the place where the graft was performed, which often happens. The psychological integration of the grafts must also be experienced by the family, who could be psychologically helped in order to accept the grafted patient's new hands more easily, and in order to prevent the patient from fearing his family circle's reactions.

CONCLUSION

By May 2003, 14 single hand transplantations had been performed:

- Lyon, France – September 1998 (1)
- Louisville, USA – January 1999 (1)
- Guangzhou, China – September 1999 (2)
- Kuala-Lumpur, Malaysia – May 2000 (1)
- Milan, Italy – October 2000 (1)
- Guangxi, China – November 2000 (2)
- Louisville, USA – February 2001 (1)
- Harbin, China – June 2001 (2)
- Milan, Italy – October 2001 (1)
- Brussels, Belgium – July 2002 (1).
- Milan, Italy – October 2002 (1)

Six double hand transplantations had been performed:

- Lyon, France – January 2000 (1)
- Innsbruck, Austria – March 2000 (1)
- Guangzhou, China – September 2000 (1)
- Harbin, China – January 2001 (1)
- Innsbruck, Austria – March 2003 (1)
- Lyon, France – April 2003 (1)

Another patient is planned for a double hand transplantation in autumn, 2002, in Lyon.

All this may open up a new era of composite tissue transplantations. Throat (larynx) and knee transplantations have already been made. Many specialists think others are to follow: for instance face transplants. We, as psychiatrists, have only one goal: to help the patients.

Any transplantation gives rise to fantasies. The first grafts of the heart aroused fantasies linked with the vital function of the organ and with the symbolic world attached to it: affectivity, courage, passions, etc. But the heart is not visible and works immediately. So the patient may invest in his or her new life and, thanks to it, 'forget' or discard the fantasies.

We tried to show that hand transplantation is very specific. Seeing on one-self the grafted part of another human body arouses thoughts and fantasies very close to being conscious and sometimes difficult to bear. Such a brief text has a condensed aspect that certainly makes it a little caricature-like. Its aim is to emphasize the importance of the patient's psychological support, before and after the hand graft. The latter is symbolic. Is the hand the organ and the tool of the brain? Or is it the other way round? It does not matter. The functional MRI shows the complicity existing between the two.[15]

Without this complicity, humans would not be what they are, as is shown by the population and media reactions that followed the first hand graft.

To conclude, we would like to quote the declaration of a patient to journalists: 'This graft is not life saving, it is life giving'.

REFERENCES

1. Barnard C Personal communication
2. Arens W 1979 The man-eating myth: anthropology and anthropophagy. Oxford University Press, Oxford
3. Carvais R, Sasportes M 2000 La greffe humaine. (In)certitudes éthiques: du don de soi à la tolérance de l'autre. Presses Universitaires de France, France
4. Trzepacz P, DiMartini A 2000 The transplant patient: biological, psychiatric and ethical issues in organs transplantation. Cambridge Unversity Press, Cambridge, UK
5. Karlson J, Sjöström L, Sullivan M 1998 Swedish obese subjects (SOS), an intervention study of obesity. Two year follow up of health related quality of life and eating behavior after gastric surgery for severe obesity. International Journal of Obesity 22: 113–126
6. Burloux G, Forestier P, Dalery J et al. 1989 Chronic pain and post traumatic stress disorders. Psychotherapy and Psychosomatics 52(1–3): 119–124
7. Rorschach H 1998 Psychodiagnostics – a diagnostic test based on perception. 10th edn. Hogrefe and Huber Publishers, Seattle
8. Kincannon JC 1968 Prediction of the standard MMPI scale scores from 71 items: the mini-mult. Journal of Consulting and Clinical Psychology 32: 319–325
9. Cassell WA 1980 Body symbolism. Aurora Publishing Co, Alaska
10. Raven J 2000 The Raven's progressive matrices: change and stability over culture and time. Cognitive Psychology 41(1): 1–48
11. Freud S 1920 Jenseits des Lustprinzips. In: Gesammelte Werke. Bd.XIII. Werke aus den Jahren 1920–1924. London 1940, S-69
12. Shelley M 1994 Frankenstein. Penguin, London
13. de Maupassant G 1974 Contes et nouvelles. Bibliothèque de la Pléiade, Paris (Tome 1: La main, p. 3; La main d'écorché, p. 1116)
14. Ray J 1961 La main de Goetz von Berlichingen. In: 25 meilleures histoires noires et fantastiques. Marabout Géant Editions Gérard et Cie Vervier
15. Giraux P, Sirigu A, Schneider F et al. 2001 Cortical reorganisation in motor cortex after graft of both hands. Nature Neuroscience 4(7): 691–692

WEBSITE OF INTEREST

International Registry on Hand and Composite Tissue Transplantation: www.handregistry.com

Petit F. Composite tissue allotransplantation and reconstructive surgery: The first clinical applications. Maîtrise Orthopédique. The French Orthopaedic Web Journal: http://www.maitrise-orthop.com/corpusmaitri/orthopaedic/111_petit/petitus.shtml

11

Implantable replacement hearts

Robert D. Dowling

SUMMARY

Millions of people suffer from heart failure, which continues to have a high mortality despite advances in medical therapy. Heart transplantation is the only approved method for replacement of the failing heart but is severely limited due to the small number of organ donors. Continued attempts to develop an artificial heart have culminated in the recent initiation of clinical trials with the AbioCor™ implantable replacement heart system. This system is totally implantable and is powered with electricity transferred across the skin. This device allows for freedom of movement that has not previously been achieved with other artificial heart systems. Patients have been discharged from the hospital with one patient being discharged to home for over 7 months. Recipients of the AbioCor™ have been able to attend sporting events, parties, resume sexual activities and spend quality time with family members. One recipient celebrated a birthday, his 50th wedding anniversary and the birth of a great-grandchild since receiving the device. The early results of this clinical trial allow a glimpse into the potential for this technology to allow physicians the ability to replace the failing heart and enable patients to markedly improve their functional status.

CASE STUDY

A 70-year-old patient was referred to our center. He had a history of myocardial infarction dating back to 1990. He was not felt to be a candidate for coronary artery bypass surgery and was managed with aggressive use of appropriate medications for heart failure. Despite this, he continued to worsen over the last few years, more markedly so in the 6 months prior to him being seen at our institution. He was initially referred to determine if he was a candidate for any clinical trials involving drug therapies or to potentially receive a biventricular pacemaker, which has been shown to improve cardiac function in select patients with heart failure. While under evaluation for these therapies, he developed worsening heart failure symptoms and eventually required transfer to the intensive care unit where he was placed on multiple inotropic medications in an attempt to maintain a normal blood pressure and normal cardiac output. Due to inadequate blood flow to his other organs, he developed evidence of kidney failure and liver failure. An intra-aortic balloon pump was placed through his femoral artery in an attempt to improve his cardiac output to the point it would allow for recovery of end organ function. At this point, it was clear that he was not a candidate for any therapies short of the placement of a total artificial heart, which had only been done previously in one other patient. Our feeling at the time was that it was very unlikely, given his age and severe heart failure, that he would improve to the point where he would be a surgical candidate. Fortunately, over the course of the next 2–3 days he demonstrated improved end organ function and did improve to the point where we felt he was an acceptable candidate for the total artificial heart. In lengthy meetings with him and his family, we discussed all the previous preclinical work with the artificial heart as well as the experience with the first patient to receive the device. The patient then underwent a CT scan followed by a virtual fit evaluation. In the virtual fit evaluation, a 3-D computerized image of the AbioCor™ thoracic unit is superimposed on the image of the patient's mediastinal and chest wall structures derived from the CT scan. The computer simulation demonstrated the position and fit of the AbioCor™ thoracic unit in this patient's chest. This virtual surgery allows us to determine whether the AbioCor™ thoracic unit can be positioned in the chest of any potential recipient without impinging on vital structures such as the left pulmonary veins and the left lower lobe bronchus. This virtual surgery predicted that the heart would easily fit into the chest of this patient. The patient was assigned an independent advocate who was made available to him and his family to assist in understanding the potential risks and benefits of entering the clinical trial. The patient advocate is able to help the patient and their family to interpret the contents of the informed consent document. After the implant procedure, the patient advocate continues to be available to the patient and family for assistance in making other important medical decisions. All the patient advocates have backgrounds in clinical medicine and all function completely independently of both the sponsoring company and the medical teams. After the patient signed an Institutional Review Board consent form, he was scheduled for implantation of the AbioCor™ total artificial heart.

The operative implant proceeded without any difficulties. The length of the surgery was just over 5 hours. The patient had excellent function of the device from the time of surgery. His postoperative course was initially uneventful. He did develop some problems with his lungs, which were not entirely surprising, given how ill he was prior to the surgery. He did have recovery of his kidney and liver function and was eventually able to be removed from the ventilator. He had a slow but progressive improvement in his strength and relatively early began aggressive physical therapy. Approximately 5 months after his surgery, his activity level had improved to the point where he was able to take short trips out of the hospital. He progressed to the point where he could be discharged to a local hotel adjacent to the hospital and then eventually discharged to his home. He has been living at home with the artificial heart system for over 7 months and continues to do quite well. He has been able to resume his normal activities including fishing trips to a nearby lake, card games with a group of friends, and a number of other activities.

INTRODUCTION

A potential complication of all forms of heart disease is the development of heart failure, which occurs when the heart is unable to pump blood at a rate to meet the body's metabolic requirements or is only able to do so at higher filling pressures.[1]

The incidence of heart failure is high and continues to increase. It is estimated that heart failure affects nearly five million people in the USA alone and 15 million people worldwide. The economic impact of this disease is quite significant. The annual expenditure on heart-failure management in the USA approached 38 billion dollars in 1991. Recent estimates for the cost of heart-failure management in 1999 is well over 50 billion dollars.[2,3]

The treatment of the majority of patients with heart failure is with aggressive medical therapy. Some patients with structural heart disease, such as valvular heart disease or coronary artery disease, may benefit from operative intervention. With progression of disease, patients often develop worsening heart failure despite appropriate aggressive medical therapy. The addition of intravenous inotropes has been used for select patients but is controversial, as some studies have shown worsening survival with intravenous inotropes. With advanced heart failure, there are often no effective therapies and the patients should be considered for some form of cardiac-replacement therapy. Currently, transplantation is the only approved form of cardiac-replacement therapy, but is quite limited by the number of available donor hearts. Though transplantation has been wonderfully successful, it is felt to be epidemiologically trivial given the small number of donor hearts available and the large number of patients who could benefit from some form of cardiac-replacement therapy. The quest to develop a mechanical device that could function as an artificial heart has been ongoing for decades. This has culminated in the development of the AbioCor™ implantable replacement heart, which was first implanted in a human on July 2, 2001.

DEVICE DESCRIPTION

The AbioCor™ implantable replacement heart system (ABIOMED, Danvers, MA) is the first artificial heart system that does not require percutaneous lines or the need for percutaneous access.[4,5] Previous experience has demonstrated that the presence of percutaneous lines will eventually lead to infection and have a significantly negative impact on patient mobility and, therefore, quality of life.

There are four internal components of the AbioCor™ implantable replacement heart – the thoracic unit, a battery, a controller, and a TET (transcutaneous energy transfer) coil (Fig. 11.1). The thoracic unit (Fig. 11.2) is placed in the chest of the recipient in the same position as the native heart after excision of the native ventricles. The thoracic unit contains two pumping chambers that function as the left and right ventricle. Between the two ventricles is an energy converter, which contains a high efficiency miniature centrifugal pump driven by a brushless direct current motor. The centrifugal pump rotates in one direction and, by doing so, pressurizes a low viscosity hydraulic fluid. A two-position switching valve is then used to alternate the direction of hydraulic fluid between the left and right pumping chambers. This results in blood being pumped alternatively into the lungs and into

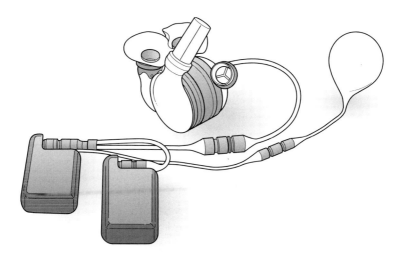

Figure 11.1 AbioCor™ implantable replacement heart system.

the systemic circulation.[6,7] The rate of the switching valve determines the beat rate of the device, which can be varied between 75 and 150 beats per minute. This results in a range of outputs from 4 to 8 liters per minute. One major engineering accomplishment has been the development of a mechanism to allow for balance between the left and right sides of circulation. This is needed because the outputs of the left and right sides of the heart are never exactly the same. This is achieved by the creation of an atrial balance chamber, which allows for decreased right-sided stroke volume to maintain this left/right balance. All the surfaces of the AbioCor™ thoracic unit that come into contact with the blood are polyether urethane. The design of the device results in a smooth continuous blood-contacting surface for the entire pathway of blood through the thoracic unit. At the time of surgery, in addition to placing the thoracic unit, an internal battery, internal controller and TET coil are also placed. The internal battery is lithium ion based and is able to power the thoracic unit for up to 20 minutes. The internal controller drives the energy converter in the thoracic unit, monitors the implanted components and transmits data regarding performance of the device to a bedside console via radiofrequency telemetry. These radiofrequency transmissions from the internal controller contain a large amount of information, which can tell the physicians how all the components are functioning at any period in time. This information can also be stored for later retrieval and analysis. The internal TET coil receives high-frequency power that is transmitted across the skin from an external TET coil. The internal TET coil is

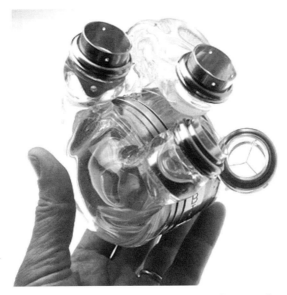

Figure 11.2   Thoracic unit of the AbioCor™ implantable replacement heart system.

able to convert this oscillating current to a direct current that is used to power the thoracic unit and recharge the internal battery.

There are also four external components of this system; an external TET coil, batteries, a TET module and a bedside console. The external TET coil transfers energy across the skin to the internal TET coil and is secured over the internal TET coil with a special adhesive dressing. When the patient is ambulatory, the external TET coil is connected to the portable TET module. The TET module delivers energy to the TET coil from external batteries and contains basic alarm systems. When the patient is not ambulatory, the external TET coil is connected to a bedside console. The bedside console is in turn plugged into a standard wall outlet, which provides energy for the artificial heart. The bedside console is used during implantation of the artificial heart, during the early recovery period and when the patient is in their primary residence. The bedside console contains a graphic user interface for control and monitoring of the implanted systems via radiofrequency communication. The external batteries are lithium ion based and are able to provide up to 1 hour on support per pound of battery. The external batteries can be carried in a vest or handbag or attached to a Velcro belt.

DISCUSSION

Heart failure constitutes a significant health problem of endemic proportion. In the USA alone, there are 250 000 deaths per year attributable to heart failure, with approximately 500 000 new patients diagnosed per year. Furthermore, the prevalence of heart failure is increasing dramatically and, is likely to double in the next 5 years.[8] Multiple studies have demonstrated the high mortality of heart failure. Cowie et al. reported a 12-month survival of 62% in a population-based study of all patients with a new diagnosis of heart failure.[9] Stewart reported a 5-year survival of 25%, and demonstrated that survival was worse for both genders when compared to all common malignancies except lung cancer.[10] The overall population rate of expected life years lost due to heart failure in men and women was 6.7 and 5.1 years per thousand years, respectively. Recent data demonstrate that patients with advanced heart failure who are dependent on intravenous inotropes have a 75% 1-year mortality.[11] The high prevalence combined with a very high mortality provides us with an urgent need to develop alternative therapies. Indeed, the Institute of Medicine has estimated that 60 000 people per year in the USA alone could benefit from some form of cardiac-replacement therapy. Currently, heart transplantation is the only approved method to replace the failing heart. However, the epidemiological impact of heart transplantation is quite limited due to the small number of donor organs. Additionally, there has been a decrease in donor hearts in the USA in 3 of the last 4 years. Transplantation is also limited by strict medical, financial and psychosocial criteria. Recent advances in the field of xenotransplantation[12] have led to renewed interest in this field. However, large immunologic hurdles remain and the demonstration of infection of multiple human cell lines by pig endogenous retrovirus has raised significant questions regarding the potential for xenotransplantation.

The AbioCor™ implantable replacement heart system has been in development for decades and has been designed to serve as a permanent replacement for the failing heart. The system has been developed to be totally implantable without the need for percutaneous lines. In addition to serving as a potential portal for infection, the presence of percutaneous lines limits patient mobility and thereby adversely impacts on quality of life. Energy transfer across the skin to power the device has been accomplished with inductive coupling. The use of radiofrequency transmission from the internal controller has allowed for the physicians and engineers to closely monitor the device performance across the intact skin barrier. Radiofrequency transmissions can also allow for the physicians to adjust the parameters of the device. The initial results of the clinical trial have been impressive.

Another design feature of the device is that it is very quiet and, therefore, does not attract attention to the recipient. This is in contrast to previous artificial heart devices and current assist devices. These other devices generate significant noise when they beat that often draws attention to the recipient. This has had a negative impact on the patient's self-image. Some patients have restricted their activities in public due to noise generated by these devices.

The heart has traditionally been felt to be involved in emotional feelings and responses. However, removal of the heart with replacement by a man-made device does not have any impact on patients' emotional makeup. Patients continued to experience the full gamut of emotional responses. Perhaps the only response that would not occur is the sensation of palpations with fear, stress or excitement. The remainder of the stress responses remain intact. We have not yet had a patient comment on the lack of palpations with stress. All of these recipients have been quite ill and have had to confront their own mortality. After recovery from operation, many patients have devoted themselves to renewing relationships with family and friends.

The patient previously described was the first patient to be discharged to home with an artificial heart. He has been able to resume normal activities and has had a marked improvement in his quality of life. The total time on support with the AbioCor™ implantable replacement heart in all recipients is over 3 years. There have been no device malfunctions with over 1.5 billion beats of the device. We have found that the internal battery has been very important for patient mobility and for allowing brief periods of untethered motion. This has been particularly helpful for allowing patients to shower without being encumbered by external components. We have also found the device to be quite user-friendly, with the patient and their families rapidly becoming well versed and familiar with the device.

In summary, there are a large and increasing number of patients who could benefit from some form of cardiac replacement therapy. Currently, cardiac transplantation is the only available option and is quite limited due to the very small number of donor hearts. However the AbioCor™ implantable replacement heart has been in development for over 4 decades with initiation of clinical trials that began in July 2001. The quiet nature of the device, the use of internal components and the unobtrusiveness of the external components have contributed to a high level of patient acceptability. The initial experience has been extremely impressive with patients being able to be discharged to home with a marked improvement in functional status. The potential role of the AbioCor™ implantable replacement heart in the treatment of end-stage heart failure is quite significant and will be determined by the results of this and future clinical trials.

REFERENCES

1. Braunwald E, Grossman W 1992 Clinical aspects of heart failure. In: Braunwald E ed. Heart disease: a textbook of cardiovascular medicine. 4th edn. Saunders, Philadelphia, 444–463
2. O'Connell JB 2000 The economic burden of heart failure. Clinical Cardiology 23(Suppl. III): 6–10
3. O'Connell JB, Bristow MR 1994 Economic impact of heart failure in the United States: time for a different approach. Journal of Heart and Lung Transplantation 13: S107–112
4. Dowling RD, Etoch SW, Stevens KA et al. 2001 Current status of the AbioCor implantable replacement heart. Annals of Thoracic Surgery 71: S147–149
5. Parnis S, Yu LS, Ochs BD et al. 1994 Chronic in vivo evaluation of an electrohydraulic total artificial heart. ASAIO Journal 40: M489–493
6. Kung RT, Ochs BD, Singh PI 1989 A unique left-right flow balance compensation scheme for an implantable total artificial heart. ASAIO Journal 35: 468–470
7. Kung RT, Yu LS, Ochs B et al. 1993 An atrial hydraulic shunt in a total artificial heart. A balance mechanism for the bronchial shunt. ASAIO Journal 39: M213–217
8. Massie BM, Shah NB 1997 Evolving trends in the epidemiologic factors of heart failure: rationale for preventive strategies and comprehensive disease management. American Heart Journal 133: 703–712
9. Cowie MR, Wood DA, Coats AJS et al. 2000 Survival of patients with a new diagnosis of heart failure: a population based study. Heart 83: 505–510
10. Stewart S, MacIntyre K, Hole D et al. 2001 More 'malignant' than cancer? Five-year survival following a first admission for heart failure. European Journal of Heart Failure 3: 315–322
11. Rose EA, Gelijns AC, Moskowitz AJ et al. 2001 Long-term use of a left ventricular assist device for end-stage heart failure. New England Journal of Medicine 345: 1435–1443
12. Patience C, Takeuchi Y, Weiss RA 1997 Infection of human cells by an endogenous retrovirus of pigs. Nature Medicine 3(3): 282–286

WEBSITES OF INTEREST

AbioCor™ Clinical Trial Information: http://www.abiomed.com/ Fabiocor.html

AbioCor™ Implantable Replacement Heart: http://www.abiomed.com/prodtech/ Fabiocor.html

The Implantable Artificial Heart Project: http://www.heartpioneers.com/

Living through technology

12

Compex Motion: neuroprosthesis for grasping applications

Milos R. Popovic   *Thierry Keller*

SUMMARY

The Compex Motion is a versatile electrical stimulation system with surface stimulation technology that can be used to develop various custom-made neuroprostheses, neurological assessment devices, muscle exercise systems, and experimental set-ups for physiological studies. This stimulator allows users to generate an arbitrary stimulation protocol that can be controlled or regulated using any external sensor, sensory system, or laboratory equipment. The Compex Motion system is modular, providing users with an unlimited number of stimulation channels, and promoting the application of complex sensory systems and user interfaces. This stimulator is specially designed to encourage sharing of stimulation protocols, sensors, and user interfaces. This feature promotes share-ware mentality, which, in our opinion, can be instrumental in accelerating technological developments in the neuroprostheses field. The Compex Motion system is especially designed for rehabilitation treatments administered during early rehabilitation (for example, immediately after stroke or spinal-cord injury), although it can also be applied as a neuroprosthetic system for patients to use in activities of daily living. In this chapter, an example is provided where the Compex Motion system was used to develop a neuroprosthesis for grasping for a 22-year-old male, C5 motor complete, C4 sensory complete, spinal-cord injured patient.

CASE STUDY

A 22-year-old male, C5 motor complete, C4 sensory complete, spinal-cord injured (SCI) patient was admitted to the Toronto Rehabilitation Institute, Lyndhurst Center, Canada, 2 months after sustaining a SCI as a result of an automobile accident. On admission, the patient could place his left hand at almost any point in the arm's workspace, but was unable to voluntarily grasp objects. The patient had good voluntary control of the left shoulder and *biceps m.*, while his left *triceps m.* was graded level 3 (patient could extend his arm against gravity when resistance was not applied to the arm). The patient had no voluntary muscle control on the left arm below the elbow. Furthermore, this right-handed patient had significant difficulty using his right arm, which could only voluntarily cover 30–40% of the right hand's workspace. The patient had limited voluntary control of the right shoulder and *biceps m.* His right *triceps m.* was graded level 2 (patient could extend the arm against gravity when resistance was not applied to the arm). The patient had no voluntary control of any muscles below the right elbow. At the time the patient was admitted to the functional electrical stimulation (FES) program at Toronto Rehabilitation Institute, he had score A on the American Spinal Injury Association (ASIA) impairment scale, which assesses sensory and motor function. Score A indicates complete injury, i.e. no sensory or motor function is preserved in the sacral segments S4-S5.

This patient was a good candidate for a left-arm grasping neuroprosthesis. A neuroprosthesis is a device that applies short, low-intensity electrical pulses to the paralyzed muscles to cause the muscles to contract on demand. By stimulating a desired group of muscles and by properly sequencing their contractions, a neuroprosthesis can generate functions such as hand opening and closing. In order to generate these functions, the muscles that need to be stimulated, must be enervated (motor neurons that project from the spinal cord towards the muscles of interest need to be intact).

This patient was fitted with a neuroprosthesis that allowed him to grasp both large and bulky objects, as well as small and light objects. The neuroprosthesis was developed using the Compex Motion electric stimulator manufactured by a Swiss-based company, Compex SA. This stimulator has four stimulation channels and is fully programmable, i.e. the stimulation protocol can be tailored to fit any patient's need. In this particular case, the stimulation protocol developed, allowed the patient to generate both lateral (to hold smaller, thinner objects) and palmar grasps (to hold bigger, heavier objects) on demand. Stimulation channel No. 1 was used to stimulate the *flexor digitorum superficialis m.* and the *flexor digitorum profundus m.* to generate finger flexion. Stimulation channel No. 2 was used to stimulate the *flexor pollicis longus m.* to generate thumb flexion. Stimulation channel No. 3 was used to stimulate the *median nerve* to produce thumb adduction. Stimulation channel No. 4 was used to stimulate the *extensor digitorium communis m.* to generate hand opening. The patient used a push button to command the neuroprosthesis. By pressing a push button for less than 0.5 s continuously, the patient would issue the lateral grasp command, and by pressing it longer than 1 s continuously, the patient would issue the palmar grasp command. Upon receiving the command, the neuroprosthesis would execute the desired grasping function instantaneously and would maintain this grasp until the next command was issued. By pressing a push button for the second time for less than 0.5 s, the patient would command hand-opening function. This system was deliberately designed so that the hand-opening function did not precede the hand-closure function. We found that the patient had more success in grasping an object if he first manipulated it with both hands and then, prior to grasping it, oriented and placed the object in his left hand. In other words, the patient used the passive stiffness of his left hand and fingers to manipulate and orient the object before the FES grasp was executed. If the patient's hand was opened with FES prior to the grasp, the patient often experienced difficulties orienting the object properly, thus had difficulties preparing the object to be grasped.

Without the neuroprosthesis, the patient was not able to grasp any object. After 2 months of FES training (three to four sessions per week, lasting less than 45 minutes per session), the patient was able to significantly increase his grasping abilities and was able to reach, grasp, and manipulate a variety of objects, such as a tea cup, paper sheet, pencil, video tape, can of coke, tooth brush, and fork. All these objects were used by the patient in the activities of daily living.

NEUROPROSTHESES AND FUNCTIONAL ELECTRICAL STIMULATION

For more than 30 years, electrical stimulation of peripheral nerves has been applied to restore or improve body functions such as walking, hearing, bladder voiding, and grasping.[1] By applying bursts of low-intensity electrical pulses, an electric stimulator creates action potentials in a stimulated nerve, which, depending on the nerve's function (nerve projected to a muscle or a part of the central nervous system), can cause muscle contractions, elicit a reflex, or help a deaf person to hear (Fig. 12.1). Since action potentials that are elicited with electric stimulation propagate along the axons, the stimulated nerves need to be intact. If a nerve is damaged, the degree of its damage will determine the efficacy with which electric stimulation elicits action potentials in the nerve. Severely injured or severed nerves prohibit the use of electric

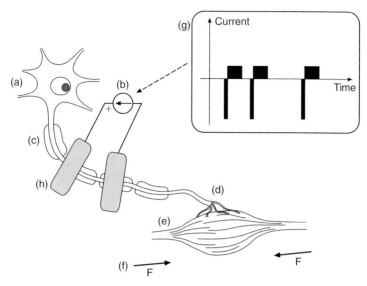

Figure 12.1 Simplified schematic diagram of functional electrical stimulation system:
a) motorneuron that projects axon from the spinal cord towards a muscle;
b) electric stimulator, i.e. current generator; c) nerve axon; d) axon terminals; e) muscle;
f) contraction forces generated by electric stimulation; g) stimulation pulses (typical
values for surface electrical stimulation are: pulse amplitude 10–100 mA, pulse frequency
20–40 Hz and pulse width 50–300 μs); and h) stimulation electrodes.

stimulation. Electric stimulators for medical applications are most frequently
applied as orthoses or neuroprostheses that are used to assist patients in performing the above-mentioned body functions in their activities of daily living
(ADL). These devices are also called functional electrical stimulation (FES)
systems. In this chapter, FES systems used for grasping will be discussed.

FES systems generate short repetitive electric pulses of 100–300 μs. Twenty
to forty such pulses per second are required to generate a tetanic muscle contraction, necessary for a functional articulation of a limb. In principle, the
nerves can be stimulated using monophasic or biphasic current or voltage
pulses.[2] Since monophasic stimulation pulses can cause skin burns and tissue damage (due to galvanic processes), the majority of electric stimulation
systems today implement either biphasic pulses or so-called monophasic
compensated pulses.[3] Many researchers and practitioners in the field prefer
to use current, instead of voltage stimulation pulses, because current stimulation pulses allow full control over the amount of electric charge induced
into the tissue. The electric stimulation pulses can be delivered to the nerve
using surface (transcutaneous), inserted (percutaneous), or implanted electrodes. The transcutaneous stimulation is performed with self-adhesive
or non-adhesive electrodes placed on the subject's skin in the vicinity of
the motor point of the muscle that needs to be stimulated. A motor point
is defined as the region of easiest excitability of a muscle. Percutaneous

electrodes, also known as intramuscular electrodes, are inserted into the muscle using epidermic needles.[4,5] Implanted electrodes are subdivided into two main categories, epimysial,[6] and cuff electrodes.[7,8] The epimysial stimulation electrodes are placed on (sutured to) the muscles, while the cuff electrodes are 'wrapped' around the nerve that is stimulated. Compared to surface stimulation electrodes, implanted and inserted electrodes can provide higher stimulation selectivity while applying lower amounts of electric charge. These are desirable characteristics of electric stimulation systems.[3,9] However, implanted electrodes, such as epimysial and cuff electrodes, require a surgical intervention to place the electrodes, and many subjects who could potentially benefit from the electric stimulation are reluctant to undergo a surgical intervention to be able to use this technology.

Neuroprostheses for grasping

In tetraplegic and stroke patients, hand function is the most important function in achieving a high level of independence in ADL. The extent to which these patients can use their hands represents a measure of their independence. In principle, the grasping function can be differentiated into holding and manipulation tasks, which again can be differentiated in mono- or bi-manual handling tasks. The main objective in applying FES in tetraplegic and stroke patients is to improve the hand function by creating a reliable and long-lasting power grasp, or a smooth pulp-pinch grasp that is needed to manipulate small objects. Regardless of the grasping strategy, it is essential that the patient can easily command the grasp and adjust the strength of grasp. In supporting the hand function, the FES system must not interfere with the patient's preserved upper-limb function, such as wrist extension or the ability to position the arm/hand at the desired place. Furthermore, the hand and arm movements generated by the FES should not oppose natural joint movements and must respect the anatomy of bone and soft-tissue composition.

The available neuroprostheses for grasping are able to restore two most frequently used grasping styles: the palmar and the lateral grasp.[10] The palmar grasp is used to hold bigger and heavier objects, such as cans and bottles, and the lateral grasp is used to hold smaller and thinner objects, such as keys, paper, and floppy disks. The lateral grasp is generated by first flexing the fingers to provide opposition, followed by the thumb flexion. The palmar grasp is generated by first forming the opposition between the thumb and the palm, followed by simultaneous flexion of both the thumb and the fingers. Finger flexion is performed by stimulating the *flexor digitorum superficialis m.* and the *flexor digitorum profundus m.* Finger extension is obtained by stimulating the *extensor digitorium communis m.* The stimulation of the thumb's *thenar muscle* or the *median nerve* produces thumb adduction, and the stimulation of the *flexor pollicis longus m.* or the *flexor pollicis brevis m.* produces thumb flexion. Typically, the stimulation sites and sequences of the neuroprosthesis for grasping have to be customized, and cannot be predicted simply from the neurological level of lesion. Therefore, various grasping strategies have to be evaluated to find the FES grasp that is functionally most useful for the patient.

The well-known neuroprostheses for grasping include the *Freehand system*,[6] *Handmaster*,[11] *Bionic Glove*,[12] *NEC-FES system*,[4] and the systems developed by Vodovnik et al.[13] and Popovic et al.[14] A few years ago, our team also developed a neuroprosthesis for grasping, better known as the *ETHZ-ParaCare neuroprosthesis*.[10] With the exception of the Freehand and NEC-FES systems, all other neuroprostheses for grasping are FES systems with surface-stimulation technology. Only the Freehand and Handmaster systems are currently available on the market while other neuroprostheses are primarily used in laboratory environments.

The Freehand system has up to eight implanted epimysial stimulation electrodes and an implanted stimulator. The stimulation electrodes are used to generate flexion and extension of the fingers and the thumb. One stimulation electrode is frequently used to provide biofeedback to the subject, i.e. to stimulate the subject's afferent nerves, informing him/her that the stimulator is working. The hand closure and the hand opening are commanded using a position sensor that is placed on the shoulder of the subject's opposite arm. The position sensor monitors two axes of shoulder motion, protraction/retraction and elevation/depression. The control strategy can be varied to fit the different shoulder motion capabilities of the subject. Typically, the protraction/retraction motion of the shoulder is used as a proportional signal for hand opening and closing. The shoulder elevation/depression motion is used to generate logic commands that are used to establish a zero level for the protraction/retraction command, and to 'freeze' the stimulation levels ('locking') until the next logic command is issued. An additional switch is also provided to allow a user to choose between palmar and lateral grasp strategies. The shoulder position sensor and the controller are not implanted. The Freehand system was the first neuroprosthesis for grasping approved by the USA Food and Drug Administration (FDA). Thus far, the Freehand system has been made available to more than 130 patients and is commercially available. One of the main advantages of the Freehand system is that it is implanted and the time needed to put on (donning) and to take of (doffing) the system is significantly shorter compared to most surface-stimulation FES systems. On the other hand, the Freehand system can be applied only 18–24 months after the injury and is only suitable for SCI subjects and not individuals suffering from stroke. Therefore, the Freehand system is not suitable for rehabilitation applications and can only be used as a permanent neuroprosthetic device. Furthermore, the patients are often subjected to additional surgery required to replace failed hardware components, or to correct the positioning of the stimulation electrodes.

The Handmaster is a neuroprosthesis for grasping with three pairs of surface-stimulation electrodes. This system can be used to generate a grasping function in tetraplegic and stroke patients. Originally, this system was envisioned as an exercise and rehabilitation tool, but it is also used as a permanent prosthetic system. The Handmaster is controlled with a push button that triggers hand opening and closing, and the patient can regulate the way in which the thumb flexes with a sliding resistor. This feature allows a patient to adjust the grasp to the size and the shape of the object they want to grasp. In addition, the subject can increase or decrease the grasping force using two additional push buttons. One of the advantages of the Handmaster is that it is easy to put on and to take off. The Handmaster is predominately used as an exercise tool for stroke subjects and is commercially available in a limited number of countries. One of the disadvantages of the Handmaster is that it does not provide the user with sufficient freedom to place the stimulation electrodes. In addition, the Handmaster's orthosis is too short and does not allow stimulation of the finger flexors at a proximal position on the forearm. This location of stimulation electrodes provides good finger-flexion with negligible wrist-flexion activity. Another limitation of this system is its stiff orthosis that restricts the range of the wrist motion. In particular, the subjects cannot perform full supination.

State of the art in the functional electrical stimulation field

Although implanted and surface electrical stimulation systems have been used extensively for more than 3 decades, the majority of these devices were developed with very specific FES applications in mind. Therefore, if one wanted to use an electric stimulator to carry out a different function (e.g. standing) other than the specific application that it was originally designed for (e.g. grasping), the user had to modify either the stimulator's hardware, software or both. Since such alterations are often impractical, many researchers and practitioners in the FES field were forced to develop their own stimulators. As a result, numerous electric stimulators have been developed, but FES practitioners and researchers continue to have overwhelming difficulties finding a standardized, programmable, reliable, and versatile electric stimulator that can be used for diverse FES applications. Thus, the level of success in the FES field is positively correlated to the amount of technical support available to the research team. In other words, rehabilitation centers, which are able to provide substantial technical support to their FES teams often have successful neuroprostheses programs, while other institutions without the necessary technical support, often close their FES programs after a brief period of experimenting with the technology. Consequently, FES technology has had limited impact on stroke and SCI rehabilitation, and is found in only a few rehabilitation centers worldwide.

Another important issue in the FES field is that many researchers believe that neuroprostheses should be used primarily as prosthetic devices. This means that each patient should have their own FES system to be used at home in ADL. This approach does have its merit, especially in the case of patients with complete SCI, and is used as the basic premise for developing implanted FES systems. However, recent studies indicate that a significant population of stroke and SCI patients could also benefit from FES rehabilitation.[15–17] In particular, it was found that stroke and incomplete SCI patients subjected to intensive FES treatment post injury were able to recover grasping or walking function faster and better than patients who did not participate in the FES treatment. These results clearly indicate the need for a reliable, portable, programmable, and versatile surface FES system. Such a system could be used in early rehabilitation to promote functional recovery rather than being used as a permanent prosthetic or orthotic device. In addition, access to a stimulator that would allow FES practitioners to freely exchange stimulation protocols in the form of libraries (e.g. a protocol for hand grasp for C5 SCI subjects that applies EMG control or a protocol for treating sub-luxation in stroke patients) would dramatically simplify and encourage the application of this technology. This strategy of knowledge sharing, combined with reliable and versatile surface FES technology, could potentially become instrumental in making a neuroprosthesis a more appealing rehabilitation tool for stroke and SCI patients.

In this chapter a new electric stimulator called Compex Motion is presented. The Compex Motion stimulator represents a further evolution and expansion of the ETHZ-ParaCare neuroprosthesis.[10] This electric stimulator exemplifies a type of technology that provides all the advanced FES application and control features, and yet, is simple to apply in a standard rehabilitation setting. The Compex Motion stimulator can be used to develop various custom-made neuroprostheses, neurological assessment devices, muscle-exercise systems, and experimental setups for physiological studies. It can be programmed to generate any arbitrary stimulation sequence that can be controlled or regulated using any external sensor, sensory system, or laboratory equipment. Each stimulator has four output channels, and any number of stimulators can be combined to form a multiple unit with a greater number of stimulation channels (8, 12, 16,...). The stimulation sequences are stored on readily exchangeable memory chip-cards. By replacing the chip-card, the function of the stimulator is changed instantaneously to provide another function or FES treatment. The Compex Motion stimulator is being manufactured by the Swiss-based company, Compex SA. A company is currently being sought to market this product.

COMPEX MOTION: FES SYSTEM WITH SURFACE STIMULATION ELECTRODES

The Compex Motion stimulator was designed to serve as a hardware platform for development of diverse FES systems that apply surface stimulation technology (Fig. 12.2). One of the main design requirements for the system was that it could be easily programmable and that even individuals with limited FES experience could generate useful stimulation protocols with the system. In addition, the stimulator is also capable of providing sophisticated stimulation protocols and control features commonly used in FES research. Furthermore, the system was designed to allow FES practitioners the ability to apply the same device to a number of different clients requiring distinct stimulation protocols, and to be able to treat one client after another with virtually zero 'transition' time between treatments. To satisfy these needs, the stimulator was designed such that it is programmed with a graphical user interface software, which is installed on a personal computer (PC). As shown in Figure 12.3, a user can program the stimulation sequence using a PC and then transfer the complete stimulation protocol to the stimulator via serial port connection. During the transfer, the stimulation protocol is programmed onto a chip-card, which is inserted into the stimulator. After the transfer is completed, the chip-card will contain all the relevant information that is needed to execute the stimulation protocol, such as stimulation parameters, stimulation sequence, data about the sensors that need to be interfaced by the stimulator, signal processing that needs to be carried out with the input signals from the sensors, control strategies that need to be applied to regulate

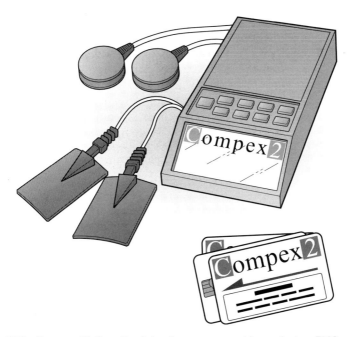

Figure 12.2 Compex Motion stimulator, three memory chip-cards, two EMG sensors and two stimulation electrodes.

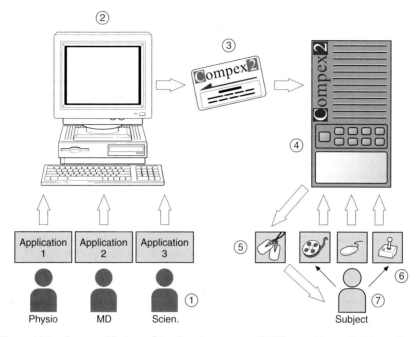

Figure 12.3 Compex Motion – Stimulator's concept: 1) FES practitioner, 2) PC used to program the stimulation protocol, 3) programmable chip-card, 4) stimulator, 5) surface stimulation electrodes, 6) sensors subject is using to trigger and control the stimulation sequences and intensity, and 7) end user.

the stimulation sequences, etc. By simply replacing the chip-card, the function of the stimulator is changed instantaneously to provide a different function or FES treatment.

The main hardware and software features of Compex Motion stimulator are:

- The unit is portable.
- Each unit has four stimulation channels, and any number of stimulators can be combined to form a multiple unit with a greater number of stimulation channels (8, 12, 16,…).
- The pulse amplitude, duration and frequency are independently controlled and can be changed during the stimulation in real time.
- The stimulation channels are galvanically separated.
- The stimulator is powered by a rechargeable battery and the only limitation in stimulation duration is imposed by the battery's capacity, which can support over 8 hours of continuous stimulation per charging.
- The stimulator can be interfaced/controlled with any external sensor, sensory system, or laboratory equipment.
- The systems reliability matches the reliability of standard consumers electronic devices.

EXAMPLES OF COMPEX MOTION APPLICATIONS

Thus far, more than 30 SCI and stroke patients have used the Compex Motion stimulator at ParaCare, University Hospital, Balgrist, located in Zurich, Switzerland and Toronto Rehabilitation Institute, located in Toronto, Canada. The system was primarily used as neuroprostheses for grasping and walking. One patient used the device to treat shoulder subluxation and a few others used it for muscle strengthening. The Compex Motion stimulator was also used to investigate muscle properties in animal studies and in closed-loop muscle-control applications at ParaCare. Other applications of the Compex Motion system, such as neuroprosthesis for standing, breathing, and sitting, are currently being explored. An example of a clinical application of Compex Motion is presented in this section. The example describes a neuroprosthesis for grasping applied to a C5, complete SCI patient. The performance and the impact of the neuroprosthesis on the patient will also be discussed in this section.

Neuroprosthesis for grasping

As discussed in the case study section of this chapter, a grasping neuroprosthesis was developed for a 22-year-old male, C5 motor complete, C4 sensory complete, SCI patient. The patient was admitted to our FES program 2 months after sustaining a SCI. The left arm was chosen for the neuroprosthesis application because the patient could place the left hand at almost any point in the arm's work space, and the muscles that needed to be stimulated were not denervated. The patient had good voluntary control of the left shoulder and *biceps m.*, while his left *triceps m.* was graded level 3. When the patient was admitted to the FES program at Toronto Rehabilitation Institute, he had ASIA score A.

The patient was fitted with a neuroprosthesis that allowed him to grasp both large and bulky objects, and small and light objects. Hence, a stimulation protocol was developed that allowed the patient to generate both lateral and palmar grasps on demand (Fig. 12.4). Stimulation channel No. 1 was used to stimulate the *flexor digitorum superficialis m.* and the *flexor digitorum profundus m.* to generate finger flexion. Stimulation channel No. 2 was used to stimulate the *flexor pollicis longus m.* to generate thumb flexion. Stimulation channel No. 3 was used to stimulate the *median nerve* to produce thumb adduction. Stimulation channel No. 4 was used to stimulate the *extensor digitorium communis m.* to generate hand opening. The patient used a push button to command the neuroprosthesis. By pressing a push button for less than 0.5 s continuously, the patient would issue user interaction A command (UI-A in Fig. 12.5) and by pressing it longer than 1 s continuously, the patient would issue user interaction B command (UI-B in Fig. 12.5). The user interaction A was used to command the lateral grasp and the user interaction B was used

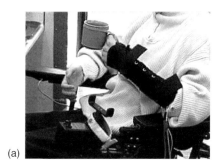 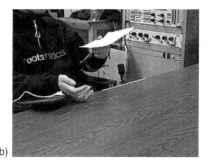

(a)   (b)

Figure 12.4 Patient with the neuroprosthesis for grasping: (a) palmar grasp, (b) lateral grasp.

to command the palmar grasp. By generating the user interaction A or B command, the neuroprosthesis would instantaneously produce the lateral or palmar grasp, respectively.

An important feature of this neuroprosthesis for grasping is that it also stimulates the *flexor pollicis longus m.*, which generates thumb flexion. An advantage of stimulating the *flexor pollicis longus m.* rather than stimulating the *median nerve* or thumb's *thenar muscle* alone, is that one can generate a proper thumb flexion. When the *median nerve* or thumb's *thenar muscle* is stimulated alone, the thumb produces opposition movement. This opposition movement combined with finger flexion is often used to generate the palmar grasp. However, this grasp is weaker and less stable than the grasp, which is generated with thumb opposition in addition to thumb flexion. Therefore, stimulation of the *flexor pollicis longus m.* is a beneficial and desirable feature. A combination of thumb flexion and opposition, together with finger flexion was used to generate the palmar grasp. The lateral grasp is generated by combining finger flexion and thumb flexion. Stimulation of the *flexor pollicis longus m.* is a common feature in implanted FES systems, such as the Freehand system,[6] but is very rarely found in surface FES systems because the *flexor pollicis longus m.* is difficult to access using surface FES due to its anatomical location in the forearm. The origin of the *flexor pollicis longus m.* is the anterior surface of body of radius below tuberosity, the interosseous membrane, medial border of coronoid process of ulna and/or medial epicondyle of humerus. The insertion of the *flexor pollicis longus m.* is the base of the distal phalanx of the thumb, palmar surface. The *flexor pollicis longus m.* in the proximal part of the forearm is a muscle located deep in the forearm and is difficult to access using surface FES. However, at the distal part of the forearm, the *flexor pollicis longus m.* comes close to the skin surface and is surrounded by the *radius, flexor digitorum superficialis m., pronator quadratus m.*, and *flexor digitorum profundus m.* on one side (covering approximately 70% of the muscle surface), and by skin and *tendon m. brachioradialis* on the other (covering approximately 30% of the muscle surface). Since skin and

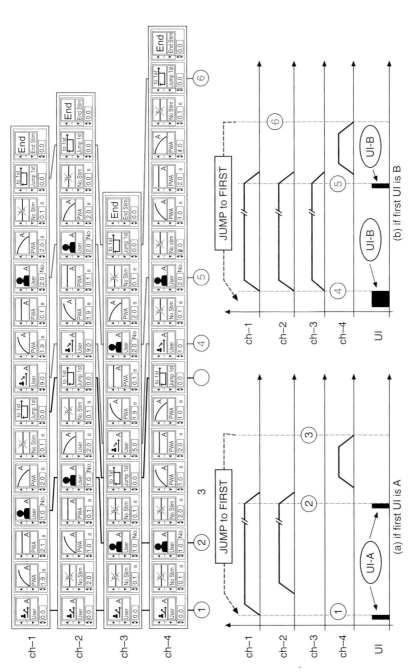

Figure 12.5 Grasping protocol that generates both a) lateral and b) palmar grasps on demand. The upper part of the figure presents primitives in time lines and the lower part represents the outputs for channels 1, 2, 3 and 4. UI-A is user interaction A which is generated if the push button is pressed less than 0.5 s; UI-B is user interaction B which is generated if the push button is pressed longer than 1 s; ch–1, 2, 3 and 4 are stimulation channels; and labels 1 to 6 are used to indicate which primitives in the time lines are responsible for certain stimulation protocol events.

tendon m. brachioradialis do not obstruct the surface electrical stimulation of the *flexor pollicis longus m.*, this site was selected for placement of the stimulation electrode. There are, however, some drawbacks to this stimulation site. When subjects perform pronation, the *flexor pollicis longus m.* and stimulation electrodes tend to shift and move with respect to one another. This movement may be problematic since it causes a reduction in the overall muscle force. In this particular case, the stimulation electrodes were positioned such that sufficient flexion force was achieved with the thumb during pronation and supination. In general, we were successful in stimulating the *flexor pollicis longus m.* in a limited number of patients (two patients out of seven).

We should point out that the stimulation of the *flexor digitorum superficialis m.* and the *flexor digitorum profundus m.* caused patients to experience weak wrist flexion. We compensated for this side effect by providing patients with a wrist retainer that was integrated into a glove which patients used in combination with the neuroprosthesis.

Achieved results with the neuroprosthesis for grasping

When the patient was first admitted to the FES program he was unable to grasp any object. As a result of the FES training, the patient significantly increased his grasping abilities and was able to reach, grasp, and manipulate a variety of objects, such as a telephone receiver, tea cup, mug, pencil, envelope, can of coke, and video tape. The patient was able to use all of these objects in ADL. However, there were some objects that the patient was unable to grasp and manipulate even while using the FES system. Typical examples of these objects include a catheter, packaged gaze, lighter, and wallet. A common factor shared among all these objects was that they required two dexterous hands in order for the objects to be manipulated properly. Since the patient had only one arm instrumented with the neuroprosthesis, it was not unexpected that he would have difficulties manipulating these objects. Despite these limitations, the patient was content with the system's performance and requested a system for home use.

An unexpected and intriguing outcome resulted from this study. As we indicated earlier, prior to the FES treatment, the patient was unable to grasp any objects voluntarily, but with the neuroprosthesis, the patient was able to manipulate a significant number of tools and objects. However, after the completion of the FES training, it was found that the patient was able to manipulate 80% of these objects, in the absence of the neuroprosthesis. This is an important result, especially since the patient's neurological condition did not change, nor did the patient experience any neurological recovery during the treatment. Thus, by the end of the treatment, the patient was still classified as a C5 motor complete and C4 sensory complete SCI. At this time, we can only offer one explanation for this finding. As a result of FES training, the patient had learned a number of tricks and techniques to effectively approach and grasp objects. These tricks were easier to learn when the patient felt a sense of security that he would not drop the objects while manipulating them. The use of FES during grasping helps patients feel more confident that objects are safe and secure in the patient's hand while using or grasping them. An additional positive side effect of FES treatment is that the patient's muscles and tendons are strengthened, which in turn provides additional passive stiffness to the hand and fingers. We have observed that stiffer hands and fingers frequently helped patients manipulate lighter objects and objects which have rougher surfaces. Our current work at Toronto Rehabilitation Institute will investigate the extent repetitive treatments with neuroprosthesis for grasping will have on C5 to C6 complete SCI patients and how this could improve grasping function. This approach represents a departure from the current trend in the FES field, where neuroprostheses for grasping were considered primarily as prosthetic systems for C5 to C6 complete SCI patients. The preliminary study results obtained from this and two additional patients are very encouraging.

Impact of neuroprosthesis for grasping on SCI patients

Over the course of 5 years, more than 20 SCI patients have used the neuroprosthesis for grasping. In general, after the first few FES sessions, all patients expressed overwhelming enthusiasm and were impressed with the movement the system helped them generate in their otherwise paralyzed hands. However, as the patients became more familiar with the neuroprosthesis technology over time, their acceptance of this technology started to differ. To date, we were able to distinguish between three patient group views regarding the neuroprosthesis for grasping technology. The first group consisted of 60–70% of the patients who remained very enthusiastic about the FES treatment and eagerly participated in the treatment until completion. These patients were all informed that FES treatments would not help them achieve neurological recovery, yet they voluntarily continued to participate in the program. In fact, some of these patients expressed interest in taking these systems home to use in ADL. Overall, these patients were content with the treatment outcome and did not express disappointment when they were not offered a system for home use. On the contrary, despite the constant reminders that FES technology would not help individuals achieve neurological recovery, the second group of patients continued to believe that FES treatment would help them regain voluntary control of their arm and hand muscles. These patients were often disappointed when they finally realized that their expectations were not rational. Due to the 'awakening', some of these patients abandoned the program all together, while others took a short break from the program and resumed it a number of weeks later. Less than 10% of our patients belonged to this group. The third group consisted of patients who were very content with the treatment and its outcomes for the first 4–6 weeks. After this time, these patients requested additional sophisticated features to be added to the system and were disappointed with the systems' overall performance. These patients were often disappointed that the system could only generate gross motor function and could not allow for more dexterous finger manipulations. These patients often got disenchanted with the treatment and after 8–10 weeks, withdrew from the program. We should point out that all individuals in this group expressed interest in resuming FES treatment once the technology became 'more advanced' and could facilitate grasping tasks, which they considered relevant. Approximately 20–30% of our patients belonged to this category.

Another interesting observation is that the majority of patients were very conscious of the aesthetic aspects of the neuroprosthesis. However, other patients were not concerned with the aesthetics at all, but were more interested with its performance. This latter group consisted of individuals who were older or who had had a SCI for 2 or 3 years prior to being admitted to the FES program. Without an exception, all patients provided good suggestions on the system design, including how to mount it on a wheelchair, and how to simplify its interfaces.

What was the overall impact of the neuroprosthesis for grasping on our patients? This is a very difficult question to answer. Our impression is that the impact is positive and significant, and we strongly believe that all our patients who participated in the program benefited considerably from the FES treatment. However, we have not yet conducted a study that confirms our subjective impressions. Our current efforts at Toronto Rehabilitation Institute and ParaCare are aimed at demonstrating how significant improvements to grasping function are, as a direct result of FES treatment, and how much this improvement correlates to the number of treatment sessions. In addition to this study, we intend to assess the consumers' perception on neuroprosthesis for grasping. This second study will be undertaken by a research team at Toronto Rehabilitation Institute, which is independent of our group. These two studies should provide quantitative and qualitative measures of the impact neuroprosthesis for grasping technology has on consumers. These data will be used to assess the effectiveness of the device and to provide suggestions for further improving the Compex Motion and the neuroprosthesis for grasping systems.

FUTURE PROSPECTS

The Compex Motion electric stimulation system represents a versatile system that can be applied as a hardware platform to develop various custom-made neuroprostheses, neurological assessment devices, muscle-exercise systems, and experimental set-ups for physiological studies. This stimulator provides all advanced FES application and control features, yet, it can be easily applied to standard rehabilitation settings. The Compex Motion stimulator can be programmed to generate any arbitrary stimulation sequence, which can be controlled or regulated using any external sensor, sensory system, or laboratory equipment. We believe that this device can potentially resolve a number of challenges that are currently facing the FES field, such as:

- The Compex Motion stimulator allows one to generate any arbitrary stimulation protocol. Developed protocols can be easily exchanged among FES practitioners. This feature would allow the users to collectively test and incrementally improve the stimulation protocols with the objective of standardizing reliable and widely accepted stimulation protocols. This would allow FES practitioners to share their stimulation protocols with other FES users, and would promote share-ware and open-source mentality in the field. This approach was instrumental in developing numerous technically challenging fields, and would most certainly be beneficial to future developments in the FES field. This is currently impossible to do with the existing FES technology.
- Since Compex Motion can be controlled by any sensor and sensory systems, the existing 'FES sensors' and man–machine interfaces can be configured to interface the stimulator. This would allow FES practitioners to share their sensor technology with other FES users as discussed above. Compex Motion user interface primitives and functions that allow regulation of stimulation amplitudes via analog input signals can dramatically simplify development of these interfaces. Thus far, our team has developed a number of sensory systems and man–machine interfaces that are reliable and can be used to control the stimulator. Some of these systems are: Gait Phase Detection System,[18] EMG measurement sensor combined with the signal processing routines for stimulation artifacts removal,[19,20] sliding resistor control strategy,[10] and voice control module (not yet published).
- FES gloves, garments and other user interfaces can be developed for the stimulator. The sharing of successful user interfaces would further simplify donning and doffing of stimulation electrodes. Our team is currently developing a glove that will be used for quicker donning and doffing of stimulation electrodes for neuroprosthesis for grasping.
- Modularity of the Compex Motion system, which allows one to have an unlimited number of stimulation channels and promotes application of complex sensory systems and user interfaces, would allow practitioners to acquire modules one by one, instead of buying an expensive complex FES system all at once. This feature would allow institutions and laboratories with limited budgets to acquire a high-quality FES system, in addition to allowing them to incorporate the system instantaneously into their research or rehabilitation environment. Later, if needed, they could add additional modules and sensory interfaces to the system, enhancing its capabilities.

- The final point is that the Compex Motion system is non-invasive and can be applied at various stages of recovery and rehabilitation. Since implanted FES systems are mainly suitable for long-term FES treatments and should be used as prosthetic devices, we believe that Compex Motion is appropriate for rehabilitation treatments, especially those treatments that are administered during early rehabilitation (for example, immediately after stroke or SCI). However, Compex Motion can also be used as a prosthetic system that the patient can apply in ADL. Often surface stimulation systems are more appealing to patients, compared to implanted systems, since their application does not involve surgical intervention.

ACKNOWLEDGEMENTS

The work on this project was supported by the Swiss Federal Committee for Technology and Innovation, the Swiss National Science Foundation, the Natural Sciences and Engineering Research Council of Canada and Toronto Rehabilitation Institute.

We would like to acknowledge the support of our colleagues Ms Marlene Adams, Ms Veronica Takes, and Mr AbdulKadir Bulsen who provided us with the neuroprosthesis for grasping example, and Ms Betty Chan and Ms Zina Bezruk for helping us with the document editing.

REFERENCES

1. Popovic D, Sinkjaer T 2000 Control of movement for the physically disabled. Springer, London
2. Baker LL, McNeal DR, Benton LA et al. 2000 Neuromuscular electrical stimulation – a practical guide, 3rd edn. USA: Rehabilitation Engineering Program, Los Amigos Research and Education Institute, Rancho Los Amigos Medical Center
3. Mortimer JT 1981 Motor prostheses. In: Brooks VB ed. Handbook of physiology – the nervous system II. American Physiological Society, 155–187
4. Hoshimiya N, Handa Y 1989 A master-slave type multichannel functional electrical stimulation (FES) system for the control of the paralyzed upper extremities. Automedica 11: 209–220
5. Cameron T, Loeb GE, Peck RA et al. 1997 Micromodular implants to provide electrical stimulation of paralyzed muscles and limbs. IEEE Transactions Biomedical Engineering 44(9): 781–790
6. Smith B, Peckham PH, Keith MW et al. 1987 An externally powered, multichannel, implantable stimulator for versatile control of paralyzed muscle. IEEE Transactions on Biomechanical Engineering 34(7): 499–508
7. Grill WM, Mortimer JT 1998 Stability of the input-output properties of chronically implanted multiple contact nerve cuff electrodes. IEEE Transactions on Rehabilitation Engineering 6: 364–373
8. Tyler DJ, Durand DM 1997 A slowly penetrating interfascicular nerve electrodes for selective activation of peripheral nerves. IEEE Transactions on Rehabilitation Engineering 5(1): 51–61

9. Kobetic R, Morsolais EB 1994 Synthesis of paraplegic gait with multichannel functional neuromuscular stimulation. IEEE Transactions on Rehabilitation Engineering 2(2): 66–78
10. Popovic MR, Keller T, Pappas IPI et al. 2001 Surface-stimulation technology for grasping and walking neuroprostheses. IEEE Engineering in Medicine and Biology Magazine 20(1): 82–93
11. Ijzerman MJ, Stoffers TS, Groen FACG et al. 1996 The NESS Handmaster orthosis: restoration of hand function in C5 and stroke patients by means of electrical stimulation. Journal of Rehabilitation Sciences 9(3): 86–89
12. Prochazka A, Gauthier M, Wieler M et al. 1997 The Bionic Glove: an electrical stimulator garment that provides controlled grasp and hand opening in quadriplegia. Archives of Physical Medicine and Rehabilitation 78(6): 608–614
13. Rebersek S, Vidovnik L 1973 Proportionally controlled functional electrical stimulation of hand. Archives of Physical Medicine and Rehabilitation 54: 168–172
14. Popovic D, Popovic M, Stojanovic A et al. 1998 Clinical evaluation of the Belgrade Grasping System. In: Proceedings of the 6th Vienna International Workshop on Functional Electrical Stimulation, September 22–24, 247–250
15. Popovic DB, Popovic MB, Sinkjaer T 2002 Neurorehabilitation of upper extremities in humans with sensory-motor impairment. Neuromodulation 5(1): 54–67
16. Field-Fote EC 2001 Combined use of body weight support, functional electrical stimulation, and treadmill training to improve walking ability in individuals with chronic incomplete spinal cord injury. Archives of Physical Medicine and Rehabilitation 82: 818–824
17. Wieler M, Stein RB, Ladouceur M et al. 1999 Multicenter evaluation of electrical stimulation systems for walking. Archives of Physical Medicine and Rehabilitation 80: 495–500
18. Pappas IPI, Popovic MR, Keller T et al. 2001 A reliable gait phase detection system. IEEE Transactions on Neural Systems and Rehabilitation Engineering 9(2): 113–125
19. Biofeedback Version 2M4456. 1996 MediCompex SA, Ecublens, Switzerland
20. Keller T, Popovic MR 2001 Stimulation artifact removal algorithm for real-time surface EMG applications. Proceedings 7th Vienna International Workshop on Functional Electrical Stimulation, September 11–13, 118–121

WEBSITES OF INTEREST

Heart and Stroke Foundation of Canada: www.heartandstroke.ca

International Functional Electrical Stimulation Society: www.ifess.org

Rehabilitation Engineering Laboratory Institute of Biomaterials and Biomedical Engineering, University of Toronto: www.utoronto.ca/IBBME/Faculty/Popovic_Milos/rel_uoft.html

Rehabilitation Engineering Group: www.aut.ee.ethz.ch/~fes

Spinal Cord Injury Resources: www.makoa.org/sci.htm

13

Technological enframing in the hemodialysis patient

Aoife Moran   Pamela Gallagher

SUMMARY

Hemodialysis as a modality of treatment for end-stage renal disease has been in existence since the 1960s. As such, it is an early example of the interface between the person and technology for life-saving purposes. The experience of hemodialysis is unique in that our blood leaves the body, is essentially cleansed and is returned in a purified state. Although hemodialysis has enabled many people to achieve aspirations that would otherwise have been impossible, there is often a cost attached. The frequent interactions that the person has with the technology, the acute and long-term physiological and psychosocial manifestations of the treatment, and the culture of the hemodialysis unit in the hospital, may enframe the person in the technology. This chapter will discuss the technological enframing that can occur with hemodialysis and pertinent issues involved in the adjustment process. Despite the fact that hemodialysis has been in existence in some form for more than 40 years, the focus remains primarily on the physical aspects of the technology and the patient, and there is relatively little focus on the psychosocial aspects, despite their potential role in adjustment. This will continue to be a potentially significant deficit in our knowledge particularly with the recent proposals of daily dialysis as a means of counteracting some of the physical effects of hemodialysis. In terms of what is known about psychosocial aspects, there is a gap between the external (i.e. empirical scientific perspective) and the internal (experiential) view. This chapter seeks to bring the two together.

CASE STUDY

Doreen is a 60-year-old lady undergoing hemodialysis therapy for the treatment of end-stage renal disease and attends the hemodialysis unit of the local hospital three times weekly for sessions lasting 4 hours. She commenced hemodialysis therapy 2 years ago following an episode of acute breathlessness caused by pulmonary edema, a symptom of renal failure. When Doreen was first admitted to hospital she felt very unwell and was unable to breathe properly. Initially, she was relieved when the doctor told her that she would need dialysis to remove the fluid and this would make her breathing improve. Doreen was optimistic that once she had dialysis the fluid would be removed from her lungs by the machine and she would be able to go home and be well again. However, when Doreen realized that she would have to have hemodialysis for the rest of her life, she refused to accept it. She heard that a kidney transplant would allow her to avoid hemodialysis and immediately asked her doctor if she could have one. Unfortunately, due to additional medical complications, transplantation was contraindicated. At this time Doreen could not believe what was happening to her, she became angry with everybody, including her husband and family, and just cried all the time. She felt her world was falling apart.

Doreen initially disliked hemodialysis as she was unwell all night afterwards and stayed in bed the following day. She felt that life on hemodialysis 'wasn't living, it was only existing'. Doreen described her first experience of hemodialysis as 'very frightening'. She was shocked and panicked that her condition would get worse and she felt extremely fragile. She would watch the blood flowing out of her body from the central venous catheter through the tubes of the hemodialysis machine and she was afraid that all her blood would be drained away and there would be none left, so she would just sit watching the machine to ensure the blood was returned. She was overwhelmed that other patients were able to read, watch television or eat while on hemodialysis, as she was afraid to move due to fear of something going wrong. In the beginning, Doreen's sons would visit her when she was having hemodialysis to provide support, but they did not enjoy it, as neither of them liked the sight of blood. Doreen became frustrated and angry because they would sit staring at the hemodialysis machine instead of talking to her. She wanted her sons to focus on her, not focus on the machine. Consequently, she decided that they should stop visiting her while she was undergoing dialysis.

While Doreen was having hemodialysis she watched the other women coming and going, and she thought that most of them were probably mothers like her. It saddened her to see how thin and worn out these women looked and she also noticed the unusual coffee color of their skin. She noticed that many patients used sticks to walk or were in wheelchairs, and this frightened and worried Doreen, as she feared she was going to end up like these people. Indeed, the complications of hemodialysis resulted in extreme weakness and an inability to perform normal activities of daily living for Doreen. Prior to commencing hemodialysis therapy Doreen loved her job working with animals. Working with animals held great significance for Doreen, as they were part of her life since childhood. However, due to the time-consuming nature and side effects of hemodialysis treatment Doreen was unable to perform the work she loved which led to frustration, sadness and depression. Initially, she even tried to avoid her own animals altogether and let her family care for them as it upset her too much to see them and reminded her of what she had lost. When Doreen was at her lowest she became very depressed and, at times, very angry and usually directed this anger at the people closest to her such as her husband and her family.

Despite this, her family, friends, healthcare team and local priest were a great source of ongoing support and made Doreen realize that she had to make an effort to cope with dialysis. Eventually, Doreen made the decision that if she was ever to move on and feel happiness again, she had to accept that hemodialysis was part of her life. She had to accept that life would never be the same again and once she did this her life began to turn around and she began to focus on the positive aspects of life; such as her husband, family and grandchildren. Due to the debilitating effects of renal bone disease and an ongoing back problem, Doreen requires a wheelchair to get around outdoors. Initially, her need to use a wheelchair caused sadness and anger, however, she soon realized that she could get out with her family more often and this has brightened her outlook on life considerably. Doreen now spends her time on hemodialysis reading, watching television, sleeping, eating and talking to other patients, all the things she was initially afraid to do. She is happy to report that she has managed to accept the changes in her life caused by hemodialysis. She is grateful to the technology of hemodialysis for alleviating breathlessness and for keeping her alive to see her grandchildren grow up. Doreen sees new patients arrive for their first hemodialysis and feels very sympathetic towards them. She talks to these patients to reassure them that, although it may be difficult at first, there is life on dialysis.

INTRODUCTION

This case study of Doreen reveals the repercussions of hemodialysis therapy on the life of the individual with end-stage renal disease. End-stage renal disease implies that the kidneys are permanently damaged and that a patient can no longer survive independently without renal-replacement therapy.[1] Renal-replacement therapy includes either a kidney transplant or dialysis. However, prior to transplantation patients are placed on a waiting list to ensure a suitable tissue match is established between donor and recipient. The majority of patients are considered suitable for transplantation, but it may be contraindicated for patients with a more complex illness trajectory and additional medical complications.[2] Consequently, it is usual for all patients to commence a modality of renal-replacement therapy.[2,3] Hemodialysis is one modality of treatment for renal disease, which involves removing the person's uremic blood from an artery and filtering it through a dialyzer, or artificial kidney, where the blood is purified and returned to the patient via the venous blood system.[4] Treatment regimes usually include sessions lasting 4 hours three times per week. Although these individuals are dependent on the technology of hemodialysis, they are encouraged to be independent and maintain some semblance of normal living between treatments.[5] As demonstrated in the case study, there are various issues influencing the individual's ability to achieve this aspiration while undergoing hemodialysis therapy and these will be discussed in more detail throughout the chapter.

Historical and philosophical perspectives on the technology of hemodialysis

The emergence of hemodialysis in the 1960s was perceived as a major life-saving therapy, as prior to its evolution the treatment of renal disease was purely palliative.[6] There were various attempts to perform hemodialysis, however, it was not until Scribner and Quinton[7] developed the arteriovenous shunt as a means of circulatory access in 1960 that long-term hemodialysis therapy for renal failure became feasible. According to Bevan,[6] in the early years the technology of hemodialysis was a 'metaphor for experimentation' due to the limited availability of hemodialysis machines. Consequently, patients were selected for treatment based on a functionalist ideology.[6] Functionalism evolved from social work theories where there was a belief that the individual should be enabled to function acceptably and appropriately in society.[8] Patients who were most likely to return to a functional role in society were selected for treatment, as this ensured the success of the technology of hemodialysis.

In 1963, at the Seattle Artificial Kidney Center, the first outpatient center was established to provide hemodialysis therapy to renal patients.[7] Home dialysis was also introduced in 1963 to decrease costs, increase accessibility and enhance social functioning in the patient.[7] Brescia and Cimino in New York developed the arteriovenous fistula in 1966, thus providing a more effective permanent access to the bloodstream.[7] As the demand for hemodialysis increased, more medical centers were established resulting in increased advances in the technology of hemodialysis including improvements in dialyzers, the introduction of disposable equipment and the development of smaller dialysis machines with monitoring equipment.[7] The integration of computer technology with hemodialysis machines and the improvements in dialyzer membranes have resulted in enhanced dialysis efficiency and decreased dialysis time.[7] The increased effectiveness of circulatory access due to innovative surgical and radiological techniques and the introduction of human recombinant erythropoeitin to treat the chronic anemia of renal disease have improved the quality of life of the hemodialysis patient over the years.[7] Subsequently, these advances have resulted in the increased availability of dialysis machines today and the liberalization of the selection criteria. Consequently, patients who would have been excluded from receiving hemodialysis previously are receiving treatment today and this has had a profound impact on the service.[9] The increasing patient numbers for treatment has developed the hemodialysis unit into a processing line of patients for treatment.[9]

Despite the increase in availability of hemodialysis, the emphasis on a functionalist ideology still remains evident today, with the primary aim of treatment being education and rehabilitation in an effort to return the patient to a normal life in society and reduce hospital admissions. However, due to the numerous complications caused by the elongation of life through hemodialysis therapy, some patients are unable to achieve this aspiration. Consequently, the life of the hemodialysis patient has been described as a fabricated existence evoked by having to live an institutionally, normalized life due to dependency on the technology of dialysis.[6] The individual undergoing hemodialysis may attempt to live a normal life, but the treatment regime and the complications of the technology of hemodialysis can mitigate against the achievement of normality. Hence, the technology of dialysis may have prolonged life and functionality, but at what cost to the individual?

Heidegger[10] indicated that technology was introduced as a reductionistic approach to ensure social control, as something to be manipulated and cause an effect on something else. This is evident in the technology of hemodialysis, as the machine must be manipulated to perform the role and functions of the kidney and cause an effect on the patient by returning them to functionality in society. In this way, the technology can be perceived as a method of ensuring social control. Heidegger also asserts that once the presence of technology is revealed to the individual, there is a requirement 'to stand reserve' in order to control the challenge it presents. When the technology of hemodialysis is introduced for the treatment of renal disease it is also imperative that the individual must 'stand reserve' or put their life on hold to abide with the demands of the technology of hemodialysis as a means of avoiding life-threatening complications, e.g. hyperkalemia, pulmonary edema and arrhythmias.

Heidegger also argues that the challenges and demands of the technological framework attempt to enclose all beings into utter availability and sheer manipulability, and in this way the presence of technology is explicitly revealed or uncovered to the individual.[10] This may be witnessed in the technology of hemodialysis as the patient's life is bound by the demands of the treatment regime. This challenging claim of technology, which causes people to 'stand reserve' or put their life on hold may be referred to as *Ge-stell* or enframing. This is the way in which the essence of modern technology is revealed or uncovered to the individual, though, paradoxically, it may be in no way technological.[10]

TECHNOLOGICAL ENFRAMING IN THE HEMODIALYSIS PATIENT

Hemodialysis therapy may lead to technological enframing in the individual. This may occur due to the physical and psychosocial manifestations of the technology of hemodialysis. Although these factors are not explicitly technological, they ensure that the presence of technology is continuously perceived by the individual, and thus contributes to their technological enframing.

Physiological manifestations

During the hemodialysis procedure excess fluid and toxic wastes, e.g. urea and creatinine, which accumulate in the body when the kidneys are no longer functioning, are removed. The physiological principles required to perform this hemodialysis procedure include diffusion, osmosis, ultrafiltration and convection. There are various physiological manifestations of hemodialysis therapy and these can be classified as acute or long term.

The most common acute complications, which occur as a result of the hemodialysis procedure, include hypotension, cramps, nausea and vomiting. Hypotension, or low blood pressure, may lead to nausea and vomiting, and is related to excessive decreases in blood volume.[11] Hypotension is usually caused by a large weight gain in the patient between treatments, resulting in substantial amounts of fluid being removed or ultrafiltrated by the hemodialysis machine.[11] Hypotension may precipitate muscle cramps, as the ultrafiltration of large amounts of fluid during hemodialysis may result in the removal of sodium by convection causing muscle cramps.[11]

Attempts to manage the long-term physiological manifestations of renal disease have become increasingly complex since the introduction of hemodialysis. Uremic symptoms affect many other systems of the body including gastrointestinal, cardiovascular, neurological, ocular, reproductive, hematological and dermatological.[12] Lancaster[13] has outlined the systemic consequences of uremic syndrome on the individual. Alterations in the patient's hematological system include anemia, caused by a reduction in erythropoetin; blood loss during hemodialysis and bleeding abnormalities caused by platelet dysfunction.

Alterations in fluid balance may result in various signs and symptoms due to excess intravascular fluid volume including weight gain, hypertension, pulmonary edema, breathlessness, cough, elevated neck veins and congestive heart failure.[13] Excess extravascular fluid volume may cause edema in such areas as the feet, ankles, hands, fingers, ascites and periorbital area.[13] Bone pain, osteodystrophy and pruritis are long-term consequences of renal disease resulting from alterations in calcium, phosphate, vitamin D, aluminium and parathyroid glands.[13] These manifestations may culminate in insomnia, poor mobility and an inability to perform the activities of daily living for the individual.[14-16] Discoloration of the skin may occur due to retained pigments that are normally excreted by the kidneys and pallor related to anemia.[13]

Alterations in the gastrointestinal system may lead to poor appetite and nausea and vomiting resulting in inadequate nutritional intake.[13] Increased insulin levels may occur due to altered insulin metabolism precipitating hypoglycemia in the hemodialysis patient.[13] Sexual dysfunction may occur due to alterations in endocrine function, poor nutrition, anxiety, side effects of drugs and reduced plasma testosterone in men.[11,17,18] Alterations in immune responsiveness may predispose the renal patient to infections[13] and this may be exacerbated by the numerous invasive procedures required to develop circulatory access for hemodialysis.

Circulatory access is required to perform hemodialysis therapy and may result in long-term complications for the hemodialysis patient. There are three types of circulatory access for hemodialysis including a central venous catheter, an arteriovenous fistula and an arteriovenous graft.[11,19] A central venous catheter involves the implantation of a cuffed dual-lumen catheter into a central vein allowing access to the blood stream for hemodialysis.[11,19] An arteriovenous fistula involves the anastamosis (joining) of an artery to a vein allowing arterial blood to flow through the vein causing enlargement and engorgement of the vein, thus allowing large-bore needles to be inserted during hemodialysis.[19] An arteriovenous graft involves the implantation of a small piece of synthetic tubing between an artery and a vein also allowing the insertion of wide-bore needles to allow the removal and return of the patients blood for hemodialysis.[19] The long-term complications caused by the insertion of circulatory access include infection and thrombosis, and may result in increased hospital admissions for the patient.

To prevent the acute and long-term physiological manifestations of hemodialysis therapy it is imperative that the patient complies with a specific treatment regime. This includes attending the hemodialysis unit three times a week, self-administering many medications and adhering to strict diet and fluid restrictions. The treatment regime arising from the technology of hemodialysis may inflict many psychosocial manifestations on the life of the individual. These manifestations serve to reinforce the all-encompassing nature of technological enframing on the individuals' life.

Psychosocial manifestations of hemodialysis

There are various psychosocial manifestations arising from hemodialysis therapy, which may culminate in the individual becoming enframed in technology. The individual's life may be completely changed due to the uncertainty about the illness trajectory, an inability to achieve life goals and changes in roles and responsibilities from independence to dependence.[20] The physiological manifestations of hemodialysis and the subsequent restrictions of this treatment modality may result in an inability to perform many activities of daily living. These issues may result in unemployment, decreased financial status, social isolation and missed activities.[2,3,21]

The environment of the hemodialysis unit indicates the presence of technology to the individual through the use and reuse of dialysis machines where demand outstrips supply and the patients' life continuously centers around the availability of the hemodialysis machine.[9] This environment also requires the individual to understand medical terminology and make decisions in stressful situations.[20] Consequently, the environment of hemodialysis may threaten to enframe the individual in technology as the presence of the technology is always revealed and raises many challenges in the individual's life.

Mapes et al.[20] identified various threats to the individual with renal disease undergoing dialysis. These included threats of bodily injury or disability, the fear of physical pain and discomfort, and the fear of the hemodialysis procedure and symptoms. Whittakker and Albee[22] also indicated various threats to the hemodialysis patient, including those to personal safety, such as the fear of needle insertion caused by the placement of an arteriovenous fistula, a fear of blood and a fear of exposure to bloodborne infection. Threats to self-identity were revealed and included a fear of depersonalization, fear of being tied to a machine and a fear of becoming an invalid.[22] Threats to body image were also indicated in the literature, including the scarring and disfigurement of repeated vascular access insertions, the skin discoloration of uremia, weight loss, premature ageing, musculoskeletal deterioration and edema.[3,17] Hemodialysis patients also have the fear of repeated hospitalizations and must learn to abide with the dehumanizing effects of the technology.[15,22,23]

Embodiment

Participants in a study by Nagle[5] described early encounters with hemodialysis as disturbing and surreal, and the shock and horror of initial encounters with the technological environment were reported. Images of the blood outside the body, the technical facets of treatment, including the noise of the hemodialysis machine and the discomfort of treatment, were also reported.[5] The participants experienced a loss of their personhood because of the dehumanizing effects of hemodialysis and the deterioration of their bodies, and they strived to remain embodied in an environment that threatened to disembody them.[5]

Embodiment evolves from a phenomenological perspective of the person where there is the assumption that all parts of the body, both physical and psychological are integral to the human being.[10,24] Based on this assumption, it is impossible for individuals to separate themselves from the technology of hemodialysis, as this has an impact on the person's sense of wholeness and embodiment. Consequently, the technology of hemodialysis introduces the individual to a new cultural system. However, it could be suggested that that this new culture may serve as another factor in the technological enframing of the hemodialysis patient.

The culture of hemodialysis

The presence of the technology of hemodialysis may introduce the individual to a new cultural system, and this must be interpreted and integrated into the life of the individual to ensure successful treatment. However, it is useful to analyze the elements that are required in the development of a cultural system to recognize how this process occurs. Argyle[25] indicates that language can play a crucial part in the development of a cultural system. People can use language so that knowledge is transmitted through the group and to the next generation.[25] Through communication and interaction, individual cooperation can be achieved, as this is essential in the formulation of culture.[25] These elements of cultural development are pronounced in the patients on hemodialysis, as these individuals must become familiar with the language of hemodialysis, such as 'ideal weight, fluid restrictions, diet restrictions, vascular access'. The use of a new language is imperative to ensure effective communication on the hemodialysis unit and cooperation with the treatment regime. Argyle[25] has also identified rules, morals, values and system of beliefs as elements of a cultural system. These morals and other values can affect the behavior of people by becoming part of their cognitive system. Therefore, development of these morals and values within a culture enforce conformity by threat of rejection or punishment.[25] These elements of culture may be demonstrated in the hemodialysis unit as it creates an environment that may coerce patients into cooperating with the treatment regime using surveillance.[6]

According to Sandelowski[26] the use of technological surveillance has been implicated as a method of exerting power over patients, and indicates a different type of watchful nursing care to the traditional approach of looking after patient's safety, comfort and well-being. Surveillance through technology as a means of exerting power and control represents a new method of gaining knowledge in healthcare. This may lead to the dehumanization of the patient caused by an inability of healthcare workers to focus on anything apart from the technological facets of treatment.[27–29] The principles of Jeremy Bentham's panopticon may exhibit how power and control are exerted legitimately on a hemodialysis unit to ensure cooperation with the treatment regime.[6]

Bentham's panopticon is a circular prison made up of individual cells open to an inner circular yard where there is an inspection tower placed in the centre.[30] The inspection tower is placed in such a way that the prisoner is unsure whether the guard is observing or not, hence the prisoner is continuously alert to 'the gaze' of the guard and this ensures co-operation.[30] The layout of many hemodialysis units positions the nurse's station in the center where a clear view of all patients is possible. The hemodialysis patient is continuously weighed, screened and monitored to ensure cooperation with the treatment regime and the success of the technology of dialysis.[6] If the patient cooperates with treatment then the technology of hemodialysis has been successful, otherwise the patient may receive a label of non-compliance.

According to Cameron[31] compliance has been described as a cognitive-motivational process of personal attitudes and intentions resulting in a set of behaviors and outcomes of patient–practitioner interactions. This is an interesting definition of compliance, as an inability to comply with the treatment regime of hemodialysis is usually perceived by healthcare professionals as a behavioral problem of the patient. Hence, the patient may receive a label of non-compliance due to an inability to cooperate with the treatment regime of hemodialysis. This incorrect labeling may subsequently result in the patient being perceived as difficult, and is, therefore, ignored and avoided by some healthcare personnel. However, there can be several reasons for non-compliance.[32–34] Consequently, this response may result in the underlying causative factors of non-compliance remaining undiagnosed, hindering the effective adjustment of the hemodialysis patient.

Heidegger[10] acknowledges that once the presence of technology is revealed, the presence of the individual may be forgotten or ignored. This may result in the inability of healthcare personnel to perceive the person as anything but an extension of the technology, thus ignoring the humanistic aspects that are essential to patient care.[9,26,28] However, these adverse effects would be reduced if the person was analyzed from a phenomeno-logical perspective and not from the reductionistic standpoint of the tech-nological framework.[10] This phenomenological view indicates that the person is someone for whom things have meaning and significance, and whose life is constituted by their interpretive understanding of the world.[10] The world, in the phenomenological sense, is the meaningful set of rela-tionships and practices, which is constituted by the person and their lin-guistic skills, cultural practices and family traditions.[35] Consequently, the individual may endure great difficulty when adjusting to hemodialysis as the technology threatens the shared skills and practices of the world on which the individual depends for meaning, identity and being.

ADJUSTMENT TO HEMODIALYSIS

It became apparent in the case study that the factors which held significance in Doreen's life were disrupted by the restrictive nature of the technology of hemodialysis and this resulted in difficulties adjusting to hemodialysis. Heidegger[36] asserts that all individuals are beings who are engaged in interpretative understanding and these interpretations are provided in the cultural and linguistic background, and make sense only when observed against this background of significance.

Loss of freedom

For many people hemodialysis is interpreted as a loss of freedom.[5] Patients indicate feelings of being trapped or tied to a machine suggesting the loss of freedom evoked by hemodialysis.[5,37,38] In a recent study, Hagren et al.[39] found that in the lives of patients on hemodialysis the main areas of suffer-ing were related to loss of freedom, expressed as dependence on the hemo-dialysis machine as a lifeline, and on caregivers. This time-consuming and tiring dependence affected marital, family and social life.

Once the individual commences hemodialysis there is a move away from the natural life towards dependency, however, for some individuals there is no substitute for the life prior to hemodialysis, and these individuals yearn for the past and the freedom they used to know.[6] However, the individual can only achieve freedom in as much as the world allows.[10] This is an import-ant viewpoint in relation to the hemodialysis patient, as the restrictive grip of the treatment regime continuously threatens the freedom of the individ-ual. Consequently, it is impossible for the individual to achieve the freedom they enjoyed prior to hemodialysis, and, as Merleau-Ponty[24] suggests, it is inconceivable to be free in some actions and at the same time be restricted to some extent in others. Consequently, from this phenomenological perspective, it is impossible for the hemodialysis patient to maintain freedom due to the restrictions induced by the technology of hemodialysis.

Inevitably, some individuals will not sacrifice their freedom and will continue to try to live the life they enjoyed before commencing hemodialysis. Although this may lead to life-threatening complications, these individuals will continue to ignore the treatment regime. This is a distressing outcome observed within patient care on a hemodialysis unit, which, as mentioned earlier, may result in the reductionistic labeling of the patient as 'non-compliant', in an effort to define and understand patient behavior. However, Merleau-Ponty[24] suggests that it may be necessary to reject the idea of causality when trying to understand the way in which individuals act. When circumstances arise that involve the individual giving up their freedom, one of two things will occur; the circumstances will be strong enough to force the individual to give up their freedom or the circumstances will not be strong enough and the individual's freedom is retained.[24] If the latter option is selected, then the demands of hemodialysis therapy may be extremely difficult and a paradox may be created for the individual.

The paradox of hemodialysis

A paradox is created for individuals undergoing hemodialysis therapy as they are expected to co-operate passively with treatment and accept dependency on the machine, while at the same time actively participate in the management of their illness.[40] Some patients, however, have great difficulty with this paradox. In a study by Nagle[5] into the meaning of technology for people with chronic renal failure, it was suggested that participants struggled to maintain a sense of wholeness and normality while undergoing hemodialysis therapy. Participants pushed their physical limits in an effort to normalize living, retain some semblance of their former selves and to avoid their lives being totally engulfed by the technology of hemodialysis.[5] Levy[40] indicated that the effort of the individual to maintain independence serves to ignore the dependency on the technology of hemodialysis; however, the reality demands of dependence run counter to the patient's independent defense and this can lead to great difficulties in adjustment to hemodialysis.

Reichsman and Levy[41] revealed the converse to this paradox in a study on adaptation of patients to maintenance hemodialysis. They found that this patient group had intense dependent needs and wanted them fulfilled in the manner which occurred when they were in a uremic state. The dependency of the hemodialysis patient may increase reliance on social support, lead to over-involvement of the family and, subsequently, increase dependency levels.[42] Individuals may use various behaviors to avoid dependency and cope with the effects of hemodialysis on their life and this was evident in the case study.

Coping with the technology of hemodialysis

The use of avoidance behaviors has been described as a method of regulating emotional distress so that destruction of moral or social functioning does not occur and dependency on dialysis is avoided.[37,42,43] In a study into coping strategies of male hemodialysis patients, Cormier-Daigle and Stewart[42] revealed that over half of the participants used avoidance behaviors to cope with the illness-related stressors of renal disease and hemodialysis. They deduced that the participants perceived little control over the illness-related stressors, which were chronic and severe, and therefore may have chosen to avoid thinking about these issues.

Denial is another term used to describe an avoidance of feelings and emotions. Denial can be a healthy mechanism, which will protect the individual from the initial threats to reality, but should eventually resolve and allow the individual to adjust effectively to the situation.[44] However, if denial is used as an avoidance of reality for a prolonged period, the patient may refuse mentally and emotionally to accept the illness and continue to live life as though nothing has changed.[44] The utilization of denial may result in the hemodialysis patient ignoring the treatment regime and, subsequently, lead to serious complications, such as pulmonary edema, hyperkalemia and cardiac arrhythmias.

The impact of hemodialysis may elicit feelings of sadness, regret, disappointment and anger in the patient.[5] These behaviors were evident in the case study of Doreen. Hemodialysis patients may develop signs of premature aging, musculoskeletal deterioration, scarring, loss of muscle tone and disfigurement.[5] Furthermore, adherence to dietary and fluid restrictions, and a strict medication and hemodialysis regime, all culminate in the realization of the impact of the technology on the individual's life.[5] This realization may elicit anger in the patient. A study by White and Grenyer[45] of patients' and their partners' experiences of hemodialysis indicated that participants responded with anger to hemodialysis therapy, as it resulted in negative changes in lifestyle, including social isolation, an inability to go on holidays and restrictions and limitations in life. Dialysis was also described in a resentful way as 'this' or 'it'.[45]

Other studies also revealed that patients may feel resentment and anger towards the restrictions of hemodialysis therapy and may displace these feelings on nursing and medical staff, and other patients.[5,18,41] Sometimes the anger may be directed at the patient's family and this was evident in the case study of Doreen. This may result in relationship problems between the patient and family members. This factor was also demonstrated in White and Grenyer's study,[45] as patients were described by their partners as selfish, inward looking and impatient. However, these difficulties may not be entirely a consequence of the patient's behavior. Daneker et al.[46] reported that spouse and patient levels of depression were related. Furthermore, a study into coping strategies of spouses of dialysis and transplant patients revealed that the coping behaviors of the patient's spouse may affect the coping ability of the patient.[16] It was apparent in the case study of Doreen that the coping behaviors of the patient's spouse can have a positive influence on the coping ability of the patient. However, in the above study the spouses of hemodialysis patients utilized more avoidance and fatalistic behaviors, e.g. expected the worse, felt that things looked hopeless, than the spouses of transplant patients, thus decreasing the patient's ability to cope effectively with hemodialysis therapy.[16] Conversely, it seems that the physical and psychosocial complications of dialysis might be alleviated by transplantation, and, at this stage, the spouses of the transplant patient may perceive themselves as living the normal, healthy life they had always hoped for and may, therefore, utilize more effective coping behaviours.[16]

The physiological and psychosocial manifestations of hemodialysis may induce depression in the patient and this was suggested in the case study of Doreen. Mittal et al.[47] reported that the self-assessed physical and mental health of hemodialysis patients was markedly diminished compared with the general population and other chronic diseases. When compared with physical manifestations, psychological manifestations are potentially more controllable by the individual, but if they are not addressed they may lead to negative outcomes, such as depression.[48] Physical manifestations may also precipitate depression, as it has been suggested that when an appraisal suggests nothing can be done to modify conditions, as in the case of physical stressors, the result may initiate behaviors such as depression.[37,49] White and Grenyer[45] revealed that moderate and severe depression in dialysis patients was due to the scarring, disfigurement and limitations of dialysis, the continuous interactions with healthcare staff and thoughts of an uncertain future. Participants in the study also made statements suggesting suicide.[45] Approximately one out of every five hundred dialysis patients commit suicide, others unsuccessfully attempt suicide and an indeterminate number of deaths caused by dietary indiscretion may also be suicide related.[50] Consequently, it is imperative that intense psychological support and therapy should be provided to patients who continue to ignore the dietary restrictions and treatment regime of hemodialysis. Labeling these individuals as non-compliant does not address the underlying difficulties, and may result in depression and attempted suicide.

Emotion-focused coping may also be associated with depressive symptoms.[48,51] Emotion-focused coping strategies are heightened by unmanageable situations and are directed at reducing or regulating emotional stress, whereas problem-solving coping strategies are directed at managing or altering a problem.[49,52] The threats of hemodialysis may appear unmanageable to some individuals and this may lead to loss of control and depression.[53] In a study on health locus of control and depression, Christensen et al.[52] revealed that hemodialysis patients who had not previously had a transplant had a greater locus of control and a lower level of depression. However, the opposite pattern was noted in hemodialysis patients who had undergone an unsuccessful transplant, as it appeared that holding a strong belief in personal or medical control over health outcomes was associated with a greater degree of depression for the failed-transplant hemodialysis patient group. For individuals who are subject to a more troubled disease trajectory, control beliefs are likely to be undermined leading to depression and maladaptive behaviours.[52] Depressed individuals may be unable to utilize a problem-solving approach, such as forming an action plan, setting goals or trying different solutions as these efforts take emotional energy that these individuals may not have.[48] Hemodialysis patients endure many complications throughout their illness and treatment, and when depression occurs, it is possible that these individuals have exhausted their repertoire of problem-solving behaviors.[48]

Depression has been described as the most common psychological complication in dialysis patients and is usually a response to real, threatened or fantasized loss.[50] Physical manifestations include sleep disorder, change in appetite and weight, and diminution of sexual interest and ability.[50] Dialysis patients, whether male or female, frequently have sexual difficulties and impotence eventually develops in approximately 70% of men on dialysis, with both men and women engaging in sexual intercourse much less frequently than they did prior to becoming uremic.[50] Fatigue is another physiological complication of end-stage renal disease and a relationship has been indicated between depression and all measures of fatigue in the hemodialysis patient.[54] Consequently, sexual dysfunction and fatigue induced by depression may be mistakenly identified as a physiological consequence of hemodialysis and treatment may not address the underlying issue.

Although adjustment to hemodialysis may be difficult, it is evident in the literature that some individuals manage to integrate the effects of technology into their life and adjust effectively. Nagle[5] indicated that this phase of coming to terms with hemodialysis involved finding a new way of living and accepting being different. An analysis of studies on the experience of chronic illness concluded that learning to accept that life will never be the same again is an essential part of coming to terms with the illness and its effects.[55] In a descriptive study of meaning of illness in chronic renal disease, it was found that patients had identifiable meanings for their illness, and these may be associated with their response to the disease, for example, they found that individuals who viewed the illness as a challenge had a more positive outlook.[56] Once the individual successfully adjusts to hemodialysis it may serve to counter the adverse effects of technology on their life. This perspective has been suggested by Rittman et al.[57] in a study of patients with renal disease, as the researchers discovered a theme of 'dwelling in dialysis', which involved the individual feeling at home in the hemodialysis unit. The initial disruption in managing daily life was gradually replaced by what came to be seen as a normal day, and as patients began to view their illness experience as a normal part of their lives, a new sense of being was adopted.[57] This was apparent in the case study as the hemodialysis unit became a normal part of Doreen's life. Participants in the above study seemed to develop a new sense of awareness as they utilized clever problem-solving approaches to overcome the effects of dietary and fluid restrictions, e.g. patients sucked ice cubes instead of having drinks and ate meals from smaller plates.[57]

This use of problem-solving coping strategies by hemodialysis patients was also indicated in other studies.[38,42,58,59] Effective problem solving addresses the use of deliberate problem-focused efforts to alter a situation combined with an analytical approach to solving the problem.[43] The literature revealed various factors, which enhanced the individual's ability to cope with the consequences of the illness and the treatment on their lives. Believers in God might have an additional coping capacity derived from various personal and/or religious practices, such as prayers and rituals.[37,43,60] The individual may utilize their relationship with God to reach a higher power and achieve self-completeness, and may also find meaning and purpose in illness resulting in self-empowerment to cope with the current stress.[60] The use of prayer as a problem-solving coping strategy was highlighted in the case study of Doreen.

The length of time on dialysis had a significant relationship with coping ability.[37,53] Patients appeared to develop a repertoire of problem-solving behaviors when on dialysis for a longer period of time, thus enabling them to adjust more effectively. However, Lok[58] indicated that the physical and psychosocial stressors might increase with length of time on hemodialysis, thus affecting the patient's ability to continuously utilize problem-solving strategies. Social support has been positively associated with effective adjustment to chronic illness and this was indicated in the case study of Doreen. Social support may occur through the provision of emotional support that reveals to the patient that they are loved and cared for, or through the provision of esteem support that involves showing the patient they are valued and held in high esteem.[61] Network support involves the patient realizing they belong to a network of mutual support that acts as a buffer to stressful events, and social acceptability enables people to focus on more positive aspects of the illness, e.g. advice and help from people with a similar experience.[61]

The effects of hemodialysis may be attenuated by hope, as this may enable individuals to cope more effectively with hemodialysis. Heidegger[36] indicated that hope is a 'potentiality for being', which tells us unambiguously that in the person there is always something still outstanding that has not yet become actual. In the hemodialysis patient this hope may lie in a transplant or, for some individuals, in the possibility of watching their family grow up.[57] Maintaining control over the situation also enables individuals on hemodialysis to cope more effectively and efforts to maintain control over the situation involve thinking through different ways to solve problems, seeking information and taking an active role in treatment.[38,48,57]

CONCLUSION AND FUTURE PROSPECTS

It is apparent from the case study of Doreen, and the supporting literature reviewed here, that the technology of hemodialysis may have a dramatic impact on the life of the individual. Although hemodialysis has evolved from the unethical selection criteria of the 1960s, it still remains an 'experiment' and there is no guarantee of its success. In fact, according to Depner,[62] due to the high mortality rates and strict controls, hemodialysis would probably not be introduced as a treatment today.[62] Despite the continuing mortality versus morbidity debate, the introduction of the technology of hemodialysis has enabled many individuals to achieve various aspirations in life that prior to its introduction would have been impossible.

However, there is a cost attached as there are many challenges imposed on the individual's life by the technology of hemodialysis. Heidegger[10] indicates that once the presence of technology is explicitly revealed or uncovered, the individual may be forced to 'stand reserve' or put their life on hold to cope with the challenges and demands imposed by technology. Heidegger refers to this phenomenon as technological enframing. There are various issues that contribute to technological enframing in the hemodialysis patient. These include, the physiological and psychosocial manifestations of treatment, the dehumanizing effects of the hemodialysis machine and the culture of the hemodialysis unit.

Hemodialysis may be interpreted as a loss of freedom and a paradox may be created as the individual is expected to accept dependency on technology, while remaining independent on the management of their treatment regime. The implications of hemodialysis may subsequently elicit various behaviors in the individual, including avoidance, denial, disappointment, regret, sadness, anger and depression. The use of emotion-focused coping strategies may elicit these behaviors in the individual, and may cause difficulties when trying to adjust to hemodialysis. However, it was also apparent in the literature that the use of problem-solving coping strategies may enable the individual to integrate the consequences of hemodialysis therapy into their life and adjust effectively. These individuals adapted a new sense of meaning and purpose in their life, which served to counter the effects of technological enframing. Certain factors enhanced the individual's ability to utilize problem-solving coping strategies, including spirituality, length of time on hemodialysis, social support, and maintaining hope and control.

It is extremely important that the renal patient adjusts effectively to hemodialysis to increase well-being. Consequently, the provision of healthcare to these patients should also focus on interventions that enhance the psychological adjustment process. The physiological status of the hemodialysis patient is assessed, monitored, screened and investigated regularly, but the psychosocial aspects of treatment do not receive the same attention.[21] This may have evolved from regarding the patient from the technological standpoint as described by Heidegger.[10] However, this problem may be overcome if the person were to be perceived from a phenomenological perspective rather than a technological one. The phenomenological perspective asserts that the person is an embodied being for whom things have significance, and this is placed in the context of the cultural and linguistic factors of the individual's life.[36] As witnessed in this chapter, the repercussions of hemodialysis threaten all these elements and, subsequently, may result in many difficulties for the individual when trying to adjust to hemodialysis.

On a final note, the physiological aspects of treatment are continuously monitored, with the most recent debates focusing on hemodialysis adequacy. Intermittent hemodialysis treatment may be inadequate as the patient is allowed more time to accumulate fluid and toxins. Therefore, according to Freitas,[63] daily hemodialysis is physiologically more beneficial for the patient and produces improved clinical outcomes. Consequently, it may become the optimal choice for treatment in the future and has already been introduced in some countries.[63] If this new approach to hemodialysis is introduced the individual will be required to accept a greater level of dependency on the technology of hemodialysis. This will have further implications on the ability of the individual to adjust to the technology of hemodialysis and will place a greater need on altering the technological focus of healthcare staff. With the advancement of technology and its implementation, there is a greater need for advancement in the understanding of its psychosocial implications, as a means of maximizing the patient's quality of life and minimizing the effects of the technology.

REFERENCES

1. Carmody M 1995 Living with renal disease, a guide for patients. Pinewood, Tipperary
2. Smith T 1997 Renal nursing. Baillière Tindall, London
3. Molzahn AE 1998 Psychosocial impact of renal disease. In: Parker J ed. Contemporary nephrology nursing. A.J. Jannetti, New Jersey, 369–382
4. Royle JA, Walsh M 1993 Watson's medical-surgical nursing and related physiology. 4th edn. Baillière Tindall, London
5. Nagle LM 1998 Meaning of technology for people with chronic renal disease. Holistic Nursing Practice 12(4): 78–92
6. Bevan MT 2000 Dialysis as 'deus ex machina': a critical analysis of hemodialysis. Journal of Advanced Nursing 31(2): 437–443
7. Hoffart N 2001 The history of nephrology nursing. In: Lancaster LE ed. ANNA Core curriculum in nephrology nursing. 4th edn. Anthony J Jannetti, New Jersey, 627–639
8. Scrambler G 1991 Sociology as applied to medicine. 3rd edn. Baillière Tindall, London

9. Bevan MT 1998 Nursing in a dialysis unit: technological enframing and a declining art, or an imperative for caring. Journal of Advanced Nursing 27(4): 730–736
10. Heidegger M 1977 The question concerning technology. In: Krell DF ed. Basic writings. Sage, London, 307–343
11. Daugirdas JT, Ing TS 1994 Handbook of dialysis. 2nd edn. Little Brown, Boston
12. Akinsanya J 1998 On being a patient. Journal of Advanced Nursing 27(2): 233–234
13. Lancaster LE 2001 Systemic manifestations of renal failure. In: Lancaster LE ed. ANNA Core curriculum for nephrology nursing. 4th edn. Anthony J Jannetti, New Jersey, 117–158
14. Putriano M 1999 The relationship between dialysis adequacy and sleep problems in hemodialysis patients. American Nephrology Nurses Association Journal 26(4): 405–407
15. Mok E, Tam B 2001 Stressors and coping methods among chronic hemodialysis patients in Hong Kong. Journal of Clinical Nursing 10(4): 503–511
16. Lindqvist R, Carlsson M, Sjoden P 2000 Coping strategies and health related quality of life among spouses of continuous ambulatory peritoneal dialysis, hemodialysis and transplant patients. Journal of Advanced Nursing 31(6): 1398–1408
17. Harries F 1996 Psychological care in end stage renal disease. Professional Nurse 12(2): 124–126
18. Molzahn AE 1991 The reported quality of life of selected home hemodialysis patients. American Nephrology Nurses Association 18(2): 173–181
19. Hartigan MF, White RB 2001 Circulatory access for hemodialysis. In: Lancaster LE ed. ANNA Core curriculum for nephrology nursing. 4th edn. Anthony J Jannetti, New Jersey, 305–330
20. Mapes DL, Callahan MB, Richie MF 2001 Psychosocial and rehabilitative aspects of renal failure and its treatment. In: Lancaster LE ed. ANNA Core curriculum for nephrology nursing. 4th edn. Anthony J Jannetti, New Jersey
21. Killingworth A, Van den Akker O 1996 The quality of life of renal dialysis patients: trying to find the missing measurement. International Journal of Nursing Studies 33(1): 107–120
22. Whittaker AA, Albee BJ 1995 Factors influencing patient selection of dialysis treatment modality. American Nephrology Nurses Association Journal 23(4): 369–374
23. Fallon M, Gould D, Wainwright S 1997 Stress and quality of life in the renal transplant patient: a preliminary investigation. Journal of Advanced Nursing 25(3): 562–570
24. Merleau-Ponty M 1962 The phenomenology of perception translated by Smith C. Routledge and Kegan Paul, London
25. Argyle M 1969 Social interaction. Tavistock, London
26. Sandelowski M 1998 Looking to care or caring to look? Technology and the rise of spectacular nursing. Holistic Nursing Practice 12(4): 1–11
27. Purnell MJ 1998 Who really makes the bed? Uncovering technologic dissonance in nursing. Holistic Nursing Practice 12(4): 12–22
28. Bernardo A 1998 Technology and the true presence in nursing. Holistic Nursing Practice 12(4): 40–49
29. McConnell EA 1998 The coalescence of technology and humanism in nursing practice: it doesn't just happen and it doesn't come easily. Holistic Nursing Practice 12(4): 23–30
30. Foucault M 1980 Power/knowledge: selected interviews and other writings 1972–1977 Harvester, Brighton
31. Cameron C 1996 Patient compliance: recognition of factors involved and suggestions for promoting compliance with therapeutic regimes. Journal of Advanced Nursing 33(6): 716–727
32. Kovac JA, Patel SS, Peterson RA et al. 2002 Patient satisfaction with care and behavioural compliance in end-stage renal disease patients treated with hemodialysis. American Journal of Kidney Diseases 39(6): 1236–1244
33. Pang SK, Ip WY, Chang AM 2001 Psychosocial correlates of fluid compliance among Chinese hemodialysis patients. Journal of Advanced Nursing 35(5): 691–698
34. Kutner NG, Zhang R, McClellan WM et al. 2002 Psychosocial predictors of non-compliance in hemodialysis and peritoneal dialysis patients. Nephrology Dialysis Tranplantation 17(1): 93–99
35. Leonard VW 1994. A Heideggerian phenomenological perspective on the concept of person. In: Benner P ed. Interpretive phenomenology. Sage, Thousand Oaks, 43–63

36. Heidegger M 1962 Being and time. Basil Blackwell, Oxford
37. Gurklis KA, Menke EM 1988 Identification of stressors and use of coping methods in chronic hemodialysis patients. Nursing Research 37(4): 236–248
38. Gurklis KA, Menke EM 1995 Chronic patients perceptions of stress, coping and social support. American Nephrology Nurses Association Journal 22(4): 381–387
39. Hagren B, Pettersen IM, Severinsson E et al. 2001 The hemodialysis machine as a lifeline: experiences of suffering from end-stage renal disease. Journal of Advanced Nursing 34(2): 196–202
40. Levy NB 1979 Psychological factors in rehabilitation of the patient undergoing maintenance hemodialysis. In: Chyatte SB ed. Rehabilitation in chronic renal failure. Williams and Wilkins, Baltimore, 46–64
41. Reichsman F, Levy NB 1972 Problems in adaptation to maintenance hemodialysis. Archives of Internal Medicine 130: 859–865
42. Cormier-Daigle M, Stewart M 1997 Support and coping of male hemodialysis-dependent patients. International Journal of Nursing Studies 34(6): 420–430
43. Gramling L, Lambert V, Pursley-Crotteau S 1998 Coping in young women: theoretical retroduction. Journal of Advanced Nursing 28(5): 1082–1091
44. Davidhizar R, Giger JN 1998 Patients use of denial. Coping with the unacceptable. Nursing Standard 12(43): 44–46
45. White Y, Grenyer B 1999 The biopsychosocial impact of end stage renal disease: the experience of dialysis patients and their partners. Journal of Advanced Nursing 30(6): 1312–1320
46. Daneker B, Kimmel PL, Ranich T et al. 2001 Depression and marital dissatisfaction in patients with end-stage renal disease and in their spouses. American Journal of Kidney Diseases 38(4): 839–846
47. Mittal SK, Ahern L, Flaster E et al. 2001 Self-assessed physical and mental function of hemodialysis patients. Nephrology Dialysis Transplantation 16(7): 1387–1394
48. Welch JL, Austin JK 2001 Stressors, coping and depression in hemodialysis patients. Journal of Advanced Nursing 33(2): 200–207
49. Lazarus P 1991 Emotion and adaptation. Oxford University Press, New York
50. Levy NB 1994 Psychology and rehabilitation. In: Daugirdas JT, Ing TS eds. Handbook of dialysis. 2nd edn. Little Brown, Boston, 369–374
51. Rohde P, Lewinson PM, Tilsonly Seely JR 1990 Dimensionality of coping and its relation to depression. Journal of Personality and Social Psychology 58: 499–511
52. Christensen AJ, Turner CW, Smith TW 1991 Health locus of control and depression in end stage renal disease. Journal of Consulting and Clinical Psychology 59(3): 419–424
53. Blake CW, Courts NF 1996 Coping strategies and styles of hemodialysis patients by gender. American Nephrology Nurses Association Journal 23(5): 477–484
54. McCann K, Boore JRP 2000 Fatigue in persons with renal failure who require maintenance hemodialysis. Journal of Advanced Nursing 35(5): 1132–1142
55. Morse JM 1997 Responding to threats to integrity of self. Advances in Nursing Science 19(4): 21–36
56. Caress AL, Luker KA, Owens RG 2001 A descriptive study of meaning of illness in chronic renal disease. Journal of Advanced Nursing 33(6): 716–727
57. Rittman M, Northsea C, Hausauer N et al. 1993 Living with renal disease. American Nephrology Nurses Association 20(3): 327–331
58. Lok P 1996 Stressors, coping mechanisms and quality of life among dialysis patients in Australia. Journal of Advanced Nursing 23: 873–881
59. Curtin RB, Mapes D, Petillo M et al. 2002 Long-term dialysis survivors: A transformational experience. Qualitative Health Research 12(5): 609–624
60. Baldacchino D, Draper P 2001 Spiritual coping strategies, a review of the nursing research literature. Journal of Advanced Nursing 34(6): 833–841
61. Niven N, Robinson J 1994 The psychology of nursing care. Macmillan Press, Hampshire
62. Depner TA 1991 Prescribing hemodialysis: a guide to urea kinetic modelling. Kluwer Academic, Boston
63. Freitas T 2002 Nursing experience with daily dialysis at El Camino hospital. Nephrology Nursing Journal 29(2): 167–169

WEBSITES OF INTEREST

American Nephrology Nurses' Association: http://anna.Inurse.com

Renal World – Renal resources from around the globe: www.renalworld.com

The Nephron Information Center: www.nephron.com

14

Critical care in high-technology environments

Ian Bennun

SUMMARY

Intensive or critical care units (ICUs) are specialist units for patients with acute life-threatening conditions. They are equipped with a complex array of technical equipment to provide patients with physiological support. Although the promise of this technology is to improve patient care and reduce mortality, the impact of this clinical environment on patients, their relatives and staff is often overlooked. This chapter explores the complex relationship between technology and those operating and benefiting from it, as well as the effect that the ICU environment has on patient's psychological status. A case study is presented at the outset, which is later reviewed in the light of the discussion on technologically sophisticated critical care units. Good-practice guidelines are considered as illustrating some of the ways of minimizing the adverse effects of providing intensive care.

CASE STUDY

Clifford, a 54-year-old married man with two children and three grandchildren, was admitted to the intensive care unit (ICU) following elective surgery. He had developed an aortic aneurysm, which required surgical intervention. While in theatre, a second aneurysm was identified that was more complicated, thus extending the duration of surgery and resulting in a more complex procedure.

When transferred to the ICU from theatre, he required very close support and monitoring. This included respiratory support, monitoring of tissue oxygenation, fluid administration, cardio-vascular monitoring, nutritional feed and intravenous drug lines. There were numerous bedside monitors to provide supportive respiratory and cardio-vascular therapy. Clifford remained sedated for 17 days, was ventilated for much of that time and was visited by his family every day. His wife remained at his bedside for approximately 9 hours each day and his sons visited regularly both to see their father and support their mother.

Clifford's three grandchildren, all under the age of 9 years, visited after school and on weekends. When they first visited their grandfather they were understandably upset even though the staff had tried to prepare them by showing hand-drawn pictures and photographs of ICUs taken from magazines. For much of his stay, the family remained present on the ward, experiencing the full range of emotions, from hope to uncertainty, from fear to resignation.

In his initial awake state, Clifford was disorientated and confused. He believed that he had been on a journey, that he had been attacked and tortured while traveling and was initially mistrusting of the clinical staff. Blood samples were regularly taken, and for some time Clifford protested believing that the blood was going to be used for some primitive ritual. His agitation was so marked that increased sedation was required. During these few days, he did not recognize his family, was unresponsive to their attention and was visibly afraid when his grandchildren first visited. He remained on the unit for 43 days, during which time his physical and psychological states slowly improved. He was transferred to the surgical ward and was later discharged from hospital after a further 8 weeks.

Clifford's case is not untypical for a man presenting with his condition. His stay in the ICU had been longer than first anticipated and his prognosis at the outset was uncertain. A relationship developed between his family and the unit staff who witnessed the full range of responses to his admission. At times his family needed a great deal of care and compassion, at other times they made managing Clifford's condition very difficult. They were admired for their courage, but also brought out staff attitudes and feelings not conducive to good holistic treatment.

TECHNOLOGY WITHIN INTENSIVE AND CRITICAL CARE

ICUs are specialist treatment units for patients with acute life-threatening conditions. They are different from normal hospital settings and are usually bustling with practitioners and technology. Beside each bed there is a complex array of technical equipment necessary for the continuous monitoring of the patient's physiological condition. Visual display monitors, bleeps, alarms and equipment noise, dominate the atmosphere. The activity within the unit does not vary with time of day and the clinical teams are constantly interacting and discussing the delivery of individual patient care.

There are few settings as evocative of health technology as the ICU (see Fig. 14.1). It needs to be pointed out, that the term 'technology' in intensive care not only includes the equipment being used to support the patient, but also the staff who are using it. This technology provides physiological support rather than curative treatment. It includes ventilators, continuous hemodynamic monitoring for measuring heart rate and rhythm, blood pressure monitoring via an arterial catheter, intracranial pressure monitoring via a small catheter placed in the subarachnoid space and monitoring of the right ventricular pressures in the heart via a pulmonary artery catheter, to name but a few. All of this technology assists in the overall care of the patient and may allow for safer interventions, but the ultimate benefit must be a reduction in mortality. Increasingly, computers are being used to integrate the physiological support and patient-monitoring systems.

Two scholarly accounts[1,2] of some of the aspects of ICU technology raise a number of paradoxes that, to some extent, make uncomfortable reading. The 'promise of technology'[1] highlights the fact that patients, their relatives and the staff depend on this technology for achieving medical success. Although units are replete with technology, few of these pieces of equipment have undergone rigorous evaluation before their dissemination, because the outcomes of improved technology are difficult to measure. When they are evaluated, some technologies considered beneficial are shown to have the potential for harm. Even though life can be prolonged, there is

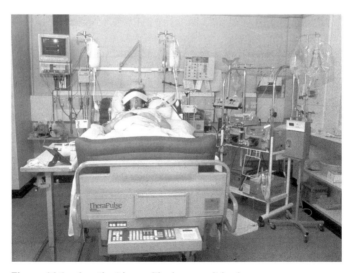

Figure 14.1   A patient in a critical care unit bed.

certainly no guarantee that the patient's quality of life can be improved. What greater dilemma can face practitioners than the preservation of a life that will ultimately be of poorer quality in the case of survival? The second account[2] notes that the use of technology is an applied science, but that there is an increasing literature concerning the philosophy of technology. Implicit in the delivery of healthcare is a personal, individualized and humanistic approach, but the advancement of medical science and technology demonstrates how our lives interact with technology to the extent that we become 'entwined with the technology'.[2]

Fundamental to the application of technology in critical and intensive care, is the role of the practitioner in using the technology to provide maximum patient benefit to ensure survival, while at the same time minimizing the adverse effects of this technology on both patients and their relatives. It is through the complex interaction of the technology and the clinical expertise that the patient–person dualism is most clearly evident. It could be argued that through the application of technical and clinical know-how, patients become discharged persons; alternatively there is the risk that the reliance on technology reduces the appreciation that the patient also has the status of a person. The technological environment within ICUs provides practitioners with many challenges. By giving primacy to the technological culture of Western biomedical science, there is the potential to render invisible humanistic clinical practice, which is linked to the notion of a 'technologically textured existence'[2] to denote how thoroughly we interact with technologies in providing intensive and critical care.

Two potential paradigms of patient care have been described, that of 'touch' and 'technology'.[3] It is argued that technology destroys human dignity by reducing people to objects. Furthermore, technology resists being assimilated into a person's individuality and its greatest impact on objectifying human life is through the experience of distance and 'otherness'. Technology is thus placed at the objective end, while the dignity of human life is placed at the subjective end of this paradigm. Dehumanization of the patient in intensive care potentially can occur; they can be referred to as bed numbers or diagnoses, during which time those caring for them can temporarily forget that the patient is someone's mother or father, daughter or son.

At issue when examining the application of technology to critical care, is the relationship between the practitioner using the technology to provide maximum benefit, while at the same time minimizing its adverse effects, and the patient. Underpinning this issue, is the fact that clinicians need to balance the demands put upon themselves by both machine and patient; the task is managing the interaction between access to technology and delivery of patient care. The implications that the use of technology has for the critically ill patient and family include not only the benefits that this technology holds for the patients, but also its adverse effects. An important aspect of critical care delivery is the minimizing of the unwanted influence that technology may have on critically ill individuals. When considering the appropriate outcomes for the assessment of this technology, the following are normally accepted: reduced numbers of patients within the unit, economic outcomes, improved safety, improved mortality, clinician comfort, and patient comfort.[4]

In two Swedish studies of patient views following their experience of being on an ICU, many respondents recalled feeling insecure and fearful, even though they were in a technologically sophisticated environment.[5,6] Patients reported not being able to trust the machinery surrounding the bed, fearing that it would break down and they would die. They felt restricted by the tubes and monitoring lines and also described feeling insecure as if they could not trust the staff caring for them. For them the experience of being connected to this equipment, which restricted their movement, seemed to result in a perception of body distortion and an altered self-concept. This latter phenomenon particularly occurred when the nurses paid more attention to the technology than to the patients. They were commonly not able to move themselves and reported being afraid of excessive movement for fear of setting off alarms. Usually in these settings, patients are lying down, possibly on their backs, and if intubated are further restricted in their movement. Limited mobility within the ICU environment causes patients to feel isolated and fearful. In these circumstances, there is the risk that they lose their integrity, body sensations and functions. Gradually, the patient may feel that their body does not exist or they develop a perceptual distortion so that they do not know where their body begins and ends.[6]

In a related study[7] critical care nurses were interviewed about the use of technology, with one finding being that a lack of knowledge about technology increased their fear. They described the expectation that they should be competent in the use of machinery and that they equated competency with feeling comfortable with the equipment. There appears to be two ways (inexperienced) critical care staff respond in these situations. One response is to become totally focused on the surrounding technology, thus failing to see the patient as their primary concern. The alternative response is to focus on the patient, thus attempting to remove the fear of the unknown by ignoring it. It has been elegantly stated, that the use of technology means that those providing care need to be psychologically fit and technologically competent.[8]

VENTILATION AND ITS EFFECT ON COMMUNICATION

The use of mechanical ventilators to support breathing is commonplace in critical care. There are three indicators for mechanical ventilation to promote the well-being of the patient: disorders of oxygenation, disorders of ventilation and disorders of oxygenation and ventilation. Oxygenation ensures that hemoglobins are saturated with oxygen from the lungs, which then circulates around the body, for example, in acute respiratory failure; ventilation will maintain appropriate breathing and clear carbon dioxide from the lungs, for example, after major surgery. A combination of oxygenation and ventilation may be required in cases of adult respiratory distress syndrome.

Patients who are mechanically ventilated are unable to speak even though they may be conscious, since air enters and leaves the tracheobronchial system via a nasotracheal, orotracheal or tracheostomy tube. Consequently, air does not come into contact with the larynx, which produces the basic sound element of speech. Even within this context, the main aims for nurse–patient communication are to establish a clinical relationship recognizing the patient's worth and individuality and determining their needs.[9]

The use of mechanical ventilators has been reported as having a negative psychological effect, particularly because of its adverse impact on the ability to communicate. Over half the patients included in one study described being worried and distressed by not being able to speak.[10] They described being misunderstood, not being able to make their needs known and fearing that they would not be able to speak again.

A qualitative investigation conducted with 12 previously ventilated patients found that when these patients failed in their attempt to mouth words, use gestures and/or write, they experienced frustration and fear.[11] Similar findings have been reported by others,[5,12] demonstrating the common communication problems experienced by ventilated patients. If it is possible to prepare patients for this prior to their admission, it may help them cope with later communication difficulties. Patients taught to use a communication board prior to open-heart surgery showed increased satisfaction with communication during the intubation period, compared with patients who did not receive the training and who relied on nurses' experience and creativity in communication.[13] Another qualitative study[14] found that postoperative ventilated patients reported shock and fear when they realized they could not speak and that the futility of trying to communicate aroused feelings of sadness, exhaustion and even a perception of torture. This perception is as a result of isolation, sleep, sensory and perceptual deprivation, which, together with the inability to communicate, are characteristics of solitary confinement.

In a study of 22 ventilated ICU patients interviewed three times over a 2-month period,[15] it was suggested that patients require greater efforts by nurses to establish functional communication. The methods most frequently used for establishing functional communication were body language, touch, lip reading, and using pen and paper. Patients reported having a preference for these somewhat simple means of communication in preference to more elaborate methods, such as a letter or word board. Relatives and patients need to have clear and unambiguous information about clinical status, treatment plans, procedures and prognosis; exploring the optimum way of sharing this goes a long way to meet their needs.

The use of touch is widely accepted and encouraged as a mode of communication with ventilated patients[16] and three definitions of touch are offered in this account. 'Comforting touch' assists the patient in coping with illness, and includes empathy and an acute awareness of their feelings and emotional needs. 'Task touch' occurs while care is being provided and constitutes the majority of touch within an ICU. 'Affectionate touch' is a tactile communication from one person to another, the primary purpose being conveying recognition, acceptance, protection and care. Touch is recommended as a form of communication in many healthcare environments, but specifically in ICUs where the patient's surroundings are predominantly impersonal technology with disorienting sounds.

SEDATION AND MEMORY

The drugs used to sedate critically ill patients can broadly be categorized as analgesics or sedatives. The sedatives most commonly used are propofol and midazolam; analgesia is provided by opioids such as morphine, fentanyl and alfentanil.

Sedation and analgesia are fundamental, but often poorly addressed aspects of critical care.[17] Patients vary widely in their response to drugs and thus require regular monitoring of plasma sedative concentrations. Many of the interventions are painful and distressing, and lying in a fixed position for prolonged periods can cause backache and discomfort. Increasingly, there is evidence to suggest that poorly controlled pain and anxiety may be associated with poorer critical illness outcome, and if the stress response can be moderated, this may be of value to patient outcome. Nevertheless, attitudes to the sedation of the critically ill have changed over the last 2 decades. In a review of trends[18] it was noted that in the 1980s there was a preference for deep sedation and occasional waking. In a later survey, these regimes had changed to one where units preferred to keep patients asleep, but easily rousable. The changes are most probably due to a greater appreciation and knowledge of the risks associated with sedative agents and the general improved clinical care. Achieving the optimal sedation level will naturally reduce the risk of over- or under-sedation. The effects of over-sedation can include, among others, respiratory depression, hypotension, bradycardia, renal dysfunction, ileus and deep-vein thrombosis. Under-sedation can result in agitation, pain and discomfort, catheter extubation or displacement, hypertension and tachycardia. Ideal sedation produces a calm, pain-free and easily rousable patient who is able to tolerate the range of frightening events characteristic of critical care.

Sedation, like anesthesia, can have marked cognitive effects on mood, psychological status and memory. In a study investigating the relationship between different sedation regimes and memory,[19] all patients 'claiming amnesia' received morphine together with propofol with none receiving alfentanil as the only opioid. Although this study had a small sample, the author concluded that it was unlikely that the choice of opioid exerted any influence on memory. Anesthetic drugs have been shown to produce amnesia of varying durations. The benzodiazepines have the least effect on memory and, indeed, this agent has a minimal effect on short-term memory. Its main effect is on long-term memory impairing the acquisition and storage of new information, but not impairing the recall of information already stored.[20] This effect is most appropriate for ICU patients and it suggests that the goal is to prevent awareness and recall of unpleasant events, while leaving the patient's prior memories unaffected. Unfortunately, emotionally charged and/or painful information is more likely to be remembered, perhaps because of the associated neuroendocrine stress responses. Of 19 critically ill patients all of whom had been ventilated, their description of the post-sedation phase was one of emptiness or, indeed, of not existing at all.[6] Some comments from patients described in this report include: '... I did not recognize my own body ... it didn't work as it used to'; another patient described his body feeling empty, that he could not feel it and that he could not feel anything, whereas another described his body as 'two opposites, sometimes very weak and at other times, very strong'.[6]

There appear to be three ICU memory reactions. Some patients will have no factual recall, but may have memories of paranoid delusions and nightmares. Even after discharge, these patients are amnesic for factual ICU events. The second patient group will have fragments of factual memories and may also recall delusions and nightmares. The third patient group will have varying amounts of recall without delusions or nightmares.

The overall recall of patients about their intensive care stay varies and no clear trend has emerged from the published literature to date. There are a number of factors that are thought to influence memory: severity of illness/injury, drug regime, length of sedation, strength of sedation and age. There are consistent reports of recollections of anxiety, pain, tiredness, weakness, thirst, the presence of catheters, intubation and intravenous lines, as well as some minor procedures, such as physiotherapy.[18] Patients may also recall dreaming, hearing conversations and noise. Many of these may be distressing and can have an effect on later psychological recovery.[21]

Even though many ICU patients report no memories of their admission, they may report distress when faced or presented with stimuli, which they associate with their illness; for example, watching medical programs on television or being alone remain unconscious reminders of their experience. Memories can be explicit and consciously remembered or implicit and remembered unconsciously. These two types of recollection can have different consequences and effects on subsequent behavior and emotion.

Most research methodologies when investigating memory have utilized questionnaires and/or interviews. There is great variation reported in these studies as to the length of time post ICU transfer that patient interviews are undertaken. Some researchers have sent out postal questionnaires 3 months following discharge,[3,10] 2 weeks after ICU discharge[21] or just 2 days following

ICU discharge.[22] Two methodological issues are noteworthy here: the time factor can affect recall as can the way patients were interviewed. Patients may be asked what they can recall or they may be presented with a list of events that may have occurred and then asked if they can recall any of them during their ICU admission. These contrasting designs have left this area of investigation with numerous problems in interpreting results. Nevertheless, the trends described above are noteworthy and have implications for clinical practice. Sedated patients may hear what clinicians say and it may be more appropriate that management plans are discussed away from the bedside. It could be postulated that these types of memory studies might, indeed, be eliciting accounts of patient awareness rather than just memory/recall.

INTENSIVE CARE SYNDROME AND DELIRIUM

The investigations of patients' memories and recollections of their ICU stay have identified a number of features, some of which have been described above. All patients admitted to hospital will have memories of their treatment, not all will be distressing and certainly not all will necessarily have adverse psychological effects. However, a significant proportion of ICU discharged patients report disturbances in psychological functioning post discharge and these rates vary from 10 to 20%.[23] There is a difference in opinion as to whether ICU patients experience hallucinations and delusions, or whether their experience can best be described as delirium resulting from a medical condition.[24–26] Hallucinations are recognized as disorders of perception that have a compelling sense of reality even in the absence of external stimuli provoking such perceptions (in this context, seeing or hearing things in the unit that do not exist). Delusions are false beliefs and are disorders of thought (in this context, a belief, for example, of being attacked by the nursing staff). Delirium is a disturbance of consciousness (i.e. reduced clarity of awareness of the environment) with reduced ability to focus, sustain or shift attention.

In a study investigating the risk factors identified as being associated with delirium in ICU,[24] patients with a history of hypertension, alcohol abuse, chronic obstructive pulmonary disease and smoking had increased episodes of delirium. Where sodium, glucose and bilirubin were in the abnormal range, and where morphine had been administered, the risk of delirium increased.[24] There is general agreement that there is a complex interaction of several contributing factors, most of which become evident when patients regain consciousness after the ventilation and sedation process.

Reports of ICU syndrome[23,27,28] have described a constellation of clinical signs that include fluctuating levels of consciousness, poor orientation, hallucinations, delusions and a number of behavioral anomalies, such as aggression and passivity. In a study where confusion was a particular focus of investigation following cardiac surgery,[29] it was noted that patients describe a variety of ways in which it occurs. Common reports include nightmares during and after an ICU stay, dreams of being imprisoned, of torture and dehumanization, as well as the unit being perceived in different ways, such as a ship or a motorized vehicle. These instances have been referred to as 'the phenomenal chaos'[29] in which patients lose touch with reality, which is then replaced by the experience of confusion and anxiety.

The diagnosis of post traumatic stress disorder (PTSD) is controversial, as there are specific criteria for such a diagnosis and it is arguable that not all of these will be present in patients within ICUs, or when transferred to other wards.[30] It is more probable that these patients have post-traumatic-related symptoms[21] rather than PTSD per se. One exception to this is the report that investigated psychological reactions to life-threatening injuries in patients admitted to an ICU.[31] These authors found that a significant proportion of patients presented with PTSD specifically linked to the seriousness of the accidents that they had experienced and the injuries sustained. The patients were pre-morbidly psychologically and physically healthy, and were then suddenly and unexpectedly exposed to an overwhelming life-threatening stressor.

The ICU syndrome has been defined as an 'acute organic brain syndrome involving impaired intellectual functioning that occurs in patients who are treated within a critical care unit'.[23] Some authors have gone further in their description and have suggested that when the patients are unable to adequately judge reality, the syndrome can controversially be termed an 'ICU psychosis'.[32] In examining the psychological consequence of an ICU admission as a distinct entity, it has been suggested that, too often, the expectation that the patient will be confused can result in an inaccurate clinical assessment and a lack of attention to the indications of delirium.[26] Failure to recognize this can have an adverse effect on patient outcomes where it is argued that early recognition of delirium and its appropriate treatment can reduce morbidity, length of stay and mortality. Transferring patients from ICU does not resolve 'ICU psychosis' because their symptoms are more similar to delirium and are not related to actual psychiatric disorders.[26] Authors and researchers in the field do not necessarily accept this claim, thus introducing a second potential area of disagreement. For the purposes of the present discussion, whether the disturbed and psychologically distressed patient is presenting with delirium or a psychotic-related condition is not the issue; what is of more concern are the symptoms, their cause and their management.

Environmental factors

The symptoms outlined thus far have been linked to potential environmental factors within intensive and critical care units. Many authors have suggested that these factors are associated with severe psychological distress, but clear causal links are yet to be established. To do so, would require a complex investigation with matched patients, and controlled and standard-ized treatments administered within a range of ergonomically contrasting environments. The status of the empirical literature to date has yet to con-clusively find environmental correlates with ICU distress.

The factors within ICU environments that are considered to contribute to the ICU syndrome have included both physiological disturbances and psy-chological stressors, such as sleep deprivation/disturbance, noise, social isol-ation, immobilization, unfamiliar surroundings, sensory monotony and an absence of diurnal light variation. Patients are simultaneously subjected to life-threatening illnesses, the awe of medical procedures and technology, an inability to communicate needs, a new and threatening environment and the loss of personal control. Windowless rooms increase the risk of developing delirium, whereas open rooms with windows have been shown to decrease the incidence of delirium, when this variable was included in a univariate analysis.[24] These authors also suggest that environmental modification may be associated with better control of psychological symptoms, without neces-sarily preventing them. This view contrasts with those who suggest that attending to these factors has little clinical or prognostic psychological influ-ence.[25] However, although in and of themselves, these factors have been found to impair functioning in healthy individuals, their effects in causing ICU-related psychological distress have yet to be conclusively proven.

Sleep

Sleep is an essential part of the 24-hour cycle and its purpose is to prevent physiological and psychological exhaustion and illness. A lack of sleep extends the recovery time from illness. There are four stages of sleep: stage I – sleep latency; stage II – slow wave sleep; stage III – rapid eye movement latency and stage IV – rapid eye movement sleep. The first stage covers the time between trying to sleep and actually falling asleep. Stages I and II together comprise non-REM sleep, stages III and IV are REM phases. Individuals normally experience at least four to six cycles of sleep each 24 hours. The average time for a normal sleep cycle is 90 minutes, but it varies from 70 to 120 minutes. REM sleep is essential for mental restoration and these become longer and more intense in later sleep cycles, occurring pri-marily in the last cycles of an interrupted night of sleep. Because of REM sleep's importance, it is likely that sleep deprivation is most significant when it occurs during this stage. Within an ICU, sleep deprivation probably results in a discontinuity of the sleep cycle, with effects such as irritability and anxiety, physical exhaustion and fatigue, and a disruption of metabolic functions, including adrenal hormone production.[22]

In a study investigating the experience of patients in an ICU,[33] 42% reported being unable to sleep, and those who did manage some sleep reported 'drifting on and off into sleep'.[33] Factors associated with sleep disturbance included noise, being in pain, and day- and night-time disorientation. This lack of sleep often results in disorientation, so that patients lose track of time, fail to recognize familiar faces and experience memory impairment.

Noise

Noise levels in hospitals, particularly in high technology wards, invariably exceed the recommended levels and can have detrimental psychological and physiological effects on both patients and staff.[34] From a review of a number of studies[35] it was noted that noise levels above 50 decibels have a 50% probability of altering the nature of an individual's sleep. Noise is universally seen as a distressing factor by both patients and staff, usually because of their perception that alarms are always a cause of concern. Ventilators and other machines supplying oxygen are invariably noisy and can affect communication, concentration and sleep. In an investigation of ICU stressors,[36] pain, followed by inability to sleep, were rated as the greatest stressors among a random sample of 50 ICU patients. Other auditory stressors included clinical staff talking too loudly, hearing other patients cry out, hearing unfamiliar and unusual sounds that could not be explained and hearing alarms. This study has been replicated with similar results.[37] When patients were asked the extent to which they experienced noise and how much of a disturbance it was, 40% reported hearing noise, 20% noted that it was very disturbing and 65% reported that it disturbed them a great deal. The 'normal egocentricity of critically ill persons'[38] causes them to interpret all surrounding conversation and action as pertaining to them. If the levels of noise exceed the limits to which the individual can comfortably adapt, then the coping system fails with the increased risk of psychological disturbance.

Sensory deprivation

Sensory input addresses the stimulation of all five senses: visual, auditory, olfactory, tactile and gustatory. Patients within ICUs have no control over the choice of their environment or most of its stimuli and, therefore, it is important to control these to avoid sensory deprivation or sensory overload. Sensory deprivation can lead to a variety of symptoms that occur after a reduction in both the quality and the quantity of sensory input. A variety of symptoms have been observed in normal adults after exposure to sensory deprivation, including a loss of sense of time, boredom, a presence of hallucinations, illusions and delusions, fear, anxiety, restlessness and psychotic symptoms.[22] Sensory overload, in contrast, involves excessive inputs into the five senses, which within a critical care context can include high noise levels, pain, continuous rhythmic sounds and an absence of diurnal light variation. Sensory overload from the environment can lead to patients becoming anxious and restless, and other excessive stimuli in the environment can influence a patient's recovery, for example, high levels of noise increasing the need for pain relief. If environmental stimuli exceed the limits to which individuals can comfortably adapt, the coping system fails and behaviors, such as anxiety, panic, confusion, delusions and hallucinations, may result.[22,23] The hospital environment often deprives patients of normal sensory input, while continuously exposing them to a continuous range of sensory stimuli not found in the average home environment. This situation, which is a combination of sensory deprivation and overload, is referred as the 'hospital phenomenon'.[22] Normal sounds from home that are familiar to patients (e.g. voices, telephones, traffic, television, appliances) usually diminish at night, whereas the sounds of the ICU (e.g. ventilators and monitors, curtain rails, suctioning, pagers) are unfamiliar and continuous throughout the day and night. These sounds and sights cause additional patient distress, and should, if possible, be reduced so that sensory and environmentally induced stress can be minimized.

Social isolation can also result in a loss of reality testing; for reality testing to occur, there must be continuous input of familiar, meaningful information from the patient's outside world. If this information is lacking, the patient's internal mental events can be mistaken for external ones, which may explain why some critical care patients appear to have hallucinations. It has been proposed that there is a process that affects memory negatively for actual external events, but enhances memory for internal events.[39] The physical constraints and social isolation experienced by ICU patients, and the life-threatening nature of the illness, may increase their experience of hypnagogic hallucinations. Attentional shift during these hypnagogic images from external stimuli to internally generated images could explain why some ICU patients have such poor recall of real external events, but can clearly remember hallucinations and vivid nightmares.

GOOD-PRACTICE GUIDELINES

There have been a number of accounts describing good-practice guidelines for technologically advanced critical care environments.[18,27,33,38] Common themes from these include:

- Reduce anxiety by attempting to facilitate communication, whether or not the patient is ventilated, by exploring the most appropriate way to convey reassurance and sensitive explanations. Similarly, explore methods to enable the patient to make their needs and fears known.
- Keep unnecessary and frightening levels of noise to a minimum.
- Collect information from those known to the patient relating to hobbies, interests, musical tastes, family photographs, and make these available in an attempt to orient the patient. Any attempt to orientate the patient in both time and place will be invaluable.

- Provide security information, such as time and place orientation, as well as an explanation of treatments and procedures.
- Ensure adequate pain relief and sedation with an appreciation of different types of pain.
- Provide physiotherapy or massage to relieve discomfort from prolonged immobility.
- Attempt to resource the unit with modern up-to-date ventilators or consider tracheotomy to allow ventilation without heavy sedation.
- Encourage friends and family to visit, and provide them with information about approaching an unresponsive patient.
- Introduce diurnal variation in an attempt to regulate day–night changes, and ensure that each patient can see a window.
- Try to provide, within reason, continuity of care by the same medical and nursing staff.
- Try, where possible, to arrange pre-admission and post-transfer visits.

CASE STUDY REVIEWED

This then describes the environment in which Clifford spent 43 days of his life. He was supported by sophisticated health technology, monitored by many machines, fed by ingenious methods of nutritional supplements and cared for by a dedicated staff and a loving family. The clinicians' teamwork that characterized this ICU, but is not always evident to patients and relatives, made choices, took decisions, and sought advice throughout his stay. Following his transfer he was seen by the outreach team and was invited back to the ICU follow-up clinic. Clifford's care highlights the fact that his admission was impacted upon to a considerable degree by physical, psychological, interpersonal and environmental factors.

When reflecting on his stay, there were times when the physical boundary between Clifford and the technology appeared to be blurred. Attempts were made to reduce the adverse effects of the technology, but, inevitably, the choices made to maintain a life outweighed some of the (psychological) consequences. At times, the staff attending to him did refer to him as 'the man in bed 7' as a quick form of communication, but equally, even when he was sedated, he was spoken to compassionately and sensitively. Although the monitoring screen was described and explained to his wife and sons, they more often than not looked at the staffs' faces as they watched the monitor, emphasizing the importance of non-verbal communication. This aspect of the relationship with relatives when in ICUs is so easily overlooked.

As a ventilated patient, Clifford had difficulties being weaned off the ventilator and this had to be done in small stages. When a speaking valve was put on his tracheostomy tube and he was able to talk, there were tears of joy from his family when they heard his voice for the first time after thinking they may never hear him speak again. He was extremely distressed and uncomfortable while on the ventilator; his mouth was dry, he could not accurately convey when he was in discomfort, his sleep was disturbed and the continuous noise, though not too intrusive, was a constant irritant.

Although sedated, Clifford was aware of some of the procedures he underwent and reported that he did hear some of the conversations. Although for the majority of his stay he was pain free, his recollections of his time in the unit were confused. He showed agitation, anxiety and at times was unable to distinguish reality from his dreams (hallucinations). Although he did not display florid psychotic symptoms, he did not recognize his family, believed he was being attacked by those providing his care and that his blood was being used for some form of ritual.

The current understanding of ICU quality of life involves an assessment and management of pain, recall of the admission, sleep disturbance, and other psychological variables, such as anxiety, confusion, agitation, delusions, hallucinations and delirium. The importance of these aspects of a patient's intensive care are too often ignored, and while good physical progress may be made, the psychological trauma that appears in conjunction with a traumatic illness or injury, is too readily neglected. Clifford experienced, among others, an emotional response to the severity of the condition that threatened his life. His experience is similar to that reported by patients facing life-threatening danger.[40] When recognizing their grave danger, these patients experienced enhanced visual imagery, panoramic memory, detachment from their bodies and altered time awareness.

There is a significant literature on providing for the needs and the support of patient's relatives.[41] Their needs can be met through the provision of accurate information and treatment explanations, agreements that they will be called immediately if the patient's condition deteriorates, allowing open visiting hours and, if possible, not being marginalized or ignored. Clifford had young grandchildren and it was important to him that they were allowed to visit. Preparing young people for this is important, as it can become an image that may linger in young memories. Debriefing for the family following the visit was extremely helpful and the youngsters were encouraged to leave pictures and mementos to familiarize him with his family relationships.

Modern technology creates tensions and potential conflict because it offers new choices, generates more information and calls for adaptive change. The problem is not necessarily with the technology itself, but the human response it so often generates. The intensity of this particular healthcare environment does not always afford patients and their relatives the privacy that they would ideally require or wish. Not only do they have to share their personal space with a continuously changing staff team, but it is also shared with potentially intrusive technology. The challenge is to master the environment rather than become one of its slaves.

ACKNOWLEDGEMENT

The author acknowledges the useful comments from Dr Mike Swart, Consultant Anesthetist, on an earlier draft of this chapter.

REFERENCES

1. Cook DJ, Sibbald WJ 1999 The promise and the paradox of technology in the intensive care unit. Canadian Medical Association Journal 161: 1118–1119, p. 1118
2. Walters AJ 1995 Technology and the lifeworld of critical care nursing. Journal of Advanced Nursing 22: 338–346, p. 338
3. Gadow S 1984 Touch and technology: two paradigms of patient care. Journal of Religion and Health 23: 63–69
4. Webb AR 2001 Assessment of medical devices. In: Sibbald WJ, Bion F eds. Evaluating critical care: using health services research to improve quality. Springer, London, 244–254
5. Bergbom-Engberg I, Haljamae H 1988 A retrospective study of patient's recall of respirator treatment: nursing care factors and feelings of security/insecurity. Intensive Care Nursing 4: 95–101
6. Granberg A, Engberg IB, Lundberg D 1998 Patients' experience of being critically ill or severely injured and cared for in an intensive care unit in relation to the ICU syndrome. Part 1. Intensive and Critical Care Nursing 14: 294–307, p. 304
7. MacConnell E 1990 The impact of machines on the work of critical care nurses. Critical Care Nursing Quarterly 12: 45–52
8. Clifford C 1986 Patients, relatives and nurses in a technological environment. Intensive Care Nursing 2: 67–72
9. Ashworth P 1987 The needs of the critically ill patient. Intensive Care Nursing 3: 182–190
10. Asbury AJ 1985 Patients' memories and reactions to intensive care. Care of the Critically Ill 1: 12–13
11. Jablonsky JS 1994 The experience of being mechanically ventilated. Qualitative Health Research 4: 186–207
12. Johnson MM, Sexton DL 1990 Distress during mechanical ventilation: patients' perception. Critical Care Nursing 10: 48–51
13. Stovsky B, Rudy E, Dragonette P 1988 Caring for ventilated patients: comparison of two types of communication methods used after cardiac surgery with patients with endotracheal tubes. Heart and Lung 17: 281–289
14. Hafsteindottir TB 1996 Patients' experience of communication during the respirator treatment period. Intensive and Critical Care Nursing 12: 261–271
15. Wojnicki-Johansson G 2001 Communication between nurse and patient during ventilator treatment: patient reports and registered nurse evaluation. Intensive and Critical Care Nursing 17: 29–39
16. Verity S 1996 Communication with sedated ventilated patients in intensive care: focusing on the use of touch. Intensive and Critical Care Nursing 12: 354–358
17. Milner QJ, Gunning MA 2000 Sedation in the intensive care unit. British Journal of Intensive Care 10: 12–16
18. Shelley MP 1998 Sedation in the ITU. Care of the Critically Ill 14: 85–88
19. Gow GL 1995 Influence of sedation regimes: effects on recall following treatment in an ICU. British Journal of Intensive Care 5: 112–116
20. Wagner BK, O'Hara DA, Hammond JS 1997 Drugs for amnesia in the ICU. American Journal of Critical Care 6: 192–201
21. Jones C, Griffiths RD, Humphris G et al. 2001 Memory, delusions and the development of acute posttraumatic stress disorder-related symptoms after intensive care. Critical Care Medicine 29: 573–580
22. Gibbons CR, Brown DJ, Shelly MP 1993 Patient memories and satisfaction with intensive care. Clinical Intensive Care 4: 222–225

23. Kleck HG 1984 ICU syndrome: onset, manifestations, treatment stressors and prevention. Critical Care Quarterly 6: 21–28, p. 23
24. Dubois MJ, Bergeron N, Dumont M et al. 2001 Delirium in an intensive care unit: a study of risk factors. Intensive Care Medicine 27: 1297–1304
25. McGuire BE, Basten CJ, Ryan CJ et al. 2000 Intensive care syndrome: a dangerous misnomer. Archives of Internal Medicine 160: 906–909
26. Justic M 2000 Does ICU psychosis really exist? Critical Care Nurse 20: 28–37
27. Bennun I 2001 Intensive care unit syndrome: a consideration of psychological interventions. British Journal of Medical Psychology 74: 369–377
28. Granberg-Axel A, Bergbom I, Lundberg D 2001 Clinical signs of ICU syndrome/delirium: an observational study. Intensive and Critical Care Nursing 17: 72–93
29. Laitenen H 1996 Patients' experience of confusion in the intensive care unit following cardiac surgery. Intensive and Critical Care Nursing 12: 79–83
30. Scragg P, Jones A, Fauvel N 2001 Psychological problems following ICU treatment. Anaesthesia 56: 9–14
31. Schnyder U, Morgeli H, Nigg C et al. 2000 Early psychological reactions to life threatening injuries. Critical Care Medicine 28: 86–92
32. Eisendrath S 1982 ICU syndrome revisited. Critical Care Update 9: 31–35
33. Green A 1996 An exploratory study of patients' memory recall of their stay in an adult intensive therapy unit. Intensive and Critical Care Nursing 12: 131–137
34. McLaughin A, McLaughin B, Elliott J et al. 1996 Noise levels in a cardiac intensive care unit: a preliminary conducted in secret. Intensive and Critical Care Nursing 12: 226–230
35. Turnick C 1994 Technology in critical care nursing. In: Millar B, Burnard P eds. Critical care nursing: caring for the critically ill adult patient. Ballière Tindall, London, 74–92
36. Novaes MA, Aronovich A, Ferraz E et al. 1997 Stressors in ICU: patients' evaluation. Intensive Care Medicine 23: 1282–1285
37. Hofhuis J, Bakker J 1998 Experiences of critically ill patients in the ICU: what do they think of us? International Journal of Intensive Care 5: 114–117
38. Hudack C 1994 Critical care nursing: a holistic approach. 6th edn. JB Lippincott, London, p. 34
39. Jones C, Griffiths RD, Humphris G 2000 Disturbed memory and amnesia related to intensive care. Memory 8: 779–794
40. Noyes R, Slymen DJ 1978 The subjective response to life threatening danger. OMEGA 9: 313–321
41. Bennun I 1999 Intensive care units: a systemic perspective. Journal of Family Therapy 21: 96–112

WEBSITE OF INTEREST

Comprehensive Critical Care (Department of Health – UK): www.doh.gov.uk/compcritcare/

Conclusion

15

Thinking through enabling technologies: guidelines for development and implementation

Pamela Gallagher   Malcolm MacLachlan

SUMMARY

Throughout this volume, implicit and sometimes quite explicit guidance on the process of technology development has been offered by the contributors. Consequently, in this concluding chapter, we offer what we consider to be the emerging important guidelines for the development, trialing and implementation of both 'user-needs-led' and 'technology-opportunity-led' enabling technologies in the hope that the potential benefits of technologies for both body image and body function can be more fully realized.

INTRODUCTION

Technology can listen to, interact with, replace or 'take over' bodily functioning. None of these are fixed or finite, and it is as a part of these dynamics that the complexity of 'the person' interplays with the potential of technology. The technology, irrespective of whether it is in the user's environment, on their person or in their body, is effectively an interface between that person and the life they wish to lead. It is, therefore, how people react to technology, and not the technology itself, that can decide just how 'enabling' or 'assistive' it is.

We can think of technology as making an important contribution to an overall system for managing life, a system also comprised of the individual using the technology, their family, social network, the social and physical environment, and the clinicians, therapists and technicians. If we fail to concentrate on all aspects of the system and only concentrate on a single aspect, for example, the technology, this may impede the overall ability of the system to achieve a desired function or goal. As the development of technology continues to grow, both in quantity and sophistication, this places a greater onus on its creators and those who prescribe and maintain it, to be aware of its impact on the psychological ways in which people understand and construct their difficulties and attempt to cope with them.

GUIDELINES

This volume has covered a wide spectrum of technologies from invasive to non-invasive, from adjunctive to integral, and from enabling to life giving. In particular, it is useful to note that the application of some technologies can be adapted to accommodate user preferences or needs, while others are fairly standard. Some technology is developed with a particular person-need in mind, that is, user-needs-led enabling technology. However, at times, technologies can come into existence and be applied to an existing need when meeting that need had never been contemplated during the development of the technology: technology-opportunity-led enabling technology.

No set of guidelines can be all encompassing. Rather, it is our aim in this chapter to bring to the reader's attention what we felt were emerging broad principles for the development and implementation of technology, both arising from within specific chapters and emerging across several chapters. We, therefore, outline issues that seem to us noteworthy for the development of technologies that truly enable, or assist their users. These guidelines are not arranged in any order of importance. They are not intended to be exhaustive, mutually exclusive, or even necessarily original, but rather to encourage people to *think through* the development and implementation of new technologies and, in so doing, to increase the likelihood of them being truly enabling for both *body image and body function.*

Utility

Beneficiary utility refers to the importance of developing technology that makes a fundamental contribution to the life of the individual using the technology. In the current climate of evidence-based practice, there is a prerequisite for identifying a definite need and fully investigating the potential impacts, outcomes and usefulness of the developed technology before a formal recommendation for implementation is made.

Clinical utility refers to the usefulness of the technology from the perspective of the therapist/clinician. Does the technology facilitate the work of the therapist/clinician by alleviating the pressure of time, facilitating in the provision of treatment, or by stimulating and accelerating further development in the field? Similarly to beneficiary utility, this should be established prior to widespread usage and implementation.

Ethical viability

Adhering to the rights of individuals must be implicit and rigorously applied in the development of technology that has personal and social repercussions. However, the influence of technology extends beyond the sphere of the user. Whatever is done to enable individuals can also have ramifications at a broader social level. Technology development may generate unease and play on the sensitivities of public opinion. Therefore, the extent to which the boundaries of technological development can be pushed is influenced not only by personal factors, but also by political, religious, societal and cultural factors.

Creating innovative environments

Technology itself cannot achieve anything, rather it is the way in which it is employed that is crucial. Therefore, an important aspect of technology development is an environment that promotes and encourages the advancement, creative use and novel application of technology.

Transferring technology know-how

Different technologies demand different characteristics in the therapists/clinicians who work with the technology and the user. Consequently, the attributes of those responsible for advising on, promoting and teaching the use of technology are an essential consideration. Furthermore, educating the promoters of technology is crucial in ensuring its use and integration. As there is a natural tendency for therapists/clinicians to use what they are familiar with and what is known to them, education is integral to the widespread use and implementation of technology.

Technological deframing

Technology has the propensity to engulf and enframe the individual, and it is important to be conscious of the factors that promote and alleviate this phenomenon. Every effort should be made to deframe the technology and enframe the human aspect; to diminish the manner in which technology can sometimes 'objectify' the individual, and instead to focus on the individual's subjective experience, needs and aspirations.

Technology reinforcement

Feedback is fundamental to the successful and continued usage of technology as it can play a critical role in acting as a reinforcement of the usefulness of the technology. This feedback may simply be the *enjoyment* and *interest* elicited through the use of the technology which, in turn, may act as an internal *motivation* to continue. Feedback may also emerge in the knowledge that one has control over the outcome of the technology, that there is a relationship between the user's actions and the functioning of the technology. Furthermore, being able to gauge outcome and progress, and to compare current achievements to the ultimate goal, can encourage and facilitate an improvement in the use of technology. However, these types of feedback are not always possible, and where this is the case other motivations and rewards must be considered in helping people to master new technologies. Furthermore, sometimes immediate reinforcement is not possible and the regaining of functionality is a slow and arduous process. In such circumstances, the realistic setting of achievable goals and sub-goals is crucial.

Impact of social support

Successful integration of technology into a person's lifestyle can often depend upon the acceptance of the technology by family and members of their social network. The technology has consequences not just for the individual, but also for their family and friends. Just as illness or injury can disrupt the physiological and psychological homeostasis of the individual, so too can technology disrupt the homeostatic balance of the family unit and social networks. Consequently, it is important that the influence of the technology on others is also considered.

User selection

This principle relates to two phases in the development of technology. Initially, the identification of appropriate people for the *pilot/clinical trial* stage is an important step, as the development of technology is driven not only by technical expertise, but also by the enthusiasm and desire for improvement of the potential user. A person participating in the clinical trial who is very clear on what he wants the technology to achieve will be a real asset to the development team. Secondly, the consideration of the individual characteristics of the average potential user of developed and *available technology* is important when reviewing the usefulness of the technology for a new user.

User's experiential world

An emphasis should be placed on the *unique circumstances* of users and an understanding of the *meanings* attributed to the technology by the potential user. What is the expectation of the user and what do they hope to achieve? Ensuring that expectations and outcomes coincide is extremely important as their incompatibility can result in discontinuance of use and disenchantment. An emphasis in future research should also be placed on what promotes optimal adjustment. It is important that research does not solely concentrate on the difficulties of using technology, but rather on what people can achieve and do. The individual's perception may have only a modest correlation with their medically defined characteristics. In addition, the degree to which impairment is a source of psychological distress will depend on the individual's personal and social resources.

Personalizing outcome benchmarks

Flexible benchmarks of success, which are largely dependent on individual factors of the user, should dictate the outcome of technology. The individual should be given the opportunity to take control of the situation as far as possible. It is important to avoid preconceived ideas about what is important in the lives of others and to not assume omniscience. There can be a tendency to concentrate on the physical aspects of the conditions and problems while grossly under-estimating the importance of the psychological, spiritual, emotional and social components that contribute to the person's quality of life. What might be considered an innocuous outcome for some might be powerful and hugely significant for others. Therefore, preconceived notions and assumptions need to be put to one side and consultation with the ultimate user is fundamental from the start. Concomitantly, we also have to be careful that the *evaluation* techniques for the implementation of technology take into consideration the potential capabilities and desires of the user, and ensure that we do not impose our own expectations onto what might otherwise be considered potentially successful outcomes.

CONCLUSION

Enabling technology is a prevalent form of intervention for people with a disability or disabling condition. The effective utilization of technology has been reported to improve the functional independence of persons with disabilities and to afford them a greater opportunity for societal participation and integration.[1] Given the estimated current number of people with a disability and the subsequent potential uptake of technology, research that maximizes the usage, and promotes the retention of enabling technology, will result in a saving of time, money and stress. More importantly, it will facilitate independent living, increase contribution to community and work and participation in society, and improve quality of life.

We are conscious that the psychological implications emerging from the work reviewed in this volume are merely the tip of the iceberg, but nonetheless at least it is now recognized that the iceberg is there! We hope our concern in this volume to address both body image and body function will spur on more research from this perspective and that the above guidelines offer a point of reference for doing so.

REFERENCE

1. Heinemann A, Pape T 2001 Coping and adjustment. In: Scherer M ed. Assistive technology: matching device and consumer for successful rehabilitation. American Psychological Association, 123–153

Biographies of Authors

Campbell Aird
Moffat, Scotland

Campbell Aird is a hotelier who owns and runs his own hotel in Moffat, Scotland. He had his right arm amputated in 1983 and has been a prosthesis wearer ever since. Over the past 10 years he has been involved in trialing, publicizing and contributing research ideas to electrically powered prosthetics.

Ned Augenblick HDipMaths
Media Lab Europe, Dublin, Ireland

Ned Augenblick graduated summa cum laude from Georgetown University in 1998, with a double major in economics and psychology. He received a higher diploma in mathematical sciences from University College Dublin as a Mitchell Scholar in 2001. He is a consultant psychologist to Media Lab Europe, Dublin, Ireland.

Danièle Bachmann MD
Hospices Civils de Lyon, France

Danièle Bachmann is a psychiatrist and psychoanalyst (Paris Psychoanalytic Society) who works for half of her time as a Practicien Hospitalier in the Hospices Civils de Lyon in France and for the other half as a private consultant.

Ian Bennun BSocSci(Hons) MPhil PhD
School of Psychology, University of Exeter and Department of Clinical Psychology, South Devon Healthcare NHS Trust, Devon, UK

Ian Bennun is a senior lecturer in the School of Psychology at the University of Exeter, UK. He is also a District Clinical Psychologist in the Department of Clinical Psychology, South Devon Healthcare NHS Trust, UK.

Niels Birbaumer PhD
Institute of Medical Psychology and Behavioral Neurobiology, University of Tübingen, Germany & Center for Cognitive Neuroscience, University of Trento, Italy

Niels Birbaumer is a full professor in the Institute of Medical Psychology and Behavioral Neurobiology, University of Tübingen, Germany and Center for Cognitive Neuroscience, University of Trento, Italy. His research interests include brain–computer interfaces and neuroprostheses, cortical reorganization and learning, psychophysiological treatment of epilepsy, Parkinson and attention-deficit disorders, and chronic pain.

Gabriel Burloux MD
Hospices Civils de Lyon, France

Gabriel Burloux is a psychiatrist and psychoanalyst (Paris Psychoanalytical Society) and has worked with hand-graft patients since the first limb transplant in Lyon, France in 1998. He is attached to the Hospices Civils de Lyon in France.

Verna Cain RN
Department of Rehabilitation Medicine, University of Washington School of Medicine, USA

Verna Cain is the nurse manager of the Burn/Plastic Clinic and is coordinator of the Outpatient Nursing Care, Burn/Plastic Center, Harborview Burn Center, Seattle. She was the first nurse in history to conduct wound care on a burn patient immersed in virtual reality, which is featured on the cover of the medical journal *Pain*, and she became an early advocate of further exploration of the use of virtual reality analgesia technology for severe burn patients' pain control.

James Condron BScEng
Media Lab Europe, Dublin, Ireland

James Condron is a research fellow in Media Lab Europe, Dublin, Ireland. He graduated from Dublin Institute of Technology (DIT), Kevin Street, in 1997 with a degree in electrical and electronic engineering. He then proceeded to do a masters in biomedical engineering, specializing in biomedical signal acquisition and analysis, with special emphasis on heart signal (ECG) analysis. In 2000 he transferred into a PhD program focusing on brainwave signal capture and analysis, which he is currently completing.

Robert D. Dowling BSc MD
Associate Professor, Department of Surgery, Division of Thoracic and
Cardiovascular Surgery, University of Louisville, Kentucky, USA

Robert D. Dowling is a professor of surgery at the University of
Louisville School of Medicine and is also the co-principal investigator for
the Jewish Hospital/University of Louisville AbioCor research team.
Dr Dowling received his bachelor of science degree in chemistry from
Allegheny College where he was inducted into Phi Beta Kappa. He
completed his MD, general surgery residency and cardiothoracic
residency at the University of Pittsburgh, Pennsylvania, USA. Having
joined the faculty and staff at the University of Louisville and Jewish
Hospital in 1994, he is now widely recognized as an expert in ventricular
remodeling (the 'Batista' procedure), transmyocardial revascularization and
mechanical heart devices. His work on these topics has been published in
the *New England Journal of Medicine, Journal for Thoracic and Cardiovascular
Surgery,* the *Annals of Thoracic Surgery,* the *Journal for Cardiothoracic Surgery*
and the *ASAIO Journal.* Dr Dowling is currently Director of the Heart
Transplant and Cardiac Assist Devices Program for the Transplant Center
at the University of Louisville Jewish Hospital, USA.

Phil Ellis PhD MA ARCM CertEd
School of Arts, Design, Media and Culture, University of Sunderland, UK

Phil Ellis is a Professor in Music within Performance Arts Studies in the
School of Arts, Design, Media and Culture at the University of
Sunderland. He was formerly Principal Research Fellow and Senior
Lecturer at the University of Warwick. His research interests have focused
on aesthetics, technology and creativity. Since 1992 his research has led to
the development of Sound Therapy for children with profound and
multiple learning difficulties, and this work is also being developed with
the elderly. This project has been awarded significant funding for a
two-year investigation. He has also been co-ordinator for an EU (European
Union) funded project in the i3 ESPRIT programme and is currently
involved in another EU project investigating tactile interactive
multimedia for blind and visually impaired children. Other activities
include being former co-chair of the International Society for Music
Education commission on Music in Special Education, Music Therapy and
Medicine programme.

Pamela Gallagher BAMod PhD DipStat
Faculty of Science and Health, School of Nursing, Dublin City University,
Dublin, Ireland

Pamela Gallagher is a lecturer of psychology in the School of Nursing at Dublin City University, Ireland. She was awarded her PhD in psychology through the University of Dublin, Trinity College, during which time she developed the 'Trinity Amputation and Prosthesis Experience Scales', which is currently being used internationally. Subsequently, her work in the Health Research Board involved the development and management of the National Physical and Sensory Disability Database, a national service-planning database, on behalf of the Irish government's Department of Health and Children. Her research areas of interest include psychosocial adjustment to illness and disability (e.g. amputation), phantom-limb pain, health service research and development, and the impact of assistive technology on the individual.

Azucena Garcia-Palacios PhD
Universidad Jaume I (Castellon Spain), and Human Interface Technology Laboratory, University of Washington, USA

Azucena Garcia-Palacios was recently promoted from assistant professor to professor of clinical psychology at Universitat Jaume I, Castellon Spain (bypassing the position of associate professor). She is a clinical psychologist who treats patients at the Anxiety Disorders Clinic in Spain, often using virtual reality exposure therapy as part of the treatment. She has worked in the USA as a visiting scientist at Harvard University, and has been collaborating with Hunter Hoffman at the University of Washington Human Interface Technology Lab for several years. In addition to studying the use of virtual reality distraction for pain control with Hunter G Hoffman and David R Patterson, she has also, along with her advisor and their virtual reality research group in Spain, helped to pioneer the use of virtual reality exposure therapy in the treatment of spider phobia (at the HITLab), anorexia and claustrophobia.

David Gow BSc PG Dip
Director, Rehabilitation Engineering Services, Eastern General Hospital, Edinburgh, Scotland

David Gow is director of Rehabilitation Engineering Services in Lothian Primary Care NHS Trust in Edinburgh, Scotland. Now based at the Eastern General Hospital, David is a prosthetics engineer who has worked in upper limb prosthetics research and development since 1981. He has led the research team at Edinburgh's Bioengineering Centre to produce leading edge prosthetics projects including the Edinburgh Modular Arm System and Prodigits.

Hunter G. Hoffman PhD
Human Interface Technology Laboratory, University of Washington, and Departments of Radiology and Psychology, University of Washington, USA

Hunter Hoffman is director of the Analgesia Neuroscience Research Center at the University of Washington Human Interface Technology Laboratory (HITLab) in Seattle, Washington. Dr Hoffman began as an experimental psychologist specializing in human memory and attention at Princeton and the University of Washington. Since joining the HITLab in 1993, Hunter has explored the medical and psychological applications of virtual reality. He is interested in techniques for maximizing presence, the use of touchable virtual spiders in 'Spider World' (a technology used in the treatment of spider phobia) and at Cornell-Presbyterian Hospital in Manhattan, with JoAnn Difede, he recently helped to develop a virtual reality exposure therapy for treating acute post-traumatic stress disorder for World Trade Center survivors. Dr Hoffman also designed and, with instrument maker Jeff Magula, implemented the construction of a unique optic fiber photonic virtual reality helmet that can be safely used by burn patients getting wound care in the scrub tank, along with a sister 'magnetically inert' system for delivery of virtual reality images to patients during fMRI scans. These helmets both use 800 000 tiny optic fibers per eye.

Darran Hughes BScEng MScEng
Media Lab Europe, Dublin, Ireland

Darran Hughes joined Media Lab Europe as a research fellow in September 2001. He completed his degree course in electronic engineering in the University College Dublin in 1996. His main outside research at this time was in language evolution and speech perception, and so he continued his studies by doing a masters in engineering science from the University College Dublin in biomedical engineering based in the National Rehabilitation Hospital in Dun Laoghaire, Dublin, Ireland. His thesis was on methods of speech enhancement for dysarthic (cerebral palsy) speech.

Bodil Jönsson PhD MA
Certec, Division of Rehabilitation Engineering Research, Department of Design Sciences, Lund University, Sweden

Bodil Jönsson is a professor of rehabilitation engineering and head of research at Certec, the Division of Rehabilitation Engineering, Department of Design Sciences at Lund University, Sweden. She founded Certec in 1987. Her background is in physics in which she received her PhD, taught and wrote textbooks. She has also contributed to public debate and written extensively on environmental concerns. Her current areas of interest are information technology and learning, especially with regard to the benefits of new technological and educational concepts for people with disabilities. She is in the process of establishing the Swedish research program, *Pacemaking,* which focuses on stress-related illnesses, their causes, consequences and cures. During the last 15 years she has received numerous awards in the areas of education and science, including the 1999 Swedish Royal Institute of Technology Prize. Throughout her career she has made a number of radio and television appearances as well as attending numerous public-speaking engagements. To the general Swedish public she is a familiar figure from the television program *Ask the Experts in Lund*. She is the author of several books including *Unwinding the Clock: Ten Thoughts on Our Relationship to Time*, 1999, Harcourt, which has been translated into nine languages.

Thierry Keller MS PhD
Rehabilitation Engineering Group, ParaCare, Paraplegic Center, University Hospital Balgrist, Zurich and Automatic Control Laboratory, Swiss Federal Institute of Technology, Zurich, Switzerland

Thierry Keller received both his doctorate (2001) and his degree in electrical engineering (1995) from the Swiss Federal Institute of Technology Zurich (ETHZ), Switzerland. He is currently working as a visiting research scholar at the Department of Physical Therapy and Human Movement Science at Northwestern University in Chicago, and the Sensory Motor Performance Program at the Rehabilitation Institute of Chicago, USA. In addition, he is in charge of the Rehabilitation Engineering Group at ETHZ and the Paraplegic Center of University Hospital Balgrist in Zurich. Since 1995 he has held the research engineer position at the Rehabilitation Engineering Group and later he was appointed as research associate. He has developed various neuroprostheses used to improve walking and grasping functions in subjects with spinal-cord injury and stroke patients. His research interests are in the development and application of rehabilitation technology. In 2002 he was awarded the Swiss National Science Foundation (SNF) fellowship for advanced researchers, and in 1997, together with Dr Milos R. Popovic, he received the Technology Transfer Award – 1st place.

Andrea Kübler PhD MSc Msc
Institute of Medical Psychology and Behavioral Neurobiology, University of Tübingen, Tübingen, Germany

Andrea Kübler is an assistant professor in the Institute of Medical Psychology and Behavioral Neurobiology at the University of Tübingen, Germany. She is currently a visiting Fellow in the Department of Psychology and Institute of Neuroscience, Trinity College Dublin. Her research focuses on the development of a brain–computer interface on the basis of neurofeedback for people with severe motor impairment, and on the maintenance of quality of life despite the physical disorder. Currently she is working as a postdoctoral fellow in the Department of Psychology, Trinity College Dublin, where she is investigating the effects of drug abuse on cognitive and neurological functioning in addicts by using functional magnetic resonance imaging.

Malcolm MacLachlan BSc MSc MA PhD DipBA FPSI FTCD
Department of Psychology, Trinity College, Dublin, Ireland

Malcolm MacLachlan is an associate professor of psychology at Trinity College Dublin, and undertakes clinical sessions at Cappagh National Orthopaedic Hospital, Dublin. His research interests include embodiment and disability; he is particularly interested in the rehabilitation of people with amputations and their experiences of phantom phenomena. He is director of the Trinity Psychoprosthetic Group, a multidisciplinary group interested in researching psychological adaptation to prosthetic devices. His other interests include the relationships between culture and health, and the organizational aspects of international aid.

Gary McDarby BE MengSc PhD
Media Lab Europe, Dublin, Ireland

Gary McDarby graduated from University College Dublin (UCD) in 1988 with a 1st class honors degree in electronic engineering. In 1995 he completed a masters degree in signal processing and mobile communications in UCD, and in 2000 he completed a PhD in biomedical engineering in the University of New South Wales, Sydney, Australia. He is a chartered engineer with the Institute of Engineers of Ireland (1995 IEI). He is now the principal investigator of the MindGames group in Media Lab Europe, a group which focuses on multi-disciplinary research combining the areas of biomedical signal processing, psychology, cognitive sciences and interactive gaming technologies.

Aoife Moran DipHE BNS(Hons)
School of Nursing, Dublin City University and Beaumont Hospital, Dublin, Ireland

Aoife Moran is co-ordinator of the graduate Diploma in Renal Nursing at Dublin City University, and Beaumont Hospital, Dublin. She has specialized in the area of hemodialysis for the past 7 years and is currently undertaking a PhD in this area.

David R. Patterson PhD ABPP ABPH
Division of Psychology, Department of Rehabilitation Medicine, University of Washington School of Medicine, USA

David R. Patterson is an internationally recognized expert on the use of hypnosis as a psychological pain control for severe acute burn pain, and for his research on patients' long-term adjustments to burn injuries and other forms of trauma. He is a professor and head of the Division of

Psychology, Department of Rehabilitation Medicine, University of Washington. His clinical activities/interests include consultation (as a liaison for trauma patients), adjustment to burn trauma, rehabilitation and pain control. Dr Patterson is a recipient of the Milton H. Erickson Award for Scientific Contributions to Hypnosis.

Milos R. Popovic PhD
Institute of Biomaterials and Biomedical Engineering, University of Toronto, Research Scientist, Toronto Rehabilitation Institute, Canada

Milos R. Popovic was appointed assistant professor at the Institute of Bio-materials and Biomedical Engineering at the University of Toronto in 2001; he is also a research scientist at the Toronto Rehabilitation Institute; both facilities are located in Toronto, Canada. From 1997 until 2001 he led the Rehabilitation Engineering Group at the Swiss Federal Institute of Technology (ETH) and the Paraplegic Center of the University Hospital Balgrist (ParaCare), both in Zurich, Switzerland. From 1996 until 1997 he worked for Honeywell Aerospace in Toronto, Canada. In 1996 he received his PhD degree in mechanical engineering from the University of Toronto, in addition to the electrical engineering degree from the University of Belgrade, Yugoslavia in 1990. Dr Popovic's interests are in neuromuscular systems, assistive technology, and neuro-rehabilitation. In 1997, together with Dr Thierry Keller, he received the Swiss National Science Foundation Technology Transfer Award – 1st place.

Anne Schmidt BA
Department of Rehabilitation Medicine, University of Washington School of Medicine, USA

Anne Schmidt is a research assistant at Harborview Burn Center, Seattle working for David R Patterson. She currently serves as research support on the use of hypnosis and the use of virtual reality for pain control in severe burn patients during wound care and physical therapy. She also conducts analog virtual reality pain-control research at the University of Washington. Human Interface Technology Laboratory and research into memory for virtual events with Hunter G Hoffman and David R Patterson. She has a BA degree in psychology from Seattle University, experience as a physical therapist's aid assisting in physical therapy sessions for children, and has helped educate children with autism, epilepsy, cerebral palsy, blindness and behavioral disorders.

John Sharry D Psych MSc(Mod)
Media Lab Europe, Dublin, and Department of Child and Family Psychiatry, Mater Misericordiae Hospital, Dublin, Ireland

John Sharry started as a consultant research scientist to Media Lab Europe in December 2001. He comes from a mixed science and humanities background, holding a degree in theoretical physics, a masters in social work and a doctorate in psychotherapy. Formerly, he has held posts in research physics and information technology, and latterly, as a social worker and psychotherapist. He is the principal social worker (job-share) in the Department of Child and Family Psychiatry, Mater Misericordiae Hospital, Dublin, Ireland; director of the Brief Therapy Group (a private practice, training and consultancy agency); trustee and co-founder of Parent Plus (a charity dedicated to developing educational materials for parents, children and professionals) and senior partner at EAP Solutions, an employee assistance program provider in Ireland.

Richard A. Sherman PhD
The Behavioral Medicine Research and Training Foundation, Washington State and Madigan Army Medical Center, Tacoma, Washington, USA

Richard A. Sherman directs the Behavioral Medicine Research and Training Foundation in Washington State and is chief research consultant for orthopedic surgery at Madigan Army Medical Center in Tacoma Washington, USA. His areas of interest, spanning over 30 years of research and clinical work in psychophysiology (PhD from New York University), include elucidating mechanisms and treatments for phantom-limb pain, determining the effectiveness of pulsed electromagnetic fields for treatment of migraine headaches and describing temporal relationships between changes in muscle tension and pain.

Emma K. Stokes BSc MSc MISCP MCSP
School of Physiotherapy, Trinity College Dublin, Ireland

Emma K. Stokes is a lecturer at the School of Physiotherapy, Trinity College Dublin. Her research interests include the role of technology in rehabilitation and physiotherapy rehabilitation for older people. She is a principal investigator on two EU-funded projects – GENTLE/s and I-Match – and she coordinates a national joint academic and clinical research group of physiotherapists (PROP) in Ireland.

Jennifer Tininenko BA
Department of Rehabilitation Medicine, University of Washington School of Medicine, USA

Jennifer Tininenko is a research assistant at Harborview Burn Center, Seattle working for David R Patterson. She currently serves as research support on the use of hypnosis and the use of virtual reality for pain control in severe burn patients during wound care and physical therapy. She also conducts analog virtual reality pain-control research at the University of Washington

Human Interface Technology Laboratory with Hunter G Hoffman and David R Patterson. She has a BA degree in psychology from Whitman College. She has previously conducted original research on the interconnection between coping styles and intelligence.

Helena Villa-Martín
Universidad Jaume I, Castellon, Spain

Helena Villa-Martín is a PhD student who is currently a research fellow with a masters in clinical psychology and a clinical psychologist at the Anxiety Disorders Clinic at the Universitat Jaume I, Castellon, Spain. She has conducted research in Spain on virtual reality exposure therapy for claustrophobia, and was a visiting scholar at the University of Washington Human Interface Technology Lab for 3 months.

Glossary

AbioCor™: a medical device developed by ABIOMED® to be the world's first fully implantable replacement heart that does not require percutaneous lines or the need for percutaneous access.

Affect: the conscious subjective aspect of feeling or emotion.

Arteriovenous fistula: a method of circulatory access for hemodialysis involving the anastamosis (joining) of an artery to a vein allowing arterial blood to flow through the vein, thus causing enlargement and engorgement of the vein allowing large-bore needles to be inserted during hemodialysis.

Arteriovenous graft: a method of circulatory access for hemodialysis involving the implantation of a small piece of synthetic tubing between an artery and a vein allowing the insertion of wide-bore needles for the removal and return of the patient's blood.

Arteriovenous shunt: a means of circulatory access consisting of two rigid tips inserted into an artery and a vein with a piece of connection tubing attached to both tips to maintain uninterrupted blood flow.

Ascites: a collection of free fluid in the peritoneal space of the abdomen.

Augmented reality: the use of virtual-reality principles to create a more authentic representation of the usually experienced world by intensifying certain parts of environmental conditions in order to heighten the sensory experience.

Autonomic ability: the part of the nervous system of vertebrates that controls involuntary actions of the smooth muscles, heart and glands. This can, however, be controlled using the conscious mind, hence autonomic ability.

Axons: these are elongated nerve fibers of neurons, which allow transmission of nerve impulses from one neuron to another neuron or muscle.

Biofeedback: providing a person with displays of real-time recordings of one or more physiological parameters with the aim of helping the person learn to recognize levels of physiological functioning and correct them to optimal levels as necessary. For example, showing a patient with pain due to tense jaw muscles a video display of jaw muscle tension, which the patient and an attending therapist would then use to monitor tension levels during a treatment.

Biphasic pulse: two consecutive monophasic pulses that have amplitudes with opposite signs.

Bi-ventricular: pertaining to the two lower chambers within the heart that receive and circulate blood.

Brain–computer interface (BCI): a direct connection between the brain and a computer. A BCI can be used as a means of communication for severely paralyzed patients and is controlled by the electrical activity of the brain.

Cardiac arrhythmias: alterations in cardiac conduction resulting from fluctuations in blood levels of a number of ions, e.g. potassium, calcium, magnesium and hydrogen, caused by renal disease and hemodialysis.

Cardiac-replacement therapy: the replacement of a failing heart with either a donor heart or an implantable mechanical system.

Central venous catheter: a method of circulatory access for hemodialysis involving the implantation of a cuffed dual-lumen catheter into a central vein allowing access to the blood stream for hemodialysis.

Chronic pain: continuous pain lasting more than 3 months.

Compliance: a cognitive–motivational process of personal attitudes and intentions resulting in a set of behaviors and outcomes of patient–practitioner interactions.

Contingency: relation between two events in which one is dependent upon another. If the contingency is greater than zero, then the probability of event A will be greater when event B is present than when it is absent.

Coronary heart disease (CHD): also known as coronary artery disease, this is an irregular thickening of the inner layer of the walls of the coronary arteries, resulting in the narrowing of the internal channel of the coronaries and a reduced blood supply to the heart muscle.

Cosmesis: a cosmetic cover placed over a prosthetic device to give it a more pleasing and, usually, naturalistic appearance. For instance, the hardware of the prosthetic arm may be covered with silicon, which is colored and textured to resemble the arm that was amputated.

Current pulse: a pulse of a current signal.

Delirium: a disturbance of consciousness and attention, a change in cognition or perceptual disturbances, such as hallucinations, a rapid onset and the assumption of an underlying medical cause.

Delusions: false beliefs characteristic of thought disorder.

Denial or disavowal: refusal of the mind to accept (or recognize) the reality of a traumatic, too painful perception. It involves a splitting of the ego.

Diffusion: the movement of a molecule from an area of higher solute concentration to an area of lower solute concentration.

Edinburgh arm: a system of electrically powered upper limb prosthetic components for the hand, wrist, elbow and shoulder. When combined together as modules they can form a complete or partial arm prosthesis.

Electroencephalogram (EEG): a graphical record of the electrical activity of the brain arising from neurons in the cerebral cortex; recorded non-invasively from the scalp.

Embodiment: a concept evolving from a phenomenological perspective of the person where there is the assumption that all parts of the body, both physical and psychological, are integral to the person's experience of the world.

Emotion-focused coping: a type of coping strategy directed at reducing or regulating emotional stress, e.g. reducing distress.

End-stage renal disease: insidious, progressive loss of renal function that is irreversible and implies that the kidneys are permanently damaged and that a patient can no longer survive independently without renal replacement therapy.

Erythropoeitin: the principal factor that stimulates red blood-cell production produced mainly by the kidneys, with a small amount being produced by the liver. The production of erythropoeitin diminishes in renal disease resulting in anemia.

Erythropoeitin therapy: a pharmacological agent that is biologically and immunologically identical to the patient's erythropoeitin and is administered to treat the anemia associated with renal disease.

Externally powered prosthesis: an artificial limb substitute which is powered by an external source such as electricity or compressed gas.

Extended physiological proprioception (EPP): extending the innate sense of proprioception present around the joints, such as the shoulder and elbow, into objects in contact with the body, such as a prosthesis or a tennis racket.

Fate neurosis: way of life characterized by the repetition of bad experiences. These repetitions are relived as if they are caused by bad luck, whereas they are determined by the unconscious repetition compulsion of the individual.

Feedback (in BCI technology): informing the user on-line about his or her current electrical brain activity.

Fully implantable: a medical device that is totally implanted in the body without any wires or tubes penetrating the skin. The elimination of skin penetration reduces the risk of patient infection.

Functional electrical stimulation: controlled, sequenced bursts of low-intensity electrical pulses that are used to create action potentials that can cause muscle contractions.

Functionalism: a concept that evolved from social-work theories specifying that the individual should be enabled to function acceptably and appropriately in society.

Galvanic skin response (GSR): non-invasive measurement of changes in the sympathetic and parasympathetic nervous systems.

Gate control heuristic: according to Melzack and Wall's gate control heuristic, the same incoming neural signal can be interpreted as more painful or less painful depending on what the patient is thinking at the time, where they focus their attention, beliefs about pain, expectations and attributions. Such psychological factors are thought to inhibit or modify signals coming into the brain from nerve endings on the skin surface.

Hemodialysis: a modality of treatment for renal disease, which involves removing the person's uremic blood from an artery and filtering it through a dialyzer or artificial kidney, where the blood is purified and returned to the patient via the venous system.

Hallucinations: perceptual disorders that have a compelling sense of reality in the absence of external stimuli.

Heart attack: technically known as an acute myocardial infarction (AMI), damage is caused to the heart muscle as a result of insufficient oxygen and nutrients. Heart attacks are frequent consequences of coronary heart disease.

Heart failure: this occurs when the heart is unable to pump blood at a rate to meet the body's metabolic requirements or is only able to do so at higher filling pressures.

Hypercalcemia: an elevated calcium level in the blood caused by the inability of the kidneys to process vitamin D needed for adequate intestinal absorption of calcium.

Hyperkalemia: an increase in the potassium level of the blood due to decreased renal excretion of potassium.

Hyperphosphatemia: an elevated phosphorus level caused by the decreased excretion of phosphorus from the blood by the kidneys due to renal disease.

Hypertension: an increase in blood pressure due to alterations in blood-pressure regulation caused by renal disease.

Hypoglycemia: a decrease in the patient's blood glucose level due to the removal of glucose during hemodialysis therapy.

Hypotension: a decrease in blood pressure that may be caused by a large interdialytic weight gain by the patient, which results in substantial amounts of fluid being removed or ultrafiltrated by the hemodialysis machine.

Illusory body experiences: experiencing the body in ways that do not coincide with our understanding of reality. For instance, a distorting mirror provides an experience of the body that is often amusing because it differs from our understanding of how it really is.

Immersive virtual reality system: this consists of 1) special 3-D graphics software, 2) head tracking sensors, 3) helmet-mounted visual display that blocks the patients view of the real world, 4) 3-D sound effects and 5) a means for patients to interact with the environment (to navigate through it, affect it, blow things up, and/or to pick up or influence virtual objects). In a typical immersive virtual reality (VR) set-up, participants wear a VR helmet that positions two goggle-sized miniature computer monitor screens near their eyes, focused at infinity. Electromagnetic position-tracking devices communicate changes in the user's head (and sometimes hand) location to the computer. The scenery in the virtual world changes as the user moves their head orientation (e.g. virtual objects in front of the patient in VR get closer as the user, wearing their VR helmet, leans forward in the real world). Sometimes the patients can physically touch the virtual objects, using real object props, or computer-generated force feedback devices like the pHanTom. The converging multisensory combination of sight, sound, touch and smell (and sometimes taste) helps give users a uniquely compelling experience of 'being there' in the virtual world. The essence of immersive VR is the illusion it gives users that they are inside the computer-generated environment. Immersive VR is different from related technologies, such as watching a video through a VR helmet; looking at 3-D objects through shutterglasses or 3-D glasses; augmented reality, where people see virtual images without blocking their view of the real world; and CAVES, where people go into rooms with rear-projection walls where VR images are projected onto the walls.

Inotropic medications: intravenous medication used in an attempt to increase the contractile strength of the heart.

Intensive care unit syndrome: a psychological reaction associated with an admission to an intensive care unit, which has the hallmark signs of fluctuating levels of consciousness, poor orientation, behavioral abnormalities, delusions and hallucinations.

Isaac: designed to be used as an aid for individuals with cognitive limitations, Isaac combined in one unit a pen-based computer, a digital camera, a global positioning system (GPS) receiver, and cellular phone channels for voice and data. You can read more about the original Isaac at http://www.english.certec.1th.se/isaac/isaac1.html. An overview of the project is available at http://www.english.certec.1th.se/isaac/. The key function of Isaac that made the difference was the managing of *many* digital pictures (with sound) and the bar-code interface to the computer. Today, Isaac is more of a framework, an *idea* about digital-pictures-as-language that can be implemented in many different ways. In August 2002, testing began of Isaac 2002, a software application for managing large collections of digital pictures, enabling simple combinations to become conveyers of meaningful language.

Lateral grasp: the lateral grasp is generated by first flexing the fingers to provide opposition, followed by the thumb flexion.

Monophasic pulse (or simply pulse): a rapid, transient change in the amplitude of a signal from a baseline value to a higher or lower value, followed by a rapid return to the baseline value.

Motor point: a motor point is defined as the region of easiest excitability of a muscle.

Musical instrument digital interface (MIDI): a standard whereby digital equipment can communicate. This typically includes equipment concerning sound, but also lighting and projection can be controlled via MIDI.

Myoelectric: pertaining to the electrical activity of muscles. Prostheses are controlled by these amplified physiological signals.

Neuroprosthesis: a system that applies functional electrical stimulation to generate body functions, such as standing, grasping and walking.

Operant conditioning: a form of learning in which a reinforcer (e.g. smiling face on the computer screen) is given only if the required response is performed. What has to be learned is the relationship between the response and the reinforcer.

Operant learning: the means whereby a person learns a skill or set of behaviors by receiving rewards (or reinforcement) for the desired behaviors and/or by experiencing 'punishment' (or the absence of reward) for mistakes or undesirable behaviors.

Osmosis: the movement of water across a membrane permeable to water from an area of lower solute concentration to an area of greater solute concentration to equalize the concentration on both sides of the membrane.

Osteodystrophy: bone disease caused by alterations in calcium, phosphate, vitamin D, aluminium, parathyroid glands as a result of renal disease.

Palmar grasp: the palmar grasp is generated by first forming the opposition between the thumb and the palm, followed by simultaneous flexion of both the thumb and the fingers.

Phenomenology: a set of beliefs, which indicate that the person is someone for whom things have meaning and significance, and this is constituted by the person and their linguistic skills, cultural practices and family traditions.

Problem-solving coping: a type of coping strategy directed at managing or altering a problem through the use of deliberate problem-focused efforts to alter a situation combined with an analytical approach to solving the problem.

Procedural and background pain: procedure pain is the pain experienced during wound care or physical therapy (and often for some minutes after such procedures). Background pain is the pain experienced while the patient is resting (i.e. not undergoing a medical procedure). Current medical practice typically includes the use of potent, short-acting opioids for treatment of procedural in-patient burn wound-care pain and long-acting agents for treatment of background pain. Opioids are morphine-related substances.

Profound and multiple learning difficulties (PMLD): a 'blanket' term which refers to people at the severe end of the disability spectrum.

Pronation: rotation of the lower forearm so that the hand faces backwards or downwards with the radius and ulna crossed.

Prosthesis: an artificial device used to replace a body part, such as a limb.

Prosthetic embodiment: identifying with a prosthetic device in such a way that it is considered to be a part of the self.

Pruritis: itching of the skin, which may be caused by circulating uremic toxins in the blood and alterations in calcium and phosphate levels caused by renal disease.

Psychophysiology: investigates the relationship between behaviour and biological processes in humans using non-invasive methodologies such as measurement of electroencephalogram, skin conductance and heart rate.

Pulmonary edema: an elevation of capillary pressure in the lungs caused by fluid-volume overload resulting in the movement of fluid into lung tissue. It is a frightening condition for the patient characterized by the rapid onset of extreme breathlessness.

Reductionistic: the reduction of the human experience into small concepts to be investigated.

Renal replacement therapy: the replacement of renal function by a kidney transplant or dialysis.

Repetition compulsion: unconscious uncontrollable process by which an individual puts himself in painful and difficult situations, repeating earlier bad experiences, although unaware he or she is doing so.

Robot: a computerized system designed to move objects through a series of programmed movements.

Robot-mediated therapy: movement-based therapy, mediated by means of a robotics system, as opposed to the traditional 'hands-on' methods.

Shaping: an operant learning procedure through which a rather difficult response is learned to be performed by reinforcing successive approximations to that response.

Sine tone: a 'pure' waveform that has a fundamental frequency and no overtones or partials.

Slow cortical potentials: shifts in the depolarization level of the apical dendrites of the cortex. Whenever a task-relevant event is expected, cortical excitation thresholds are lowered in the corresponding cortical cell assemblies to facilitate neuronal firing, resulting in negative slow cortical potential amplitudes. Positive slow cortical potential amplitudes can be caused during periods in which no motor or cognitive operations are performed and, therefore, no neuronal resources are required.

Soundbeam: developed by Edward Williams in Bristol, the Soundbeam is a device that converts physical movement into sound via MIDI. The Soundbeam emits an ultrasonic beam. Any physical movement in this beam is converted into MIDI code that is typically then converted into sound.

Sound processor: a digital device that is used with a microphone in sound therapy. Effects such as reverberation, echo and changing the pitch of a voice are available with this device.

Sound therapy: developed by Phil Ellis during the 1990s, this combines aspects of music technology, sound, vibroacoustic techniques and esthetics in an approach that empowers even the most profoundly handicapped.

Splitting (of the ego): coexistence in the mind of two different attitudes towards outer reality. One part of the mind takes this reality into account (because it is perceived), but another part denies this reality because of its traumatic nature and replaces it with its own desire. 'I know it, but I do not want to know it'.

Stimulation: see functional electrical stimulation

Subluxation: partial dislocation of a joint, so that the bone ends are misaligned but still in contact.

Supination: rotation of the lower forearm so that the hand faces forwards or upwards with the radius and ulna parallel.

Surface electromyogram: a signal recorded from sensors mounted on the skin, which is highly correlated with tension in muscles under the recording sensors.

Surface stimulation technology: functional electrical stimulation applied using surface stimulation electrodes.

Technological enframing: a term that describes the all encompassing way in which modern technology is revealed or uncovered to the individual causing them to 'stand reserve' or put their life on hold to abide with the challenges it presents in their life. This may be witnessed in the technology of hemodialysis as the patient's life is bound by the demands of the treatment regime.

Technological surveillance: a method of exerting power by continuously watching and monitoring patients to ensure they abide with the technology of hemodialysis.

Thoracic unit: this is placed in the chest of the recipient of the AbioCor™ in the same position as the native heart after excision of the native ventricles. The thoracic unit contains two pumping chambers that function as the left and right ventricle.

Tracheostomy: tracheotomy/tracheostomy is a surgical procedure in which an incision is made into the trachea (windpipe) that forms a temporary or permanent opening to allow the passage of air and removal of secretions. Instead of breathing through the nose and mouth, the patient will breath through the tracheostomy tube, which is attached to a ventilator.

Transcutaneous energy transfer (TET) coil: there is an internal and external TET coil in the AbioCor™. The internal TET coil receives high-frequency power that is transmitted across the skin from an external TET coil. The internal TET coil is able to convert this oscillating current to a direct current that is used to power the thoracic unit and recharge the internal battery.

Trauma: a life event, which is defined by its intensity and the incapacity of the subject faced with it, to respond or to deal with it. What is felt is beyond ordinary anxiety and becomes fright.

Traumatic neurosis: the symptoms are mental enfeeblement, low spirits, intrusive recurrent visions of the event, bad dreams and nightmares following a trauma. Moreover, the patient is sometimes liable to have other accidents, resembling (i.e. repeating) the former one.

Ultrafiltration: the process by which plasma water is removed because of a pressure gradient that is applied between the blood and dialysate compartment during dialysis. The actual pressure that forces water out of the blood compartment can be accomplished with positive pressure on the blood compartment and negative pressure on the dialysate compartment.

Ultrasonic beam: the Soundbeam has from one to four sensors. These emit a beam at a frequency higher than human hearing (50 khz).

Uremic syndrome: the collective term for the signs and symptoms that occur as a result of renal disease.

Voltage pulse: a pulse of a voltage signal.

Working through: a process, which permits mental integration of elements that had been repressed or denied.

Xenotransplantation: transplantation of an organ or tissue from one species into a recipient from another species (e.g. pig donor heart into a human recipient).

Index